Breastfeeding: Problems and Solutions

Breastfeeding: Problems and Solutions

Editor: Johanna Watts

AMERICAN MEDICAL PUBLISHERS
www.americanmedicalpublishers.com

AMERICAN
MEDICAL PUBLISHERS
www.americanmedicalpublishers.com

Cataloging-in-Publication Data

Breastfeeding : problems and solutions / edited by Johanna Watts.
p. cm.
Includes bibliographical references and index.
ISBN 978-1-63927-608-0
1. Breastfeeding. 2. Breast milk. 3. Infants--Nutrition. 4. Lactation--Nutritional aspects.
5. Breastfeeding--Physiological aspects. I. Watts, Johanna.
RJ216 .B743 2023
649.33--dc23

American Medical Publishers,
41 Flatbush Avenue,
1st Floor, New York,
NY 11217, USA

ISBN 978-1-63927-608-0 (Hardback)

Contents

Preface

I am honored to present to you this unique book which encompasses the most up-to-date data in the field. I was extremely pleased to get this opportunity of editing the work of experts from across the globe. I have also written papers in this field and researched the various aspects revolving around the progress of the discipline. I have tried to unify my knowledge along with that of stalwarts from every corner of the world, to produce a text which not only benefits the readers but also facilitates the growth of the field.

Breastfeeding refers to the act of feeding an infant with breast milk. There are several problems associated with breastfeeding including nipple soreness, breast engorgement, plugged milk duct, breast infection, thrush, and inability to produce enough milk for the needs of the baby. Some factors such as poor feeding techniques, wrong position of the baby while breastfeeding and not taking care of the nipples contribute to the development of nipple soreness. It can be prevented by simply changing the position of the baby while breastfeeding. Breast engorgement is the gradual buildup of milk and blood in the breast after a few days of birth. This leads to hard, swollen and painful breasts. The treatment for this condition involves performing a gentle massage to breasts, reducing distractions in the duration of breastfeeding, and providing heat treatment to the breasts. This book outlines the problems of breastfeeding along with their solutions. It presents researches and studies performed by experts across the globe. This book will prove to be immensely beneficial to students and researchers in this field.

Finally, I would like to thank all the contributing authors for their valuable time and contributions. This book would not have been possible without their efforts. I would also like to thank my friends and family for their constant support.

Editor

1

Prevalence and Associated Factors of Caesarean Section and its Impact on Early Initiation of Breastfeeding in Abu Dhabi, United Arab Emirates

Zainab Taha [1,*], Ahmed Ali Hassan [2], Ludmilla Wikkeling-Scott [1] and Dimitrios Papandreou [1]

1 Department of Health Sciences, College of Natural and Health Sciences, Zayed University, Abu Dhabi, P.O. Box 144534, UAE; ludmilla.scott@gmail.com (L.W.-S.); Dimitrios.Papandreou@zu.ac.ae (D.P.)
2 Taami for Agricultural and Animal Production, Khartoum, Sudan; aa801181@gmail.com
* Correspondence: Zainab.taha@zu.ac.ae

Abstract: The World Health Organization (WHO) recommends the early initiation of breastfeeding. Research shows that factors such as mode of delivery may interfere with the early initiation of breastfeeding. However, data in the United Arab Emirates (UAE) on these findings is limited. Thus, the aim of this study was to describe the prevalence of caesarean sections (CSs) and evaluate their effect on breastfeeding initiation among mothers of children under the age of two years in Abu Dhabi. Data were collected in clinical and non-clinical settings across various geographical areas in Abu Dhabi during 2017 using consent and structured questionnaires for interviews with mothers. Data analysis included both descriptive and inferential statistics. Among the 1624 participants, one-third (30.2%) reportedly delivered by CS, of which 71.1% were planned, while 28.9% were emergency CS. More than half of all mothers (62.5%) initiated early breastfeeding. Multivariable logistic regression indicated factors that were associated positively with CS included advanced maternal age, nationality, and obesity. However, gestational age (GA) was negatively associated with CS. This study shows that the prevalence of CS is high in Abu Dhabi, UAE. CS is associated with lower early initiation rates of breastfeeding. The early initiation rates of breastfeeding were 804 (79.2%) 95% confidence interval (CI) (76.4, 82.0), 162 (16.0%) 95% CI (10.4, 21.6), and 49 (4.8%) 95% CI (1.2, 10.8) among vaginal delivery, planned CS, and emergency CS, respectively. Regarding the mode of delivery, vaginal were 2.78 (Adjusted Odd Ratio (AOR)): CI (95%), (2.17–3.56, $p < 0.001$) times more likely related to an early initiation of breastfeeding. CS in general, and emergency CS, was the main risk factor for the delayed initiation of breastfeeding. The study provides valuable information to develop appropriate strategies to reduce the CS rate in UAE. Maternal literacy on CS choices, the importance of breastfeeding for child health, and additional guidance for mothers and their families are necessary to achieve better breastfeeding outcomes.

Keywords: caesarean section; initiation of breastfeeding; maternal age; gestational age; United Arab Emirates

1. Introduction

The rate of caesarean section (CS) in the United Arab Emirates (UAE) has increased from 10% in 1995 [1] to 24% in 2014 [2]. The World Health Organization (WHO) [3] suggests a CS rate of 10%–15% of all live births, which is significantly lower than those reported in the UAE. Researchers suggest that the mode of delivery influences breastfeeding initiation and duration [4,5], and may influence subsequent breastfeeding and duration [6].

CS is well documented to be associated with suboptimal consequences related to both the mother and her infant's health [7,8]. Among those consequences reported, endometritis, hemorrhage, cystitis, infant respiratory complications, and hypoglycemia [8,9] may have negative effects on breastfeeding. The effect of CS on the initiation of breastfeeding may be related to the adverse effects of anesthesia for both mothers and their newborns. Maternal distress, which often accompanies CS, may negatively affect the baby's feeding behaviors and breastfeeding outcomes.

An abundance of studies have shown that mothers who give birth via CS delivery may be less likely to breastfeed, and or more likely to delay breastfeeding initiation [10–12]. An early initiation of breastfeeding, i.e., within the first hour after delivery, has been recommended by the WHO as an important factor to extend breastfeeding duration [13–15]. An important practice recommended by the WHO, as part of the 10 steps of the Baby-Friendly Hospital Initiative (BFHI), is skin-to-skin contact [16]. To ensure this practice, the mother and her newborn infant must be conscious and fully awake. Therefore, babies born by CS may not benefit from skin-to-skin contact immediately after birth, and may be more susceptible to delayed breastfeeding [16]. Previous studies have found that delaying breastfeeding initiation that co-occurs with CS delivery is associated with factors such as mother–baby separation, impaired suckling skills, and insufficient milk production. This will ultimately impact the continuation of breastfeeding [10,17,18].

The health benefits of breastfeeding for mother and child have been well documented. Mothers who breastfeed their babies have a reduced incidence of type 2 diabetes mellitus, as well as breast and ovarian cancers [19]. Moreover, breastfed babies are less likely to develop childhood illnesses and obesity, and have higher levels of intelligence as an adult [20,21].

Following the WHO recommendations [14], the UAE has incorporated the Global Strategy for Infant and Young Child Feeding, and the Ministry of Health (MOH) has issued a national infant feeding policy [22]. This policy states that infants should be breast fed exclusively until six months of age and continue breastfeeding up to or beyond two years of age [22]. A previous study by Taha et al. revealed a breastfeeding initiation rate of 95.6% and early initiation of 62.5% [23]. However, only 7% of babies were still breastfeeding at six months of age, which prompted the authors to further investigate these findings.

Multiple studies from different countries on the effects of CS versus vaginal delivery on breastfeeding practices have shown contradicting results [24–27]. While some research has documented major barriers to breastfeeding after CS [28–30], other studies have indicated that CS had no effect on breastfeeding initiation [31,32] and duration [33]. Some studies reported that planned CS was associated with delayed breastfeeding [25,34] while others concluded the opposite [35].

Regardless of the discrepancies in previous results, CS will remain a significant and alarming concern, as it influences the initiation of breastfeeding. For a country such as the UAE, which follows the WHO recommendations of infants' and young children's feeding, but still encounters increased rates of CS deliveries, further investigation and more implementation is required to improve knowledge about predictive breastfeeding factors. Thus, the aim of this study was to describe the prevalence of CS and evaluate its effect on breastfeeding initiation among mothers of children under the age of two years in Abu Dhabi.

2. Materials and Methods

2.1. Participants and Data Collection

The sample for this study is based on secondary data from an original sample of clinical and non-clinical data obtained from mothers with at least one infant under the age of two years. Participants for the original study included UAE nationals and non-nationals in the Emirate of Abu Dhabi, which represents 87% of the geographical landmass of the UAE [36]. All data were collected between March and September 2017. The subjects were randomly selected from the community and seven out of a total of 11 maternal and child health centers serving children in Abu Dhabi Capital City (two rural, one suburban, four urban), which provided the possibility of data collection across various areas of Abu Dhabi. Among the 1578 mothers from the clinics who were invited to participate, 1555 mothers agreed and were included in the study. Another 267 mothers from the community also agreed to participate in the study, resulting in a total sample size of 1822 mothers. The geographical distribution of the sample was 54%, 10.8%, and 35.2% of mothers recruited from rural areas, suburban areas, and urban areas respectively.

Mothers with young children attending the centers were approached by the trained bilingual (Arabic and English) female research assistants, who provided oral and written information about the study. Consenting mothers who met the inclusion criteria of having at least one child under two years of age were interviewed by the research assistants using a structured questionnaire.

2.2. *Study Instrument*

A pre-tested questionnaire included family demographics (e.g., education, age, nationality, occupation), child's information (e.g., birth weight and height, delivery mode), and infant feeding practices (e.g., initiation of breastfeeding, and rooming-in). Details of the methodology of the primary data have been previously described [23].

2.3. *Study Inclusion and Exclusion Criteria*

From the 1822 mother–child pairs, there were 1624 with complete data on all the variables of interest that were included in the analysis.

2.4. *Statistical Analysis*

Data analysis was conducted using Statistical Package for the Social Science (IBM SPSS Statistics for Windows, Version 20.0. Armonk, NY: IBM Corp.). Both descriptive and inferential statistics were used to analyze the data. T-tests and chi-square tests were applied to analyze continuous and categorical data, respectively. Variables with significant *p*-value (<0.05) in univariate analysis were entered in multivariable logistic analysis with mode of delivery (vaginal delivery was coded as 0 and CS was coded as 1) as the dependent variable. In addition, body mass index (BMI) was categorized to underweight, normal, overweight, and obese in order to establish which category was associated with CS. Other variables such as sociodemographic characteristic (e.g., age, parent education, occupation, child gender, etc.) were considered as the independent variables. Odds ratio (OR) and 95% confidence intervals (CIs) were calculated with a significance level of p-value < 0.05. Furthermore, multinomial logistic regression analysis was used to investigate the impact of each mode of delivery (vaginal delivery, planned and emergency CS) on the early initiation of breastfeeding.

2.5. *Ethics*

The original study from which this data was extracted was approved by the Research Ethics Committee at Zayed University UAE (ZU17_006_F). Additional clearance was obtained from the Abu Dhabi Health Services Company. Informed consent was obtained from all participants prior to any data collection. Several measures were taken to ensure privacy and confidentiality throughout the study period by excluding personal identifiers during data collection.

2.6. *Definitions*

Early initiation of breastfeeding: when the infant initiated breastfeeding within one hour after birth [37].

Delayed initiation of breastfeeding: when the infant initiated breastfeeding within more than one hour after birth.

Rooming-in: the child stays with mother in the same room during hospital stay.

Exclusive breastfeeding: the infant being fed only breast milk without any other oral intake, except medications and vitamins, for the first six months of life; it was calculated based on the last 24 h.

Breastfeeding support: the support and encouragement from family (mother, husband, other relatives, and other non-relatives) on breastfeeding

Breastfeeding advice and or discussion: any received information, positive or negative things about breastfeeding before or after delivery

Gestational age: a measure of the age of a pregnancy that is taken from the beginning of the woman's last menstrual period

Preterm birth: the birth of a baby at <37 weeks GA

Arab nationality: all Emirati mothers and other Arab ones

Non-Arab nationality: Asian mothers and other nationalities

Cesarean section: a surgical procedure in which incisions are made through a woman's abdomen and uterus to deliver her baby

3. Results

Secondary data analysis included 1624 samples from the original study, of which 491 (30.2%) participants reportedly delivered by CS, of which 349 (71.1%) delivered by planned CS, and 142 (28.9%) delivered by emergency CS (Figure 1).

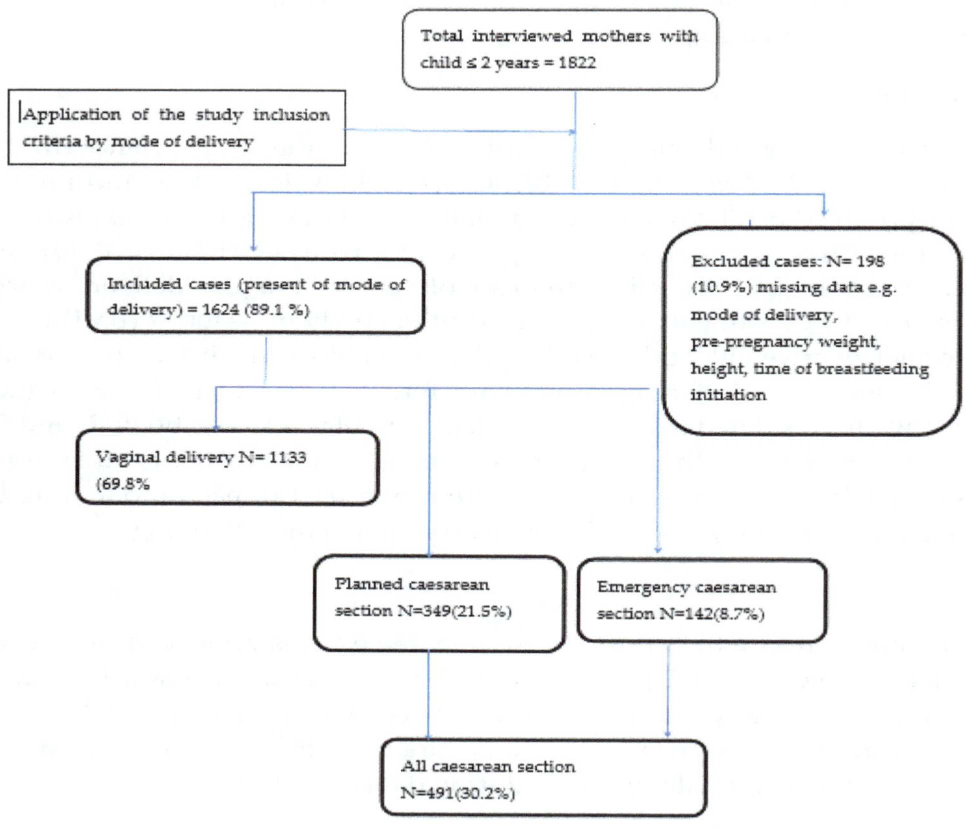

Figure 1. Study participants flow chart and main findings.

The mean and standard deviation (SD) of the mothers' age and children's age were 30.1 (5.2) years and 8.1 months (5.9), respectively. The mean (SD) gestational age at delivery was 39.1 (1.9) weeks, and 6.5% of infants were preterm (GA <37 weeks). More than half (62.5%) of the mothers initiated early breastfeeding. Bivariate analysis showed that child age, birth weight, pre-pregnancy BMI, maternal education, initiation of breastfeeding, and rooming-in were associated with the mode of delivery (Table 1). Exclusive breastfeeding among infants between 0–6 months was 46.5% (332/710).

Table 1. Bivariate analysis of factors associated with caesarean section among mothers with children two years old and younger in Abu Dhabi, United Arab Emirates (UAE).

Variables	Mode of Delivery						
	Total ($n = 1624$)		Vaginal ($n = 1133$)		CS ($n = 491$)		
	Mean (SD), range		Mean (SD)		Mean (SD)		*p*-Value
Maternal age, years		30.1(5.2)		29.9(5.3)		31.0(4.8)	<0.001
Child age, months (median 6, interquartile range 9)		8.1(5.9)		8.3(6.0)		7.6(5.7)	0.042
Gestational age, weeks		39.1(1.9)		39.4(1.7)		38.6(2.1)	<0.001
Birth weight, grams		3079(518)		3110(463)		3008(621)	<0.001
Mother pre-pregnancy BMI		23.9(3.8), (15.2, 64.9)		23.7(3.7)		24.3(4.2)	0.002
	N	%	N	%	N	%	
Child Gender							
Male	799	49.2	560	49.4	239	48.7	0.781
Female	825	50.8	573	50.6	252	51.3	
Nationality by category							
Arab	1056	65.0	757	66.7	299	60.9	0.049
Non-Arab	568	35.0	376	33.3	192	39.1	
Marital status							
Married	1602	98.6	1116	98.5	486	99.0	0.440
Unmarried	22	1.4	17	1.5	5	1.0	
Initiation of breastfeeding							
Delayed initiated	609	37.5	329	29.0	280	57.0	< 0.001
Early initiated	1015	62.5	804	71.0	211	43.0	
Rooming-in							
Yes	1562	96.2	1101	97.2	461	93.9	0.002
No	62	3.8	32	2.8	30	6.1	
Mother's education							
Secondary level	65	4.0	53	4.7	12	2.4	0.035
≥secondary level	1559	96.0	1080	95.3	479	97.6	
Father's education							
<Secondary level	31	1.9	23	2.0	8	1.6	0.588
≥secondary level	1593	98.1	1110	98.0	483	98.4	
Mother occupation							
Housewives	1008	62.1	695	61.3	313	63.7	0.533
Employed	616	37.9	438	38.7	178	36.3	
Child order							
1st order	1038	63.9	399	35.2	187	38.1	0.269
>1st order	1038	63.9	304	61.9	304	61.9	

Multivariable logistic regression analysis indicated that several factors were positively associated with caesarean section (CS). These included: advanced maternal age (Adjusted Odd Ratio (AOR) = 1.04, 95% confidence interval (CI) = 1.02, 1.07), nationality (non-Arab) (AOR = 1.30, 95% CI = 1.02, 1.65), and body mass index (BMI) status (obesity) (AOR = 1.79, 95% CI = 1.15, 2.79). Gestational age (GA); however, (AOR = 0.80, 95% CI = 0.75, 0.86) was found to be negatively associated with CS (Table 2).

Table 2. Multivariable logistic regression analyses of factors associated with caesarean section among mothers with children two years old and younger in Abu Dhabi, UAE.

Variable		Adjusted Odds Ratio	95% Confidence Interval	*p*-Value
Advanced maternal age, years		1.04	1.02, 1.07	< 0.001
Gestational age, weeks		0.80	0.75, 0.86	<0.001
Child's birth weight, grams		1.00	1.00, 1.00	0.283
Nationality	Non-Arab	1.36	1.08, 1.71	0.009
	Arab	Reference		
Maternal education	≥Secondary	1.88	0.94, 3.75	0.072
	<Secondary	Reference		
Mother pre-pregnancy BMI	Underweight (<18.5)	1.12	0.56, 2.26	0.746
	Normal (18.5–24.9)	Reference		
	Overweight (25–29.9)	1.10	0.85, 1.42	0.477
	Obese (≥30)	1.79	1.15, 2.79	0.010

From the total (1624), 1133 (69.8%), 349 (21.5%), and 142 (8.7%) delivered vaginally, by planned CS and by emergency CS, respectively. Among mothers who initiated breastfeeding early (1015), the rates of an early initiation of breastfeeding were 804 (79.2%) 95% CI (76.4, 82.0), 162 (16.0%) 95% CI (10.4, 21.6), and 49 (4.8%) 95% CI (1.2, 10.8) for vaginal deliveries, planned CS, and emergency CS, respectively.

By using logistic regression analysis, the different impacts of each mode of delivery (vaginal, planned CS, and emergency CS), and their impact on early initiation of breastfeeding, the study findings showed that vaginal delivery mothers were most likely to initiate early breastfeeding, followed by planned CS and emergency CS delivery (Table 3).

Table 3. Impact of mode of delivery (vaginal delivery, planned CS, and emergency CS) in comparison to each other on an early initiation of breastfeeding using logistic regression analysis.

Mode of Delivery	95% Confidence Interval (CI)	*p*-Value	AOR [1] (95% CI)	*p*-Value	AOR (95% CI)	*p*-Value
Vaginal delivery	4.5 (3.16, 6.61)	< 0.001	2.78 (2.17, 3.56)	< 0.001	Reference	
Planned CS	1.64 (1.09, 2.46)	0.017	Reference		0.36 (0.28, 046)	< 0.001
Emergency CS	Reference		0.61 (0.41, 0.91)	0.017	0.22 (0.15, 0.32)	< 0.001

[1] AOR: Adjusted for advance maternal age, gestational age, and mother's BMI.

4. Discussion

One of the main findings was the high rate of CS (30.2%). This rate is more than double in comparison to the WHO set upper limit of 15% [3], and three times that of rates previously reported in the UAE (10% in 1995%) [1]. These data support the WHO reports that the rate of CS is increasing [2]. The results from this study exceed those for other Arab nations such as Saudi Arabia where a low rate of CS was reported (13.7%) [38] and Sudan (17.8%) [39]. Researchers attributed the varying trend of CS rate among nations to multiple factors including affluence [40], urbanization [40], and increases in preterm births [41]. For example, Boatin et al. [42] reported a low CS rate in South Sudan of 0.6% in comparison to the Dominican Republic, which reported 58.9%. CS rates also vary between public and private hospitals [43,44], which may be attributed to access to care.

This study indicated that non-Arab mothers were 1.3 times more likely to deliver by CS compared to Arab mothers. In multinational countries such as the UAE, the interpretation of such differences requires additional research. It should be noted that maternal age among non-Arab mothers was higher than Arab mothers, which may have contributed to the increased rates of CS in this group.

Advanced GA was found to be a protective factor for CS, (AOR 0.80, 95% CI = 0.75, 0.86) i.e., full-term babies were less likely to have been delivered by CS in comparison to preterm babies, which is a finding that is supported by previous research [41,45]. In addition, advanced maternal age was found to be associated with preterm birth [46–48]. Thus, we can conclude that factors such as advanced maternal age, preterm birth, and nationality are correlated.

In contrast to our results, previous studies have found birth weight [43,49] and maternal education [40,49] to be associated with mode of delivery. Differences in the scope and approach to data collection may limit the ability to adequately compare current results with previous studies and warrant additional research.

As with previous findings [50–52], the current study found an increased risk of CS in obese women. However, overweight was not associated with CS, and the findings of the current study were confined to the obese mothers. Regardless of the association between obesity and CS, it is well documented that maternal obesity is associated with a decreased intention and initiation of breastfeeding, a shortened duration of breastfeeding, a less adequate milk supply, and a delayed onset of lactogenesis II, and can thus be considered as a risk factor for adverse breastfeeding outcomes [53–55].

In addition to the CS prevalence and its associated factors, including the breastfeeding ones, the study also documented the impact of each mode of delivery on breastfeeding initiation. In line with others, the present results documented CS as a key risk factor for the delayed initiation of breastfeeding [24,28,56,57]. The researchers attributed the delay to many reasons, including pain [28], delayed lactogenesis [56], and feeding the newborn with formula [28,57].

The current study found that women who had a vaginal delivery 4.57 (3.16, 6.61) versus planned CS delivery 1.64 (1.09, 2.46) were four times more likely to initiate breastfeeding early. This finding is in line with several studies that documented vaginal delivery to be associated with an early initiation of breastfeeding [26,28–30]. This finding supports previous research that suggests rooming-in as a factor for the early initiation of breastfeeding, and CS decreases that opportunity.

However, controversy exists between planned CS and emergency CS. Some researchers propose that planned CS is associated with a delayed initiation of breastfeeding [34] while others report that emergency CS is associated with a delayed initiation of breastfeeding [35], similar to our findings. The delayed initiation of breastfeeding after emergency CS could be attributed to the stress accompanying the labor and delivery, which is associated with a delayed onset of lactation [35].

Our study is the first of this kind in the UAE, using clinical and non-clinical data to describe CS and the initiation of breastfeeding. Several limitations should be noted. First, maternal indications and/or fetal indications of CS such as fetal distress, the type of anesthesia (general or regional) used during CS, and maternal and child condition such as morbidity and history of hospitalization after delivery by CS were not reported. These issues can affect the mode of delivery and its effect on breastfeeding practices. Future studies are needed to better describe the factors associated with CS in UAE populations.

5. Conclusions

This study suggests that the prevalence of CS is high in Abu Dhabi, UAE and that CS is associated with advanced maternal age, GA, nationality, and obesity. CS, and emergency CS in particular, was the main risk factor for a delayed initiation of breastfeeding. The study provides valuable information to aid with the development of appropriate strategies to reduce the CS rate in the UAE. Maternal literacy on CS choices, the importance of breastfeeding for child health, and additional guidance so that mothers and their families can achieve better breastfeeding outcomes are recommended to ensure successful breastfeeding practices.

Author Contributions: Z.T. designed the study and recruited the participants. Z.T. and A.A.H. analyzed the data and wrote the manuscript. L.S. and D.P. contributed to the design of the study, data collection, and manuscript writing. All contributing authors of this original manuscript authorized the final version of the manuscript. All authors read and approved the final manuscript.

Acknowledgments: The authors are grateful to the Abu Dhabi Health Services Company (SEHA) for granting access and approval to seven public ambulatory health care centers across the capital city of Abu Dhabi. We would like to express our gratitude to the mothers for their sincere cooperation and the provision of valuable information. Furthermore, we would like to thank the research assistants Amira Badr Eldin, Razan Abdelrahman, Nahed Yaghi, Nour Mohammed, Dhuha Abdulla Naser, Ayesha Rashed, and Jawaher Saeed for their time and commitment. We appreciate the work done by Teresa Arora on improving the English language. Special thanks go to Malin Garemo and Joy Nanda for their technical assistance in the study design.

References

1. World Health Organization. *The World Health Report 2005 Statistical Annex*; World Health Organization: Geneva, Switzerland, 2005.
2. World Health Organization. *World health Statistics 2015*; World Health Organization: Geneva, Switzerland, 2015.
3. World Health Organization. *WHO Statement on Caesarean Section Rates*; World Health Organization: Geneva, Switzerland, 2015.
4. Smith, L.J. Impact of birthing practices on the breastfeeding dyad. *J. Midwifery Womens Health* **2007**, *52*, 621–630. [CrossRef]
5. Procianoy, R.S.; Fernandes-Filho, P.H.; Lazaro, L.; Sartori, N.C. Factors affecting breastfeeding: The influence of caesarean section. *J. Trop. Pediatr.* **1984**, *30*, 39–42. [CrossRef]
6. Jaafar, S.H.; Ho, J.J.; Lee, K.S. Rooming-in for new mother and infant versus separate care for increasing the duration of breastfeeding. *Cochrane Database Syst. Rev.* **2016**, Cd006641. [CrossRef]
7. Bodner, K.; Wierrani, F.; Grunberger, W.; Bodner-Adler, B. Influence of the mode of delivery on maternal and neonatal outcomes: A comparison between elective cesarean section and planned vaginal delivery in a low-risk obstetric population. *Arch. Gynecol. Obstet.* **2011**, *283*, 1193–1198. [CrossRef]
8. Wax, J.R. Maternal request cesarean versus planned spontaneous vaginal delivery: Maternal morbidity and short term outcomes. *Semin. Perinatol.* **2006**, *30*, 247–252. [CrossRef]
9. Karlstrom, A.; Lindgren, H.; Hildingsson, I. Maternal and infant outcome after caesarean section without recorded medical indication: Findings from a Swedish case-control study. *BJOG Int. J. Obstet. Gynaecol.* **2013**, *120*, 479–486; discussion 486. [CrossRef]
10. Rowe-Murray, H.J.; Fisher, J.R. Baby friendly hospital practices: Cesarean section is a persistent barrier to early initiation of breastfeeding. *Birth* **2002**, *29*, 124–131. [CrossRef]
11. Watt, S.; Sword, W.; Sheehan, D.; Foster, G.; Thabane, L.; Krueger, P.; Landy, C.K. The effect of delivery method on breastfeeding initiation from the The Ontario Mother and Infant Study (TOMIS) III. *J. Obstet. Gynecol. Neonatal Nurs.* **2012**, *41*, 728–737. [CrossRef]
12. Esteves, T.M.; Daumas, R.P.; Oliveira, M.I.; Andrade, C.A.; Leite, I.C. Factors associated to breastfeeding in the first hour of life: Systematic review. *Rev. Saude Publica* **2014**, *48*, 697–708. [CrossRef]
13. Meedya, S.; Fahy, K.; Kable, A. Factors that positively influence breastfeeding duration to 6 months: A literature review. *Women Birth* **2010**, *23*, 135–145. [CrossRef]
14. World Health Organization and United Nations Children's Fund (UNICEF). *Baby-Friendly Hospital Initiative Revised, Updated and Expanded for Integrated Care*; World Health Organization and United Nations Children's Fund: Geneva, Switzerland, 2009.
15. World Health Organization. *Global Strategy for Infant and Young Child Feeding*; World Health Organization: Geneva, Switzerland, 2003; pp. 1–30.
16. Moore, E.R.; Bergman, N.; Anderson, G.C.; Medley, N. Early skin-to-skin contact for mothers and their healthy newborn infants. *Cochrane Database Syst. Rev.* **2016**, *11*, Cd003519. [CrossRef]
17. Patel, R.R.; Liebling, R.E.; Murphy, D.J. Effect of operative delivery in the second stage of labor on breastfeeding success. *Birth* **2003**, *30*, 255–260. [CrossRef]
18. Zanardo, V.; Pigozzo, A.; Wainer, G.; Marchesoni, D.; Gasparoni, A.; Di Fabio, S.; Cavallin, F.; Giustardi, A.; Trevisanuto, D. Early lactation failure and formula adoption after elective caesarean delivery: Cohort study. *Arch. Dis. Child. Fetal Neonatal Ed.* **2013**, *98*, F37–F41. [CrossRef]
19. Ip, S.; Chung, M.; Raman, G.; Chew, P.; Magula, N.; DeVine, D.; Trikalinos, T.; Lau, J. Breastfeeding and maternal and infant health outcomes in developed countries. *Evid. Rep. Technol. Assess.* **2007**, *153*, 1–186.

20. Yan, J.; Liu, L.; Zhu, Y.; Huang, G.; Wang, P.P. The association between breastfeeding and childhood obesity: A meta-analysis. *BMC Public Health* **2014**, *14*, 1267. [CrossRef]
21. Victora, C.G.; Horta, B.L.; Loret de Mola, C.; Quevedo, L.; Pinheiro, R.T.; Gigante, D.P.; Goncalves, H.; Barros, F.C. Association between breastfeeding and intelligence, educational attainment, and income at 30 years of age: A prospective birth cohort study from Brazil. *Lancet Glob. Health* **2015**, *3*, e199–e205. [CrossRef]
22. Taha, Z. Trends of breastfeeding in the United Arab Emirates (UAE). *Arab. J. Nutr. Exerc.* **2017**, *2*, 152–159. [CrossRef]
23. Taha, Z.; Garemo, M.; Nanda, J. Patterns of breastfeeding practices among infants and young children in Abu Dhabi, United Arab Emirates. *Int Breastfeed. J.* **2018**, *13*, 48. [CrossRef]
24. Perez-Rios, N.; Ramos-Valencia, G.; Ortiz, A.P. Cesarean delivery as a barrier for breastfeeding initiation: The Puerto Rican experience. *J. Hum. Lact.* **2008**, *24*, 293–302. [CrossRef]
25. Prior, E.; Santhakumaran, S.; Gale, C.; Philipps, L.H.; Modi, N.; Hyde, M.J. Breastfeeding after cesarean delivery: A systematic review and meta-analysis of world literature. *Am. J. Clin. Nutr.* **2012**, *95*, 1113–1135. [CrossRef]
26. Perez-Escamilla, R.; Maulen-Radovan, I.; Dewey, K.G. The association between cesarean delivery and breast-feeding outcomes among Mexican women. *Am. J. Public Health* **1996**, *86*, 832–836. [CrossRef] [PubMed]
27. Brown, A.; Jordan, S. Impact of birth complications on breastfeeding duration: An internet survey. *J. Adv. Nurs.* **2013**, *69*, 828–839. [CrossRef] [PubMed]
28. Albokhary, A.A.; James, J.P. Does cesarean section have an impact on the successful initiation of breastfeeding in Saudi Arabia? *Saudi. Med. J.* **2014**, *35*, 1400–1403. [PubMed]
29. Badaya, N.; Jain, S.; Kumar, N. Time of initiation of breastfeeding in various modes of delivery and to observe the effect of low birth weight and period of gestation on initiation of breastfeeding. *Int. J. Contemp. Pediatr.* **2018**, *5*, 1509–1517. [CrossRef]
30. Regan, J.; Thompson, A.; DeFranco, E. The influence of mode of delivery on breastfeeding initiation in women with a prior cesarean delivery: A population-based study. *Breastfeed. Med.* **2013**, *8*, 181–186. [CrossRef] [PubMed]
31. Kiani, S.N.; Rich, K.M.; Herkert, D.; Safon, C.; Perez-Escamilla, R. Delivery mode and breastfeeding outcomes among new mothers in Nicaragua. *Matern. Child. Nutr.* **2018**, *14*, e12474. [CrossRef] [PubMed]
32. Hassan, A.A.; Taha, Z.; Ahmed, M.A.A.; Ali, A.A.A.; Adam, I. Assessment of initiation of breastfeeding practice in Kassala, Eastern Sudan: A community-based study. *Int. Breastfeed. J.* **2018**, *13*, 34. [CrossRef]
33. Rabiepoor, S.; Sadeghi, E.; Hamidiazar, P. The relationship between type of delivery and successful breastfeeding. *Int. J. Paediatr.* **2017**, *5*, 4899–4907.
34. Palla, H.; Kitsantas, P. Mode of delivery and breastfeeding practices. *Int. J. Pregnancy Child Birth* **2017**, *2*, 167–172.
35. Grajeda, R.; Perez-Escamilla, R. Stress during labor and delivery is associated with delayed onset of lactation among urban Guatemalan women. *J. Nutr.* **2002**, *132*, 3055–3060. [CrossRef]
36. Abu Dhabi Government. *Abu Dhabi Emirate: Facts and Figures*; Abu Dhabi Government: Abu Dhabi, UAE, 2018.
37. World Health Organization. *Protecting, Promoting and Supporting Breastfeeding in Facilities Providing Maternity and Newborn Services*; World Health Organization: Geneva, Switzerland, 2017.
38. Ghadeer, Z.; Abdullah, A.; Afnan, B.; Abdullah, A.; Abrar, H.; Hanoof, A.; Aeshah, A.; Fatimah, A.; Duaa, F.; Amair, A. Prevalence of caesarean section and its indicating factors among pregnant women attending delivery at King Abdulaziz University Hospital, Jeddah city during 2016. *EC Gynaecol.* **2018**, *7*, 43–51.
39. Elmugabil, A.; Rayis, D.A.; Hassan, A.A.; Ali, A.A.A.; Adam, I. Epidemiology of cesarean delivery in Kassala, Eastern Sudan: A community-based study 2014–2015. *Sudan JMS* **2016**, *11*, 49–54.
40. Khan, M.N.; Islam, M.M.; Shariff, A.A.; Alam, M.M.; Rahman, M.M. Socio-demographic predictors and average annual rates of caesarean section in Bangladesh between 2004 and 2014. *PLoS ONE* **2017**, *12*, e0177579. [CrossRef] [PubMed]
41. Barros, F.C.; Rabello Neto, D.L.; Villar, J.; Kennedy, S.H.; Silveira, M.F.; Diaz-Rossello, J.L.; Victora, C.G. Caesarean sections and the prevalence of preterm and early-term births in Brazil: Secondary analyses of national birth registration. *BMJ Open* **2018**, *8*, e021538. [CrossRef]

42. Boatin, A.A.; Schlotheuber, A.; Betran, A.P.; Moller, A.B.; Barros, A.J.D.; Boerma, T.; Torloni, M.R.; Victora, C.G.; Hosseinpoor, A.R. Within country inequalities in caesarean section rates: Observational study of 72 low and middle income countries. *BMJ* **2018**, *360*, k55. [CrossRef]
43. Al Rifai, R. Rising cesarean deliveries among apparently low-risk mothers at university teaching hospitals in Jordan: Analysis of population survey data, 2002–2012. *Glob. Health Sci. Pract.* **2014**, *2*, 195–209. [CrossRef]
44. Einarsdottir, K.; Haggar, F.; Pereira, G.; Leonard, H.; de Klerk, N.; Stanley, F.J.; Stock, S. Role of public and private funding in the rising caesarean section rate: A cohort study. *BMJ Open* **2013**, *3*, e002789. [CrossRef]
45. Delnord, M.; Blondel, B.; Drewniak, N.; Klungsoyr, K.; Bolumar, F.; Mohangoo, A.; Gissler, M.; Szamotulska, K.; Lack, N.; Nijhuis, J.; et al. Varying gestational age patterns in cesarean delivery: An international comparison. *BMC Pregnancy Childbirth* **2014**, *14*, 321. [CrossRef]
46. Cavazos-Rehg, P.A.; Krauss, M.J.; Spitznagel, E.L.; Bommarito, K.; Madden, T.; Olsen, M.A.; Subramaniam, H.; Peipert, J.F.; Bierut, L.J. Maternal age and risk of labor and delivery complications. *Matern. Child. Health J.* **2015**, *19*, 1202–1211. [CrossRef]
47. Fuchs, F.; Monet, B.; Ducruet, T.; Chaillet, N.; Audibert, F. Effect of maternal age on the risk of preterm birth: A large cohort study. *PLoS ONE* **2018**, *13*, e0191002. [CrossRef]
48. Waldenstrom, U.; Cnattingius, S.; Vixner, L.; Norman, M. Advanced maternal age increases the risk of very preterm birth, irrespective of parity: A population-based register study. *BJOG Int. J. Obstet. Gynaecol.* **2017**, *124*, 1235–1244. [CrossRef] [PubMed]
49. Apanga, P.A.; Awoonor-Williams, J.K. Predictors of caesarean section in northern Ghana: A case-control study. *Pan Afr. Med. J.* **2018**, *29*, 20. [CrossRef] [PubMed]
50. Cresswell, J.A.; Campbell, O.M.; De Silva, M.J.; Slaymaker, E.; Filippi, V. Maternal obesity and Caesarean delivery in sub-Saharan Africa. *Trop. Med. Int. Health* **2016**, *21*, 879–885. [CrossRef] [PubMed]
51. Ovesen, P.; Rasmussen, S.; Kesmodel, U. Effect of prepregnancy maternal overweight and obesity on pregnancy outcome. *Obstet. Gynecol.* **2011**, *118*, 305–312. [CrossRef]
52. Tsvieli, O.; Sergienko, R.; Sheiner, E. Risk factors and perinatal outcome of pregnancies complicated with cephalopelvic disproportion: A population-based study. *Arch. Gynecol. Obstet.* **2012**, *285*, 931–936. [CrossRef]
53. Donath, S.M.; Amir, L.H. Maternal obesity and initiation and duration of breastfeeding: Data from the longitudinal study of Australian children. *Matern. Child. Nutr.* **2008**, *4*, 163–170. [CrossRef]
54. Ramji, N.; Quinlan, J.; Murphy, P.; Crane, J.M. The impact of maternal obesity on breastfeeding. *J. Obstet. Gynaecol. Can.* **2016**, *38*, 703–711. [CrossRef]
55. Verret-Chalifour, J.; Giguere, Y.; Forest, J.-C.; Croteau, J.; Zhang, P.; Marc, I. Breastfeeding initiation: Impact of obesity in a large Canadian perinatal cohort study. *PLoS ONE* **2015**, *10*, e0117512. [CrossRef]
56. Isik, Y.; Dag, Z.O.; Tulmac, O.B.; Pek, E. Early postpartum lactation effects of cesarean and vaginal birth. *Ginekol. Pol.* **2016**, *87*, 426–430. [CrossRef]
57. Chen, C.; Yan, Y.; Gao, X.; Xiang, S.; He, Q.; Zeng, G.; Liu, S.; Sha, T.; Li, L. Influences of Cesarean Delivery on Breastfeeding Practices and Duration: A Prospective Cohort Study. *J. Hum. Lact.* **2018**, *34*, 526–534. [CrossRef]

2

Lactation Duration and Long-Term Thyroid Function: A Study among Women with Gestational Diabetes

Pranati L. Panuganti [1,2], Stefanie N. Hinkle [1], Shristi Rawal [1,3], Louise G. Grunnet [4,5,6], Yuan Lin [1,7], Aiyi Liu [1], Anne C. B. Thuesen [5], Sylvia H. Ley [8,9], Sjurdur F. Olesen [4] and Cuilin Zhang [1,*]

1 Epidemiology Branch, Division of Intramural Population Health Research, Eunice Kennedy Shriver National Institute of Child Health and Human Development, National Institutes of Health, Bethesda, MD 20817, USA; pranati_panuganti@brown.edu (P.L.P.); hinklesn@mail.nih.gov (S.N.H.); shristi.rawal@rutgers.edu (S.R.); linyy@iu.edu (Y.L.); liua@mail.nih.gov (A.L.)

2 The Warren Alpert Medical School of Brown University, Providence, RI 02903, USA

3 Department of Nutritional Sciences, School of Health Professions, Rutgers University, Newark, NJ 07107, USA

4 Centre for Fetal Programming, Department of Epidemiology Research, Statens Serum Institut, DK-2300 Copenhagen, Denmark; Louise.Groth.Grunnet@regionh.dk (L.G.G.); SFO@ssi.dk (S.F.O.)

5 Department of Endocrinology, Rigshospitalet University Hospital, DK-2200 Copenhagen, Denmark; anne.cathrine.baun.thuesen@regionh.dk

6 The Danish Diabetes Academy, DK-5000 Odense, Denmark

7 Department of Epidemiology, Richard M. Fairbanks School of Public Health, Indiana University, Indianapolis, IN 46202, USA

8 Harvard T.H. Chan School of Public Health, Harvard University, Boston, MA 02115, USA; sylvia.ley@channing.harvard.edu

9 Channing Division of Network Medicine, Harvard Medical School and Brigham and Women's Hospital, Boston, MA 02115, USA

* Correspondence: zhangcu@mail.nih.gov

Abstract: Lactation is associated with reduced postpartum weight retention and a lower risk of several cardiometabolic disorders in population-based studies. We examined the association between lactation and long-term thyroid function among women with history of gestational diabetes mellitus (GDM), a high-risk population for subsequent metabolic complications. The study included 550 women who developed GDM in the Danish National Birth Cohort (1996–2002) and followed-up in the Diabetes & Women's Health Study (2012–2014). We assessed adjusted associations between cumulative lactation duration and concentrations of thyroid stimulating hormone (TSH), free triiodothyronine (fT3), and free thyroxine (fT4) measured at follow-up. Women with longer cumulative lactation duration tended to have higher fT3 levels (adjusted β and 95% confidence interval (CI) for $\geq$12 months vs. none: 0.19 (0.03–0.36); p-trend = 0.05). When restricted to women with a single lifetime pregnancy to control for parity (n = 70), women who lactated for >6 months (vs. none) had higher fT3 levels (0.46 pmol/L (0.12–0.80); p-trend = 0.02) and a higher fT3:fT4 ratio (0.61 (0.17–1.05); p-trend = 0.007). Our findings suggested that a longer duration of lactation may be related to greater serum fT3 levels and fT3:fT4 ratio 9–16 years postpartum among Danish women with a history of GDM. The association was particularly pronounced among women who only had one lifetime pregnancy.

Keywords: GDM; lactation; thyroid; triiodothyronine; thyroxine; thyroid antibodies

---

1. Introduction

The thyroid gland is involved in several physiological processes, including glucose metabolism, muscle repair, cardiovascular function, and thermogenesis [1]. Thyroid dysfunction may be manifested as clinical, subclinical, or autoimmune, depending on the levels of thyroid hormones (thyroid stimulating hormone (TSH), free triiodothyronine (fT3), and free thyroxine (fT4)) and anti-thyroid antibodies (e.g., thyroperoxidase antibody (anti-TPO), and thyroglobulin antibody (anti-TG)). Women who develop diabetes in pregnancy, or gestational diabetes mellitus (GDM), are particularly subject to a substantially increased risk for cardiometabolic disorders [2]. Given the importance of thyroid hormones in maintaining the function of multiple systems and regulatory pathways related to cardiometabolic functions, the identification of potentially modifiable factors related to thyroid function among GDM women is of important clinical and public health significance.

Lactation has been associated with several health benefits in women [3]. Foremost, postpartum weight retention is reduced in women who breastfed their children [3]. In addition, women with a longer lifetime duration of lactation are at lower risk for cardiometabolic disorders, including cardiovascular disease, type 2 diabetes mellitus (T2DM), and hypertension [3]. Interestingly, animal data also demonstrate that increasing lactation duration is associated with heightened thyroid activity, resulting in increased levels of biologically active thyroid hormone, triiodothyronine (T3) [4]. Specifically, in bovine models, mRNA transcripts for the enzyme responsible for generating T3 were 6-fold greater with 90 days of lactation compared to levels preceding birth [4]. A link between lactation and thyroid function may lie in the reduction of postpartum weight retention, as weight gain was previously highly associated with TSH and fT4 humans [5]. However, human data are lacking for the influence of lactation on long-term thyroid function among both the general population and women with a history of GDM in particular.

The objective of this study was to examine the association between lactation duration and long-term thyroid function among a high-risk cohort of women with a history of GDM [6–13]. We hypothesize that a longer cumulative lactation duration is associated with improved thyroid function, approximately 9–16 years after the index GDM pregnancy.

2. Materials and Methods

2.1. Study Design

In the Diabetes & Women's Health (DWH) Study [14], we followed up women identified as having GDM during the index pregnancy of the Danish National Birth Cohort (DNBC) [15]. The DNBC collected data on maternal demographics, perinatal exposures, and health conditions through four telephone interviews conducted at gestational weeks 12 and 30, and 6 and 18 months postpartum (1996–2002). The DWH Study (2012–2014) enrolled 790 women who had GDM during their index pregnancy, 9–16 years after their enrollment in the DNBC. This analysis was limited to women who completed the DWH Study clinical exam in which biospecimens were collected ($n = 619$) and for whom thyroid markers were available ($n = 611$; 99.0%). Women reporting thyroid disease before the index DNBC pregnancy ($n = 18$; 3.0%) were excluded. We further excluded participants with missing data on breastfeeding duration ($n = 43$; 7.3%) to arrive at the final analytic sample ($n = 550$). All participants provided informed consent. The study was approved by the Regional Scientific Ethical Committee (VEK) of the Capital Region of Denmark (record No. H-4-2013-129).

2.2. Ascertainment of Cumulative Lactation History after Index GDM Pregnancy

At the DWH Study follow-up, women retrospectively reported the duration of lactation for each of their pregnancies. The cumulative duration of lactation was calculated by summing the number of lactating months following each birth and was categorized as: none, <6, 6 to <12, or $\geq$12 months. Because we lacked covariate information for pregnancies before the index DNBC pregnancy, we calculated lifetime lactation duration starting at the index pregnancy and thus, adjusted for parity at the index pregnancy and performed further analyses limited to women who were nulliparous at the index pregnancy.

To assess the validity of recalled lactation duration, we examined the correlation between lactation duration proximally reported for the index DNBC pregnancy at 6 and 18 months postpartum interviews, and the duration recalled for the corresponding pregnancy on the DWH Study follow-up questionnaire 9–16 years postpartum. The correlation was high ($r = 0.81$), and 69.9% of women accurately reported the duration within 1 month. In our analyses, we use the retrospectively reported lactation data as it captured the lactation history over all pregnancies as opposed to only the index pregnancy.

2.3. Thyroid Function

At the DWH Study follow-up clinical exam, fasting venous blood samples were collected, processed within 1 h, and stored at −80 °C until being analyzed by a central laboratory following a standardized protocol. All samples were assayed in a single batch by a certified clinical laboratory at the University of Minnesota. Concentrations of thyroid stimulating hormone (TSH) (mIU/L) were measured using a sandwich immunoassay (Roche Diagnostics, Indianapolis, IN, USA). Concentrations of free triiodothyronine (fT3) (pmol/L), free thyroxine (fT4) (ng/dL), anti-TPO (IU/mL), and anti-TG (thyroglobulin antibody; IU/mL) were measured using a competitive immunoassay (Roche Diagnostics, Indianapolis, IN, USA). The fT3:fT4 ratio was calculated by dividing serum concentrations of fT3 (pmol/L) by fT4 (ng/dL). The inter-assay coefficients of variance (CV) were all <6.2% for fT3, fT4, and TSH and <15.1% for the anti-TPO and anti-TG antibodies.

Thyroid function was assessed based on continuous levels of thyroid hormones (TSH, fT3, fT4, fT3:fT4). Additionally, following the American Thyroid Association guidelines, subclinical hypothyroidism (SCH) was defined as having an elevated TSH (normal range 0.45–4.12 mIU/L) with normal fT4 levels (0.93–1.7 ng/dL) [16]. Subclinical hyperthyroidism was defined as having low to undetectable TSH with normal levels of fT3 (normal range 3.53–6.45 pmol/L) and fT4 (normal range 0.93–1.7 ng/dL) [16,17]. Women with both TSH and fT4 levels within the normal range were classified as euthyroid. Participants who did not meet the criteria for euthyroid, SCH, or subclinical hyperthyroidism were classified as "other". Lastly, participants were categorized as positive for anti-TPO and anti-TG if their antibody levels were above lab reference ranges (anti-TPO: ≥35 IU/mL; anti-TG: ≥115 IU/mL).

2.4. Covariates

Data on potential confounders were available from interview responses at the baseline index DNBC pregnancy. Covariates selected a priori included age (years), socioeconomic status (high or medium level professional, skilled worker, other (student, unskilled, unemployed)), nulliparity (yes, no), smoking during pregnancy (any, none), alcohol during pregnancy (any, none) and pre-pregnancy body mass index (BMI) (<25, 25–29.9, ≥30.0 kg/m^2) calculated from self-reported height and pre-pregnancy weight. Pre-pregnancy weight was not reported at the time of the index pregnancy for a small sub-set of women ($n = 41$), however, pre-pregnancy weight was reported on the DWH Study follow-up questionnaire. For women who reported a pre-pregnancy weight at both instances the weight was highly correlated ($r = 0.89$) and thus, was used to supplement the missing data when available ($n = 40$).

We considered effect modification by several key variables at the DWH Study follow-up, including T2DM status, age, menopausal status, and long-term weight change since the index pregnancy. T2DM status was classified based on HbA1c levels ≥6.5%, fasting glucose ≥7 mmol/L, 2 h glucose after 75 g oral glucose tolerance test ≥11.1 mmol/L, or self-report of physician diagnosis at follow-up [18]. Type 1 diabetes at follow-up was based on self-report of physician diagnosis. Women self-reported their menopausal status (yes, no). Age was categorized according to the median age in the cohort at follow-up (<45 years vs. ≥45 years). Long-term weight change was calculated as the difference in measured weight at the DWH follow-up and self-reported pre-pregnancy weight at the DNBC index pregnancy and was categorized according to the median level (<4.1 kg vs. ≥4.1 kg).

2.5. *Statistical Analysis*

Characteristics of study participants were presented overall and by cumulative lactation duration after the index pregnancy. Differences across lactation duration were described as mean (standard deviation, SD) for continuous variables and frequency (%) for categorical variables. Bivariate associations were evaluated using the one-way Analysis of Variance (ANOVA) for continuous variables and the χ^2 test for categorical variables.

For each lactation category, we used generalized linear models to estimate the unadjusted and adjusted differences in concentrations of TSH, fT3, fT4 and fT3:fT4, by categories of cumulative lactation duration, with no lactation as the reference group. We assessed linear trends (p-trend) by using the median for each category of lactation duration as a continuous exposure. We used logistic regression to estimate unadjusted and adjusted odds ratios (ORs) for SCH, anti-TG positivity, and anti-TPO positivity. All multivariable models were adjusted for potential confounders measured at the index pregnancy and included age, socioeconomic status, pre-pregnancy BMI, parity, smoking during pregnancy, and alcohol consumption during pregnancy. An unknown category was used to account for the small proportion of missing covariate data. Due to a small number of women with SCH (n = 17), the models were unstable and results for SCH are not reported.

To ensure that our findings were not biased by pregnancy or lactation characteristics prior to the index DNBC pregnancy and to remove the effect of parity, we repeated our analyses with only women who had one pregnancy overall and thus, were nulliparous at the index pregnancy. By limiting our sample, we also reduced recall bias from women with multiple pregnancies. In this subset of women, lactation was based on only a single pregnancy and was categorized as none, >0 to 6 months, and >6 months.

To understand whether the observed findings differed across several clinically distinct subgroups of individuals, we tested for a multiplicative interaction with the following characteristics measured at the DWH Study follow-up: age, menopausal status, T2DM status, and long-term weight change.

Two-tailed p-values < 0.05 were considered significant. All statistical analyses were performed using SAS version 9.4 (SAS Institute, Cary, NC, USA).

3. Results

Overall, the median cumulative duration of lactation after a median of one (interquartile range 1–2) pregnancy was 9 (interquartile range 4–15) months, including a lactation duration of 0 months for women who reported never lactating (n = 62, 11.3%). With an increasing duration of lactation, women tended to be lower in pre-pregnancy BMI, of older age, multiparous, and report no alcohol consumption during the index pregnancy. Thyroid biomarkers for most participants were within the euthyroid range (n = 476, 86.6%), while the remainder were classified as SCH (n = 19, 3.5%), hyperthyroid (n = 7, 1.3%), or other (n = 48, 8.7%). Participants in the "other" category did not meet the criteria for SCH, hyperthyroidism, or euthyroid. Several participants were positive for anti-TPO (n = 78, 14.2%) and anti-TG (n = 69, 12.6%) (Table 1).

There was no significant association between lactation and odds of anti-TG positivity or anti-TPO positivity (Table 2). Table 3 shows the unadjusted and adjusted differences in women's thyroid marker levels for each category of cumulative lactation, compared to women who never lactated. Women with a longer lactation duration had higher fT3 levels at follow-up, (adjusted β and 95% confidence interval (CI) for ≥12 months vs. none: 0.19 (0.03, 0.36); p-trend = 0.05). No significant associations were observed between lactation and concentrations of TSH, fT4, or the fT3:fT4 ratio at follow-up.

Table 1. Participant characteristics overall and by lactation history from the Diabetes & Women's Health Study.

Characteristics Ascertained at Index Pregnancy (1996–2002)	Overall (n = 550)	Cumulative Lactation Duration, Months				p *
		None (n = 62)	>0 to < 6 (n = 106)	6 to < 12 (n = 171)	≥12 (n = 211)	
Age, years	31.5 (4.5)	31.1 (4.5)	31.8 (4.0)	32.2 (4.6)	30.8 (4.4)	**0.01**
Pre-pregnancy BMI, kg/m^2						**<0.001**
Unknown	30 (5.5)	6 (9.7)	8 (7.6)	6 (3.5)	10 (4.7)	
<25.0	221 (40.2)	13 (21.0)	30 (28.3)	76 (44.4)	102 (48.3)	
25.0–29.9	143 (26.0)	16 (25.8)	26 (24.5)	45 (26.3)	56 (26.5)	
≥30.0	156 (28.4)	27 (43.6)	42 (39.6)	44 (25.7)	43 (20.4)	
Occupation						**<0.001**
Unknown	49 (8.9)	13 (21.0)	12 (11.3)	9 (5.3)	15 (7.1)	
Professional	254 (46.2)	20 (32.3)	31 (29.3)	82 (48.0)	121 (57.4)	
Skilled worker	152 (27.6)	16 (25.8)	41 (38.7)	47 (27.5)	48 (22.8)	
Other (unskilled worker, unemployed, student)	95 (17.3)	13 (21.0)	22 (20.8)	33 (19.3)	27 (12.8)	
Parity						**<0.001**
Unknown	46 (8.4)	13 (21.0)	11 (10.4)	8 (4.7)	14 (6.6)	
0	200 (36.4)	26 (41.9)	32 (30.2)	41 (24.0)	101 (47.9)	
≥1	304 (55.3)	23 (37.1)	63 (59.4)	122 (71.4)	96 (45.5)	
Drank any alcohol while pregnant						**<0.001**
Unknown	21 (3.8)	8 (12.9)	4 (3.8)	3 (1.8)	6 (2.8)	
No	244 (44.4)	33 (53.2)	42 (39.6)	68 (39.8)	101 (47.9)	
Yes	285 (51.8)	21 (33.9)	60 (56.6)	100 (58.5)	104 (49.3)	
Smoked while pregnant						**0.002**
Unknown	21 (3.8)	8 (12.9)	4 (3.8)	3 (1.8)	6 (2.8)	
No	383 (69.6)	34 (54.8)	69 (65.1)	124 (72.5)	156 (73.9)	
Yes	146 (26.6)	20 (32.3)	33 (31.1)	44 (25.7)	49 (23.2)	
Characteristics ascertained at follow-up (2012–2014)						
Age, year	43.6 (4.6)	43 (4.6)	43.9 (4.3)	44.3 (4.7)	43.1 (4.6)	
Weight change, kg						0.36
Unknown	8 (1.5)	2 (3.2)	2 (1.9)	2 (1.2)	2 (1.0)	
<4.1	269 (48.9)	35 (56.5)	52 (49.1)	89 (52.1)	93 (44.1)	
≥4.1	273 (49.6)	25 (40.3)	52 (49.1)	80 (46.8)	116 (55.0)	
Diabetes						**0.02**
Unknown	6 (1.1)	2 (3.2)	2 (1.9)	1 (0.6)	1 (0.5)	
No	388 (70.6)	37 (59.7)	65 (61.3)	120 (70.2)	166 (78.7)	
Type 1	14 (2.6)	1 (1.6)	5 (4.7)	4 (2.3)	4 (1.9)	
Type 2	142 (25.8)	22 (35.5)	34 (32.1)	46 (26.9)	40 (19)	
Post-Menopausal						**0.047**
Unknown	6 (1.1)	2 (3.2)	2 (1.9)	1 (0.6)	1 (0.5)	
No	463 (84.2)	49 (79)	87 (82.1)	137 (80.1)	190 (90.1)	
Yes	81 (14.7)	11 (17.7)	17 (16)	33 (19.3)	20 (9.5)	
TSH (mIU/L)	2.1 (1.5)	2.2 (1.5)	2 (1.3)	2.1 (1.3)	2.2 (1.8)	0.90
fT3 (pmol/L)	4.6 (0.6)	4.5 (0.6)	4.6 (0.7)	4.6 (0.5)	4.7 (0.6)	0.16
fT4 (ng/dL)	1.1 (0.2)	1.1 (0.2)	1.2 (0.2)	1.1 (0.2)	1.2 (0.2)	0.67
fT3:fT4 ratio	4.1 (0.6)	4.1 (0.7)	4 (0.6)	4.1 (0.7)	4.1 (0.6)	0.59
Anti-TPO positive	78 (14.2)	8 (12.9)	13 (12.3)	30 (17.5)	27 (12.8)	0.51
Anti-TG Positive	69 (12.6)	5 (8.1)	9 (8.5)	26 (15.2)	29 (13.7)	0.25

Data are presented as mean (standard deviation; SD) for continuous variables and n (%) for categorical variables. * Bolded p values represent significant global differences in participant characteristics across lactation duration categories. Abbreviations: BMI, body mass index; TSH, thyroid stimulating hormone; fT3, free triiodothyronine; fT4, free thyroxine; anti-TOP, thyroperoxidase antibody; anti-TG, thyroglobulin antibody.

Table 2. Odds of thyroid autoimmunity 9 to 16 years postpartum according to lactation history among women with a history of gestational diabetes, Diabetes & Women's Health Study.

Outcome	n	Unadjusted OR (95% CI)	p *	Adjusted OR [1] (95% CI)	p *
TG-positive [2]					
≥12 months	211	1.82 (0.67, 4.91)	0.23	2.63 (0.74, 9.37)	0.13
6 to <12 months	171	2.04 (0.75, 5.58)	0.16	2.88 (0.80, 10.27)	0.10
<6 months	106	1.06 (0.34, 3.31)	0.92	1.72 (0.44, 6.82)	0.43
None	62	1.00 (reference)		1.00 (reference)	
TPO-positive [2]					
≥12 months	211	0.99 (0.43, 2.31)	0.98	0.93 (0.36, 2.39)	0.88
6 to <12 months	171	1.44 (0.62, 3.33)	0.40	1.17 (0.46, 2.99)	0.74
<6 months	106	0.94 (0.37, 2.42)	0.90	0.70 (0.24, 2.03)	0.52
None	62	1.00 (reference)		1.00 (reference)	

[1] Model was adjusted for the following covariates, measured at the index pregnancy: age, pre-pregnancy body mass index (unknown, <25, 25–29.9, ≥30.0 kg/m^2), occupation (unknown, professional, skilled worker, unskilled/unemployed/student), nulliparity (unknown, yes, no), smoking during pregnancy (unknown, any, none), and alcohol consumption during pregnancy (unknown, any, none). [2] TG, thyroglobulin antibody; TPO, thyroid peroxidase antibody. * p-values represent significance in the difference in odds of TG- or TPO- positivity for each category of lactation duration compared to no lactation.

Table 3. Thyroid biomarker levels 9 to 16 years postpartum according to lactation history among women with a history of gestational diabetes, Diabetes & Women's Health Study.

Thyroid Biomarker	n	Unadjusted β Estimate (95% CI)	*p-Trend* *	Adjusted [1] β Estimate (95% CI)	*p-Trend* *
TSH (mIU/L)			0.79		0.87
≥12 months	211	−0.05 (−0.48, 0.38)		−0.03 (−0.47, 0.41)	
6 to <12 months	171	−0.07 (−0.51, 0.37)		−0.03 (−0.49, 0.43)	
<6 months	106	−0.17 (−0.64, 0.31)		−0.13 (−0.61, 0.35)	
None	62	Reference		Reference	
fT3 (pmol/L)			**0.03**		0.05
≥12 months	211	**0.18 (0.01, 0.34)**		**0.19 (0.03, 0.36)**	
6 to <12 months	171	0.10 (−0.07, 0.27)		0.15 (−0.02, 0.32)	
<6 months	106	0.10 (−0.08, 0.28)		0.13 (−0.05, 0.31)	
None	62	Reference		Reference	
fT4 (ng/dL)			0.65		0.55
≥12 months	211	0.03 (−0.02, 0.07)		0.03 (−0.02, 0.07)	
6 to <12 months	171	0.02 (−0.03, 0.07)		0.03 (−0.02, 0.07)	
<6 months	106	0.03 (−0.02, 0.08)		0.04 (−0.01, 0.09)	
None	62	Reference		Reference	
fT3:fT4 ratio			0.24		0.30
≥12 months	211	0.04 −0.14, 0.23)		0.06 (−0.13, 0.25)	
6 to <12 months	171	−0.01 (−0.20, 0.18)		0.03 (−0.16, 0.23)	
<6 months	106	−0.06 (−0.26, 0.14)		−0.05 (−0.25, 0.15)	
None	62	Reference		Reference	

[1] Model was adjusted for the following covariates, measured at the index pregnancy: age, pre-pregnancy body mass index (unknown, <25, 25–29.9, ≥30.0 kg/m^2), occupation (unknown, professional, skilled worker, unskilled/unemployed/student), nulliparity (unknown, yes, no), smoking during pregnancy (unknown, any, none), and alcohol during pregnancy (unknown, any, none). * Bolded p-trend values represent significant linear trends in thyroid biomarker levels with increasing lactation duration. We assessed p-trends by using the median for each category of lactation duration as a continuous exposure.

Although there were significant differences in mean levels of several thyroid biomarkers according to long-term weight change and diabetes status at follow-up (Table A1), there was no variation in the lactation duration–thyroid function association according to maternal weight change, diabetes status, or age at follow-up (p for interaction >0.05). There was a significant interaction between lactation duration and menopause status for the outcomes of fT3 (p = 0.02) and the fT3:fT4 ratio (p = 0.03).

The results were null among pre-menopausal women, but stronger among post-menopausal women such that a lactation duration of ≥12 months was associated with higher fT3 levels by 0.47 pmol/L compared to women who never lactated (Table A2).

To tease apart the effect of lactation from the number of pregnancies, we restricted the analyses to women with a single lifetime pregnancy (n = 70). Women with a cumulative lactation duration >6 months had significantly higher levels of fT3 (0.46 pmol/L (0.12, 0.80); p-trend = 0.02) and a higher fT3:fT4 ratio (0.61 (0.17, 1.05); p-trend = 0.007) than women who had never lactated (Table 4). In addition, there was a significant trend (p = 0.04) of increasing TSH with increasing lactation duration.

Table 4. Thyroid biomarker levels 9 to 16 years postpartum according to lactation history among women with a history of gestational diabetes who had a single lifetime pregnancy, Diabetes & Women's Health Study.

Thyroid Biomarker	n	Unadjusted β Estimate (95% CI)	p-Trend *	Adjusted [1] β Estimate (95% CI)	p-Trend *
TSH (mIU/L)			**0.045**		**0.04**
>6 months	24	0.67 (−0.09, 1.44)		0.78 (−0.03, 1.58)	
>0 to 6 months	26	−0.04 (−0.79, 0.71)		0.14 (−0.65, 0.94)	
None	20	Reference		Reference	
fT3 (pmol/L)			0.17		**0.02**
>6 months	24	0.22 (−0.12, 0.56)		**0.46 (0.12, 0.80)**	
>0 to 6 months	26	0.04 (−0.29, 0.38)		0.27 (−0.06, 0.60)	
None	20	Reference		Reference	
fT4 (ng/dL)			0.07		0.36
>6 months	24	−0.09 (−0.20, 0.01)		−0.05 (−0.15, 0.06)	
>0 to 6 months	26	−0.03 (−0.14, 0.07)		−0.02 (−0.12, 0.09)	
None	20	Reference		Reference	
fT3:fT4 ratio			**0.009**		**0.007**
>6 months	24	**0.55 (0.12, 0.99)**		**0.61 (0.17, 1.05)**	
>0 to 6 months	26	0.12 (−0.31, 0.55)		0.25 (−0.18, 0.69)	
None	20	Reference		Reference	

[1] Model was adjusted for the following covariates, measured at the index pregnancy: age, pre-pregnancy body mass index (unknown, <25, 25–29.9, ≥30.0 kg/m^2), occupation (unknown, professional, skilled worker, unskilled/unemployed/student), nulliparity (unknown, yes, no), smoking during pregnancy (unknown, any, none), and alcohol during pregnancy (unknown, any, none). * Bolded p-trend values represent significant linear trends in thyroid biomarker levels with increasing lactation duration. We assessed p-trends by using the median for each category of lactation duration as a continuous exposure.

4. Discussion

In the present study following women 9–16 years after GDM pregnancy, a high-risk population for cardiometabolic complications, we examined whether cumulative duration of lactation is associated with long-term thyroid function. Findings from this study suggested that a longer cumulative lactation duration is associated with higher serum fT3 levels and fT3:fT4 ratio approximately 9–16 years after the index pregnancy. The positive association between lactation duration and fT3 levels was more pronounced among nulliparous women at the index pregnancy. While the strengths of these associations are modest, they highlight novel findings, extending the existing literature which demonstrates long-term associations between women's lifetime duration of lactation and cardiometabolic health to potentially include thyroid function as a novel endpoint [19–21].

An important feature of our study was distinguishing the effect of cumulative duration of lactation from parity, as these variables are highly correlated. We accomplished this by restricting the study specifically to women who were nulliparous at the index pregnancy and had only a single lifetime pregnancy. The results of our analyses were more robust among this subset, as we removed any residual confounding due to parity. It was meaningful to analyze this subset, as we observed an association between lactation and thyroid biomarker levels even within the shorter lactation periods following only a single birth.

Prior studies have observed that a longer lactation duration is related to lower levels of risk for breast and ovarian cancer, cardiovascular disease, diabetes, hypertension, and hyperlipidemia [3]. There has been limited clinical or epidemiologic research on lactation and long-term maternal thyroid function. Our study adds an intriguing piece to the prior work by linking lactation duration with long-term thyroid function, as we provide suggestive evidence that women who lactated for longer durations of time had higher levels of serum fT3 later in life. Interestingly, we observed that women with even 6 months of lactation, compared to none, had higher levels of fT3 and the fT3:fT4 ratio.

Several hypotheses may explain the biological mechanisms associating lactation with long-term maternal metabolic health. To support the developing fetus and prepare the mother for lactation, there is an increase in visceral adiposity, circulating lipids, and insulin levels during pregnancy [22]. It is hypothesized that a prolonged duration of lactation helps to rapidly and more completely reverse these metabolic changes by mobilizing the fat stores accumulated during pregnancy [22]. This "reset" to the maternal metabolism may reduce women's risk for future metabolic diseases, possibly including thyroid dysfunction. Animal models also offer unique insight into the biological pathways linking lactation and thyroid function. In bovine models, the quantity of mRNA transcripts in the mammary gland for iodothyronine deiodinase type II (DIO2), the enzyme responsible for generating T3, the biologically active thyroid hormone, from inactive T4, increased with lactation duration [4]. This observation is consistent with our findings that a longer duration of lactation is associated with greater fT3 levels and fT3:fT4, as fT3 is the form of T3 that is in circulation, and the fT3:fT4 ratio is a proxy for the conversion from T4 to T3. Furthermore, we hypothesized that a potential mechanism for the association between lactation and thyroid function may have been through weight change, yet we did not observe any evidence for this. Lastly, the association between GDM and T2DM has been previously studied and served as the impetus for this research to look beyond cardiometabolic disorders and extend to thyroid metabolism. However, it should be noted that the results were consistent regardless of T2DM status at follow-up. Further research into the mechanisms is warranted.

Although the effect sizes observed in our study do not clinically alter euthyroid status, prior research has demonstrated an association between small changes in thyroid hormone levels and clinical outcomes, even within the euthyroid range. Specifically, the importance of T3 in overall health and metabolic function has been demonstrated among patients with end-stage renal disease, hemodialysis, chronic heart failure, and cerebral infarction who also had clinically low T3 (i.e., low T3 syndrome) and were receiving T3 replacement therapy [23–26]. Conversely, higher fT3 levels have been associated with several parameters of metabolic syndrome, non-alcoholic fatty liver disease (NAFLD), and insulin resistance among cohorts of healthy euthyroid individuals [27–30]. The conflicting results from these studies warrant further investigation of lifetime lactation and thyroid disease, beyond clinical biomarkers. Lactation was not associated with thyroid autoimmunity status (i.e., TGO-positivity and TG-positivity); however, the sample size in the current study may have been too small to detect an association. Further research, with a larger sample and longer follow-up time, may be necessary to understand the clinical significance of higher fT3 levels associated with a longer duration of cumulative lactation.

There are several strengths to our study, including the hybrid study design, combining DNBC pregnancy data with follow-up data from the DWH Study. This study design provided the unique opportunity to follow a large high-risk cohort of women with a history of GDM for over a decade, and to understand their long-term health consequences and modifiable risk factors for specific health outcomes. Additionally, lactation duration, which was reported by women immediately following the index DNBC pregnancy, was highly correlated with women's reported duration at the DWH

Study follow-up 9–16 years later. This also helped to validate women's recall of lactation duration for the additional births. Our study was further strengthened by consideration of several risk factors for thyroid function reported during the index DNBC pregnancy, including pre-pregnancy BMI, age, socioeconomic status, smoking during pregnancy, and alcohol consumption during pregnancy. Finally, our study is generalizable to Danish women with a history of GDM. While our findings may not be generalizable to all women, women with GDM represent a unique high-risk model for metabolic dysfunction.

Several limitations warrant discussion. First, the cumulative duration of lactation was calculated following the index pregnancy because we did not have detailed lactation data and related covariates before the index pregnancy. However, to account for potential confounding from previous lactation history, we adjusted for the number of pregnancies before the index pregnancy (i.e., parity at the index pregnancy). In addition, we conducted an analysis restricted to women for whom the index pregnancy was their first pregnancy and thus had no prior lactation history. In these analyses, we observed a similar, but stronger positive association between lactation duration and thyroid marker levels. Second, we did not have clear data on how many additional pregnancies were complicated by GDM. Third, we assessed thyroid biomarkers only at a single follow-up and we were unaware of baseline thyroid marker levels before pregnancy or during the interim between the index GDM pregnancy and follow up. While we excluded women with known thyroid disorders prior to pregnancy, we did not have information on the development of, and treatment for, thyroid disease during the period between the index GDM pregnancy and follow up. Fourth, we did not have the power to test for associations between lactation and clinical end points related to thyroid function, such as SCH and other thyroid diseases. Lastly, we did not have data from women on reasons for discontinuing breastfeeding or choosing not to breastfeed, and thus we cannot tease out confounding from other factors (i.e., social factors, milk supply, etc.) that may have contributed to lactation duration.

5. Conclusions

In Danish women with a history of GDM, our findings suggest a positive association between 'onger duration of lactation and higher levels of thyroid hormone 9–16 years postpartum, even ɔng women with a single lifetime pregnancy. Here we identified lactation as a novel potential ifiable factor for thyroid function, and with replication, these findings may add thyroid function wide-array of long-term cardiometabolic outcomes associated with increased lactation duration. the findings related to metabolic health, more research is needed to understand the mechanisms ur findings. A longer follow-up period may help further understanding of the clinical impact d fT3 levels associated with longer lactation duration.

butions: The study was conceived and designed by C.Z. The data were analyzed by P.L.P. and was obtained by C.Z. The first draft of the manuscript was prepared by P.L.P. and S.N.H., which the input from the writing team (S.N.H., S.R., L.G.G., S.H.L., Y.L., A.L., A.C.B.T., S.F.O., C.Z.). d the manuscript critically for important intellectual content. All authors gave final approval of ublished and have contributed to the manuscript. C.Z. and S.N.H. are the guarantors.

Appendix A

Table A1. Thyroid biomarkers according to participant characteristics at follow-up (2012–2014).

Characteristics Ascertained at Follow-Up (2012–2014)	*n*	Thyroid Biomarkers			
		TSH (mIU/L)	fT3 (pmol/L)	fT4 (ng/dL)	fT3:fT4 Ratio
Age					
Unknown	6	1.73 (1.10)	4.0 (1.38)	1.09 (0.41)	3.74 (0.46)
<45	314	2.09 (1.66)	4.65 (0.60)	1.14 (0.15)	4.12 (0.66)
≥45	230	2.20 (1.32)	4.62 (0.52)	1.15 (0.17)	4.07 (0.62)
p *		0.41	0.51	0.47	0.32
Weight change, kg					
Unknown	8	2.31 (1.73)	4.19 (1.22)	1.10 (0.35)	3.84 (0.45)
<4.1	265	2.09 (1.31)	4.53 (0.56)	1.17 (0.16)	3.94 (0.62)
≥4.1	277	2.17 (1.70)	4.74 (0.56)	1.13 (0.15)	4.25 (0.64)
p *		0.57	**<0.01**	**0.01**	**<0.01**
Diabetes					
Unknown	6	1.73 (1.10)	4.0 (1.38)	1.09 (0.41)	3.74 (0.46)
No	388	2.15 (1.63)	4.61 (0.57)	1.14 (0.15)	4.09 (0.60)
Type 1	14	2.69 (1.44)	4.55 (0.48)	1.04 (0.09)	4.37 (0.43)
Type 2	142	2.04 (1.19)	4.72 (0.58)	1.18 (0.18)	4.09 (0.76)
p *		0.29	0.13	**<0.01**	0.28
Post-menopausal					
Unknown	6	1.73 (1.10)	4.0 (1.38)	1.09 (0.41)	3.74 (0.46)
No	463	2.14 (1.55)	4.63 (0.56)	1.14 (0.15)	4.11 (0.65)
Yes	81	2.13 (1.36)	4.70 (0.59)	1.18 (0.19)	4.05 (0.62)
p *		0.99	0.29	0.05	0.43

Data are presented as the mean (standard deviation; SD) of each thyroid biomarker (i.e., TSH, fT3, fT4, fT3:fT4), according to categories of participant characteristics (i.e., age, weight change, diabetes status, menopause status). * Bolded *p*-values represent significant global differences in the levels of each thyroid biomarker across non-missing categories of participant characteristics.

Table A2. Associations between lactation duration and fT3 and the fT3:fT4 ratio by menopausal status among women with a history of gestational diabetes, Diabetes & Women's Health Study.

Thyroid Biomarker	Pre-Menopausal Women (*n* = 463)		*p-Trend* *	Post-Menopausal Women (*n* = 81)		*p-Trend* *
	n	Adjusted [1] β Estimate (95% CI)		*n*	Adjusted [1] β Estimate (95% CI)	
fT3 (pmol/L)			0.29			0.22
≥12 months	190	0.10 (−0.08, 0.28)		20	**0.47 (0.04, 0.90)**	
6 to <12 months	137	0.12 (−0.07, 0.03)		33	0.10 (−0.30, 0.50)	
<6 months	87	0.02 (−0.17, 0.22)		17	**0.46 (0.03, 0.90)**	
None	49	Reference		11	Reference	
fT3:fT4 ratio			0.43			0.33
≥12 months	190	0.00 (−0.20, 0.21)		20	0.38 (−0.06, 0.82)	
6 to <12 months	137	0.05 (−0.17, 0.27)		33	−0.12 (−0.53, 0.29)	
<6 months	87	−0.11 (−0.34, 0.12)		17	0.14 (−0.30, 0.59)	
None	49	Reference		11	Reference	

[1] Model was adjusted for the following covariates, measured at the index pregnancy: age, pre-pregnancy body mass index (unknown, <25, 25–29.9, ≥30.0 kg/m^2), occupation (unknown, professional, skilled worker unskilled/unemployed/student), nulliparity (unknown, yes, no), smoking during pregnancy (unknown, any, none and alcohol during pregnancy (unknown, any, none). * *p*-trend values represent linear trends in thyroid biomark levels with increasing lactation duration. We assessed *p*-trends by using the median for each category of lactatic duration as a continuous exposure.

References

1. Yen, P.M. Physiological and molecular basis of thyroid hormone action. *Physiol. Rev.* **2001**, *81*, 1097–1142. [CrossRef] [PubMed]
2. Reece, E.A. The fetal and maternal consequences of gestational diabetes mellitus. *J. Matern. Fetal Neonatal Med.* **2010**, *23*, 199–203. [CrossRef] [PubMed]
3. Stuebe, A.M.; Schwarz, E.B. The risks and benefits of infant feeding practices for women and their children. *J. Perinatol.* **2010**, *30*, 155–162. [CrossRef] [PubMed]
4. Capuco, A.V.; Connor, E.E.; Wood, D.L. Regulation of mammary gland sensitivity to thyroid hormones during the transition from pregnancy to lactation. *Exp. Biol. Med.* **2008**, *233*, 1309–1314. [CrossRef] [PubMed]
5. Knudsen, N.; Laurberg, P.; Rasmussen, L.B.; Bulow, I.; Perrild, H.; Ovesen, L.; Jorgensen, T. Small differences in thyroid function may be important for body mass index and the occurrence of obesity in the population. *J. Clin. Endocrinol. Metab.* **2005**, *90*, 4019–4024. [CrossRef] [PubMed]
6. Baker, J.L.; Gamborg, M.; Heitmann, B.L.; Lissner, L.; Sorensen, T.I.; Rasmussen, K.M. Breastfeeding reduces postpartum weight retention. *Am. J. Clin. Nutr.* **2008**, *88*, 1543–1551. [CrossRef] [PubMed]
7. Bano, A.; Dhana, K.; Chaker, L.; Kavousi, M.; Ikram, M.A.; Mattace-Raso, F.U.S.; Peeters, R.P.; Franco, O.H. Association of thyroid function with life expectancy with and without cardiovascular disease: The rotterdam study. *JAMA Intern. Med.* **2017**, *177*, 1650–1657. [CrossRef] [PubMed]
8. Fatima, S.S.; Rehman, R.; Butt, Z.; Tauni, M.A.; Munim, T.F.; Chaudhry, B.; Khan, T.A. Screening of subclinical hypothyroidism during gestational diabetes in pakistani population. *J. Matern. Fetal Neonatal Med.* **2016**, *29*, 2166–2170. [CrossRef] [PubMed]
9. Shahbazian, H.; Shahbazian, N.; Baniani, M.R.; Yazdanpanah, L.; Latifi, S.M. Evaluation of thyroid dysfunction in pregnant women with gestational and pre-gestational diabetes. *Pak. J. Med. Sci.* **2013**, *29*, 638–641. [CrossRef] [PubMed]
10. Speller, E.; Brodribb, W. Breastfeeding and thyroid disease: A literature review. *Breastfeed. Rev.* **2012**, *20*, 41–47. [PubMed]
11. Vafaeimanesh, J.; Asgarani, F.; Bagherzadeh, M.; Ebrahimi, G.; Parham, M. Thyroid function in pregnant women with gestational diabetes: Is screening necessary? *Thyroid Res. Pract.* **2015**, *12*, 3–7. [CrossRef]
12. Vitacolonna, E.; Lapolla, A.; Di Nenno, B.; Passante, A.; Bucci, I.; Giuliani, C.; Cerrone, D.; Capani, F.; Monaco, F.; Napolitano, G. Gestational diabetes and thyroid autoimmunity. *Int. J. Endocrinol.* **2012**, *2012*, 867415. [CrossRef] [PubMed]
13. Yang, S.; Shi, F.T.; Leung, P.C.; Huang, H.F.; Fan, J. Low thyroid hormone in early pregnancy is associated with an increased risk of gestational diabetes mellitus. *J. Clin. Endocrinol. Metab.* **2016**, *101*, 4237–4243. [CrossRef] [PubMed]
14. Zhang, C.; Hu, F.B.; Olsen, S.F.; Vaag, A.; Gore-Langton, R.; Chavarro, J.E.; Bao, W.; Yeung, E.; Bowers, K.; Grunnet, L.G.; et al. Rationale, design, and method of the diabetes & women's health study—A study of long-term health implications of glucose intolerance in pregnancy and their determinants. *Acta Obstet. Gynecol. Scand.* **2014**, *93*, 1123–1130. [CrossRef] [PubMed]
15. Olsen, J.; Melbye, M.; Olsen, S.F.; Sorensen, T.I.; Aaby, P.; Andersen, A.M.; Taxbol, D.; Hansen, K.D.; Juhl, M.; Schow, T.B.; et al. The danish national birth cohort—Its background, structure and aim. *Scand. J. Public Health* **2001**, *29*, 300–307. [CrossRef] [PubMed]
16. Garber, J.R.; Cobin, R.H.; Gharib, H.; Hennessey, J.V.; Klein, I.; Mechanick, J.I.; Pessah-Pollack, R.; Singer, P.A.; Woeber, K.A. Clinical practice guidelines for hypothyroidism in adults: Cosponsored by the american association of clinical endocrinologists and the american thyroid association. *Endocr. Pract.* **2012**, *18*, 988–1028. [CrossRef] [PubMed]
17. Hollowell, J.G.; Staehling, N.W.; Flanders, W.D.; Hannon, W.H.; Gunter, E.W.; Spencer, C.A.; Braverman, L.E. Serum TSH, T_4, and thyroid antibodies in the united states population (1988 to 1994): National health and nutrition examination survey (NHANES III). *J. Clin. Endocrinol. Metab.* **2002**, *87*, 489–499. [CrossRef] [PubMed]
18. Association, A.D. Diagnosis and classification of diabetes mellitus. *Diabetes Care* **2011**, *34*, S62–S69. [CrossRef] [PubMed]
19. Bianco, A.C.; Kim, B.W. Deiodinases: Implications of the local control of thyroid hormone action. *J. Clin. Investig.* **2006**, *116*, 2571–2579. [CrossRef] [PubMed]

20. Hyatt, H.W.; Zhang, Y.; Hood, W.R.; Kavazis, A.N. Lactation has persistent effects on a mother's metabolism and mitochondrial function. *Sci. Rep.* **2017**, *7*, 17118. [CrossRef] [PubMed]
21. Stuebe, A.M.; Michels, K.B.; Willett, W.C.; Manson, J.E.; Rexrode, K.; Rich-Edwards, J.W. Duration of lactation and incidence of myocardial infarction in middle to late adulthood. *Am. J. Obstet. Gynecol.* **2009**, *200*, 138.e1–138.e8. [CrossRef] [PubMed]
22. Stuebe, A.M.; Rich-Edwards, J.W. The reset hypothesis: Lactation and maternal metabolism. *Am. J. Perinatol.* **2009**, *26*, 81–88. [CrossRef] [PubMed]
23. Chang, T.I.; Nam, J.Y.; Shin, S.K.; Kang, E.W. Low triiodothyronine syndrome and long-term cardiovascular outcome in incident peritoneal dialysis patients. *Clin. J. Am. Soc. Nephrol.* **2015**, *10*, 975–982. [CrossRef] [PubMed]
24. Fragidis, S.; Sombolos, K.; Thodis, E.; Panagoutsos, S.; Mourvati, E.; Pikilidou, M.; Papagianni, A.; Pasadakis, P.; Vargemezis, V. Low T3 syndrome and long-term mortality in chronic hemodialysis patients. *World J. Nephrol.* **2015**, *4*, 415–422. [CrossRef] [PubMed]
25. Wu, G.H.; Kong, F.Z.; Cheng, Q.Z.; Luo, W.F.; Du, X.D. Low T3 syndrome predicts severe neurological deficits of cerebral infarction inpatients with large artery artherosclerosis in internal carotid artery system. *Neuro Endocrinol. Lett.* **2014**, *35*, 149–153. [PubMed]
26. Zoccali, C.; Mallamaci, F.; Tripepi, G.; Cutrupi, S.; Pizzini, P. Low triiodothyronine and survival in end-stage renal disease. *Kidney Int.* **2006**, *70*, 523–528. [CrossRef] [PubMed]
27. Ferrannini, E.; Iervasi, G.; Cobb, J.; Ndreu, R.; Nannipieri, M. Insulin resistance and normal thyroid hormone levels: Prospective study and metabolomic analysis. *Am. J. Physiol. Endocrinol. Metab.* **2017**, *312*, E429–E436. [CrossRef] [PubMed]
28. Roef, G.L.; Rietzschel, E.R.; Van Daele, C.M.; Taes, Y.E.; De Buyzere, M.L.; Gillebert, T.C.; Kaufman, J.M. Triiodothyronine and free thyroxine levels are differentially associated with metabolic profile and adiposity-related cardiovascular risk markers in euthyroid middle-aged subjects. *Thyroid* **2014**, *24*, 223–231. [CrossRef] [PubMed]
29. Tarcin, O.; Abanonu, G.B.; Yazici, D.; Tarcin, O. Association of metabolic syndrome parameters with TT3 and FT3/FT4 ratio in obese turkish population. *Metab. Syndr. Relat. Disord.* **2012**, *10*, 137–142. [CrossRef] [PubMed]
30. Van den Berg, E.H.; van Tienhoven-Wind, L.J.; Amini, M.; Schreuder, T.C.; Faber, K.N.; Blokzijl, H.; Dullaart, R.P. Higher free triiodothyronine is associated with non-alcoholic fatty liver disease in euthyroid subjects: The lifelines cohort study. *Metabolism* **2017**, *67*, 62–71. [CrossRef] [PubMed]

3

Variability of Serum Proteins in Chinese and Dutch Human Milk during Lactation

Mohèb Elwakiel [1,2], Sjef Boeren [3], Jos A. Hageman [4], Ignatius M. Szeto [5], Henk A. Schols [2] and Kasper A. Hettinga [1,*]

1 Food Quality and Design Group, Wageningen University & Research, Bornse Weilanden 9, 6708 WG Wageningen, The Netherlands; moheb.elwakiel@wur.nl
2 Laboratory of Food Chemistry, Wageningen University & Research, Bornse Weilanden 9, 6708 WG Wageningen, The Netherlands; henk.schols@wur.nl
3 Laboratory of Biochemistry, Wageningen University & Research, Stippeneng 4, 6708 WE Wageningen, The Netherlands; sjef.boeren@wur.nl
4 Biometris-Applied Statistics, Wageningen University & Research, Droevendaalsesteeg 1, 6708 PB Wageningen, The Netherlands; jos.hageman@wur.nl
5 Inner Mongolia Yili Industrial Group Co., Ltd., Jinshan Road 8, Hohhot 010110, China; szeto@yili.com
* Correspondence: kasper.hettinga@wur.nl

Abstract: To better understand the variability of the type and level of serum proteins in human milk, the milk serum proteome of Chinese mothers during lactation was investigated using proteomic techniques and compared to the milk serum proteome of Dutch mothers. This showed that total milk serum protein concentrations in Chinese human milk decreased over a 20-week lactation period, although with variation between mothers in the rate of decrease. Variation was also found in the composition of serum proteins in both colostrum and mature milk, although immune-active proteins, enzymes, and transport proteins were the most abundant for all mothers. These three protein groups account for many of the 15 most abundant proteins, with these 15 proteins covering more than 95% of the total protein concentrations, in both the Chinese and Dutch milk serum proteome. The Dutch and Chinese milk serum proteome were also compared based on 166 common milk serum proteins, which showed that 22% of the 166 serum proteins differed in level. These differences were observed mainly in colostrum and concern several highly abundant proteins. This study also showed that protease inhibitors, which are highly correlated to immune-active proteins, are present in variable amounts in human milk and could be relevant during digestion.

Keywords: mammary gland; immune-active proteins; proteases; protease inhibitors; digestive tract

---

1. Introduction

Human milk is the best source of nutrition for babies, enhances children's immune system and influences the microbiota [1–3]. Health benefits have been linked to the presence and concentration of human milk components like oligosaccharides and proteins [4,5]. There are two distinct groups of proteins in human milk; caseins and milk serum proteins [6]. Human milk in early lactation consists of approximately 30% caseins and 70% serum proteins, with a 50:50 ratio typically found after a six month lactation period [6].

Serum proteins in human milk have been categorized according to their main and highly diverse biological functions [7,8]. It was found that immune-related proteins, transport proteins, and enzymes were present in the largest quantities, and their concentrations generally decrease over lactation [7,8]. Immune-active proteins not only protect infants against pathogenic microorganisms, but also confer passive immunity to the neonate until its own immune system has been fully developed [9–11].

Serum proteins in human milk also include an array of blood coagulation proteins, membrane proteins, signaling proteins, and protease inhibitors [9–11]. Protease inhibitors play a key role in the blood coagulation cascade and complement pathway [12–14], and might protect proteins against degradation by proteases in the mammary gland and even in the infant's gastrointestinal tract [12–18].

There is a wide range of proteins (e.g., α_{S1}-, β-, and κ-casein, lactoferrin, immunoglobulins, serum albumin, and α-lactalbumin) in relatively high concentrations in human milk [19]. Most milk proteins are synthesized in the mammary gland, except for immunoglobulins and serum albumin [19]. Serum albumin can enter milk via the paracellular pathway and immunoglobulins are transported from blood through mammary epithelial cells by a receptor-mediated mechanism [19]. Caseins are transport proteins that form micelles, and these micelles are capable of binding—and thereby transporting—minerals. Caseins can easily be digested in the infant's gastrointestinal tract [15–18], being a valuable source of amino acids and minerals, which can easily be absorbed. Milk serum proteins such as lactoferrin, immunoglobulins, serum albumin, and α-lactalbumin cover 90% of the milk serum proteome in abundance [20]. The milk serum protein α-lactalbumin is required for the synthesis of lactose, supplies infants with large amounts of tryptophan, and facilitates the absorption of essential minerals [21]. Several other milk serum proteins, like lactoferrin and immunoglobulins, protect infants against pathogens and decrease the risk of having acute or chronic diseases [21,22]. Lactoferrin, a globular glycoprotein of the transferrin family, ends up in the infant's feces, and was shown to influence the microbiota composition of neonates [22]. Human milk is also a rich source of antibodies or immunoglobulins, which are able to recognize and bind to unique epitopes of pathogens, preventing their colonization [23–25]. Serum albumin is a protein mainly involved in the transportation of hormones, fatty acids, and other milk components [21].

Individual differences in milk serum proteins between mothers have been reported, where it was found that there was a large overlap in identified proteins in human milk among mothers, whereas there were also major quantitative changes, both between mothers and over time [7]. Given the various potential benefits of milk serum proteins, it would be of interest to obtain insights in the variability of serum proteins in human milk from mothers from other geographical and ethnic origin.

Therefore, the main objective of this study was to investigate the milk serum proteome of seven Chinese mothers and to investigate the variability in type and level of serum proteins in Chinese human milk over a 20-week lactation period using liquid chromatography and mass spectrometry (LC-MS/MS). Additionally, the type and level of serum proteins in Chinese human milk were compared to those in colostrum and mature milk from Dutch mothers.

2. Materials and Methods

2.1. Study Setup and Sample Collection

Chinese participants were recruited in the Hohhot region, China, between August 2014 and November 2015 by the Yili Innovation Center (Hohhot, China). Yili organized the collection of the human milk, including sampling using a human milk pump. For every time point, a volume of 10 mL was collected in a polypropylene bottles. Milk bottles were shaken gently, aliquoted directly into 2 mL Eppendorf tubes, and stored at −20 °C. Milk samples from seven healthy mothers who delivered term (38–42 weeks) infants were assessed in weeks 1, 2, 4, 8, 12, and 20 postpartum. Human milk collection was approved by the Chinese Ethics Committee of Registering Clinical Trials (ChiECRCT-20150017). Written informed consent was obtained from all mothers. Milk collection and analysis of the milk of four Dutch mothers over a 24-week lactation period was described preciously and was a collaboration with the Dutch Human Milk Bank (Amsterdam, The Netherlands) [7]. Healthy women who delivered singleton term infants (38–42 weeks) were eligible for that study. The data from these analyses were re-used and made compatible with the Chinese data within this research to facilitate direct comparison, as explained further in Section 2.4 (Data Analysis).

2.2. *Milk Serum Preparation and Concentrations*

Human milk samples (5 mL) were fractionated, as described previously [10]. Briefly, the milk fat was removed by centrifugation (10 min, 1500 *g*, 4 °C) and the obtained skim milk was transferred to ultracentrifuge tubes. After ultracentrifugation (90 min, 100,000 *g*, 4 °C), the top layer represented the remaining milk fat still present, the middle layer was milk serum (with some free soluble caseins), and the bottom layer consisted of micellar casein. The free soluble caseins are part of the milk serum proteome. A comparative study previously showed that ultracentrifugation is the most effective method to separate caseins from serum proteins [26], although it is not possible to rule out low amounts of serum proteins in the casein pellet [6]. Milk serum concentrations were measured in duplicate using the bicinchoninic acid (BCA) protein assay kit (Thermo Scientific Pierce, Massachusetts, U.S.), to ensure that the same amount of protein (10 μg) was used for further sample preparation. Bovine serum albumin was used as standard for making a BCA calibration curve.

2.3. *Sample Preparation, Dimethyl Labeling, Protein Digestion, and Peptide Analysis*

Milk serum samples were prepared for protein analysis using filter-aided sample preparation and dimethyl labeling, as described previously [27]. Milk serum (20 μL) was mixed with a buffer containing sodium dodecyl sulfate (SDS) for protein denaturation and dithiothreitol (DTT) to reduce the disulfide bridges in proteins, after which the samples were loaded on a Pall 3 K omega filter (10–20 kDa cutoff, OD003C34, Pall, Washington, U.S.) for protein digestion. The lysis buffer contained 0.1 M Tris/HCl pH 8.0 + 4% SDS + 0.1 M DTT to get a 1 μg/μL protein solution. Next, 180 μL of 0.05 M iodoacetamide/urea (0.1 M Tris/HCl pH 8 + 8 M urea) was used for protein alkylation. Samples were washed three times with 100 μL of 8 M urea, using centrifugation, followed by 110 μL of 50 mM ammonium bicarbonate (ABC). Then 0.5 μg trypsin in 100 μL ABC was added, followed by overnight incubation at room temperature while mildly shaking, and centrifuged to separate peptides from undigested material. The trypsin digested samples were then labeled, using distinct combinations of isotopic isomers of formaldehyde and cyanoborohydride, leading to a unique stable isotope composition of labeled peptide doublets with different masses [27]. After dimethyl labeling, the prepared samples were analyzed using LC-MS/MS, as described before [7]. For LC-MS/MS, a Prontosil 300-3-C18Hmagic C18AQ 200 Å analytical column was used, and the full scan FTMS spectra were measured in positive mode between m/z 380 and 1400 on a Thermo LTQ-Orbitrap XL. CID fragmented MS/MS scans of the four most abundant doubly- and triply-charged peaks in the FTMS scan were recorded in data-dependent mode in the linear trap (MS/MS threshold = 5.000).

2.4. *Data Analysis*

The MS/MS spectra obtained were processed by the software package Maxquant 1.3.0.5 with the Andromeda search engine, as described previously [28]. Protein identification and quantification was done according to the literature [7]. Maxquant created a decoy database consisting of reversed sequences to calculate the false discovery rate (FDR). The FDR was set to 0.01 at the peptide and protein levels. The minimum required peptide length was six amino acids, and proteins were identified based on a minimum of two distinct peptides. The intensity–based absolute quantification (iBAQ) values were selected, representing the total peak intensity as determined by Maxquant for each protein and their values were corrected for the number of measurable peptides [7]. The iBAQ values have been reported to have a good correlation with known absolute protein amounts over at least four orders of magnitude [29]. For data normalization, iBAQ values for each protein were transformed into BCA equivalent milk serum protein concentrations, by dividing the iBAQ values of each protein in a sample by the summed iBAQ values of all protein within a sample, there were then multiplied with the corresponding milk serum protein concentration based on the BCA assay. To facilitate direct comparison between Chinese and Dutch data within this research, BCA equivalent values at time points 12 and 20 weeks postpartum were compared to weeks 16 and 24, respectively. Biological functions were assigned to all the serum proteins using the online UniprotKB database, as done previously [7]. To assign a specific function to multifunctional proteins, DAVID Bioinformatics Resource 6.7 was used additionally for further protein biological function classification and clarification [30].

2.5. Statistical Analysis

Statistical analysis was performed based upon previously described methods [7], with modifications. For the BCA equivalent values of each protein in Chinese and Dutch human milk over lactation, a regression line was fitted using R (Lucent Technologies, New York, NY, U.S.A.), summarizing the profile over time for each protein into an intercept and slope. The calculated intercepts are the protein BCA equivalent values at week 1, while the calculated slopes indicate the decrease or increase in BCA equivalent values per week. To determine the significant different milk serum proteins over the course of lactation per country, a comparison was made based on the calculated slope. Only BCA equivalent values of the common serum proteins found in both Chinese and Dutch human milk were used for comparison. The common serum proteins in Chinese and Dutch human milk were then evaluated based on the calculated intercept and slope using a two-tailed *t*-test, with a significance level set at $\alpha = 0.05$. Next, these common milk serum proteins were compared in Chinese and Dutch human milk using a two-tailed *t*-test in Perseus [31], separately for each lactation week, with correction for multiple testing based on permutation-based FDR. The BCA equivalent values of serum proteins in Chinese and Dutch human milk were also summed per function and were then compared using a two-tailed *t*-test. To quantify the relation between biological function groups, Pearson correlation coefficients were calculated for summed BCA equivalent values and visualized in correlation matrix plots. Pearson correlation coefficients of >0.5 were considered good. All the serum proteins in Chinese and Dutch human milk were plotted in a graph in order to visualize the differences in serum proteins over the course of lactation.

3. Results

The objective of this study was to investigate the variability in the type and level of serum proteins in Chinese human milk over a 20-week lactation period. For this, the milk serum proteome of seven mothers over the course of lactation was investigated using LC-MS/MS.

3.1. Level and Type of Milk Serum Proteins in Chinese Human Milk

The total milk serum protein concentrations in Chinese human milk of the seven mothers over the course of lactation are presented in Figure 1. Concentrations ranging from 12 to 25 g/L decreased significantly ($\alpha < 0.05$) over a 20-week lactation period, although with large individual variations (Figure 1).

Serum proteins in human milk were grouped based on their main biological functions (Supplementary Supporting information, data file). Not only the total protein concentrations, but also the protein composition differed among mothers and over lactation as measured after protein digestion and subsequent LC-MS/MS analysis (Figure 2). The figure shows that immune-active proteins, transport proteins, and enzymes were the most abundant for all mothers (Figure 2). The percentage of total protein attributable to these main biological functions, however, varied widely among mothers (Figure 2). Although the BCA equivalent values were always higher in colostrum than in mature milk, the rate of decline for the three main groups varied among mothers (Figure 2).

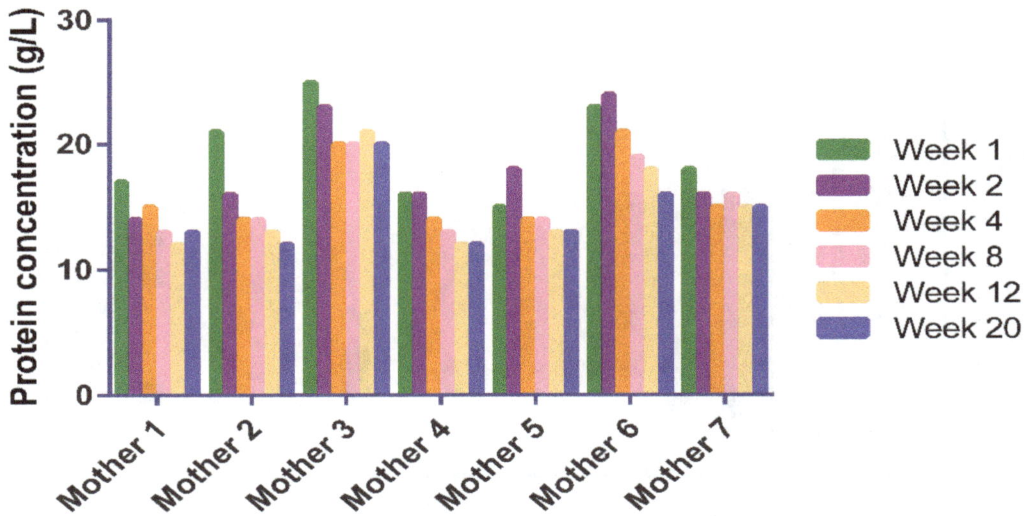

Figure 1. Total bicinchoninic acid (BCA) serum protein concentrations (g/L) in Chinese human milk per mother over a 20-week lactation period.

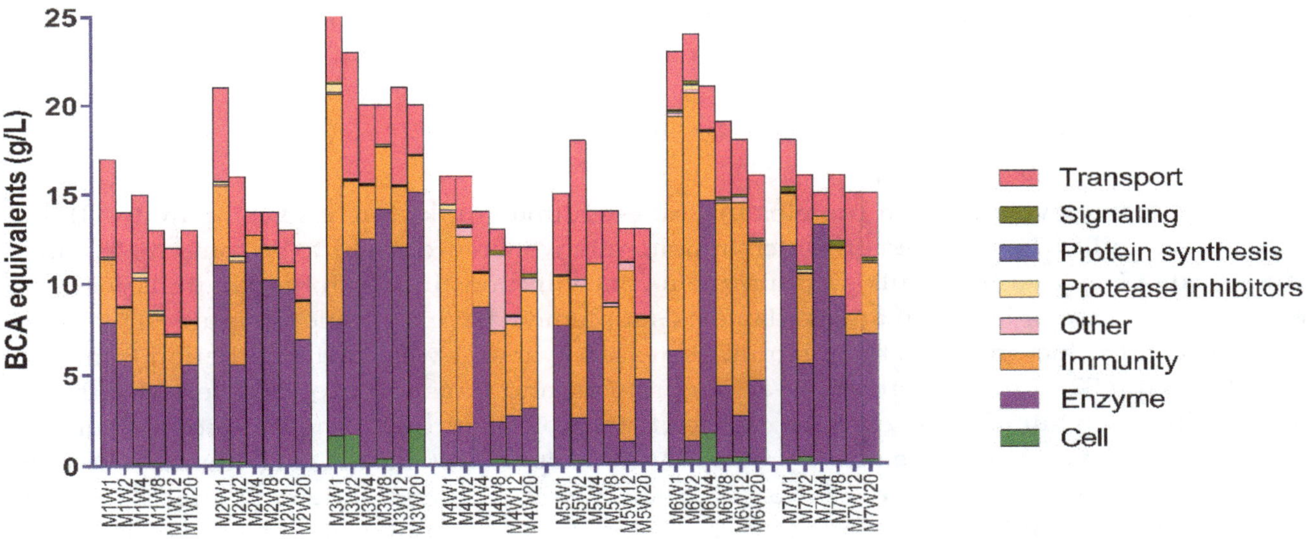

Figure 2. Serum protein composition in human milk of seven Chinese mothers over a 20-week lactation period, based on BCA equivalent values (g/L). The number after the M indicates the mother, and the numbers after the W (1 to 20) indicates the number of weeks postpartum.

To facilitate the comparison between Chinese and Dutch human milk, data were averaged among mothers, as shown in Figure 3. The average total BCA equivalent values in Chinese human milk for enzymes, immune-active proteins, and transport proteins ranged over 4.5–10.0 g/L, 2.9–7.8 g/L, and 2.9–5.0 g/L, respectively (Figure 3).

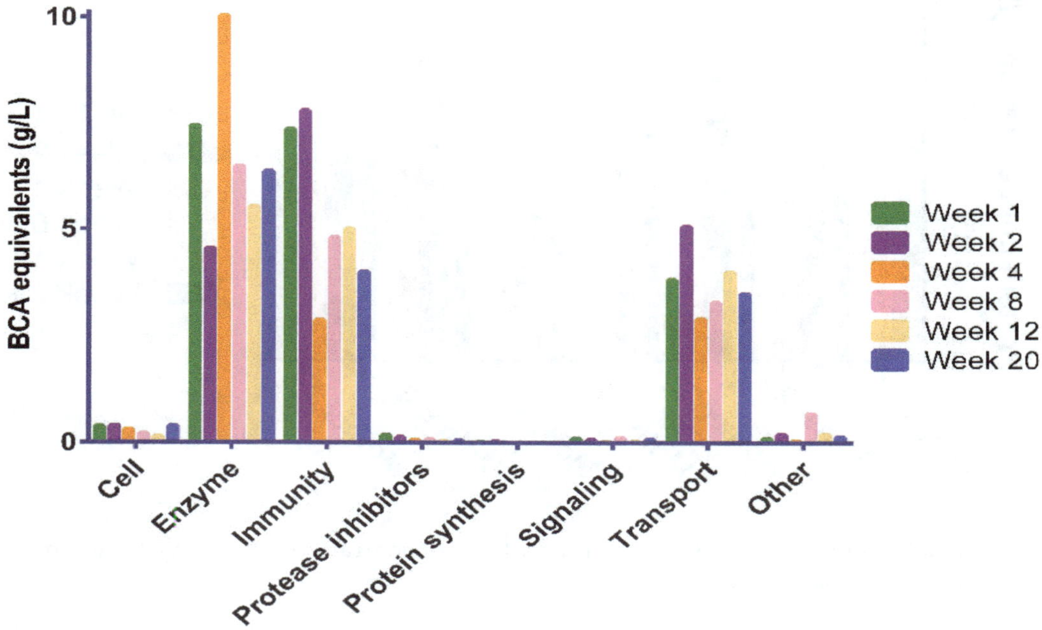

Figure 3. Averaged BCA equivalent values (g/L) of serum proteins for human milk from seven Chinese mothers categorized per biological function over a 20-week lactation period.

3.2. Comparison of the Chinese and Dutch Milk Serum Proteomes

The type and level of serum proteins in Chinese human milk were also compared to those in Dutch human milk. The raw data on Dutch human milk were reprocessed to be compatible with the Chinese data. The total BCA milk serum protein concentrations in Dutch human milk per mother and over the course of lactation are available as supplementary information (Figure S1). The total BCA equivalent values in Dutch human milk decreased over a 24-week lactation period from 21.6 to 13.6 g/L (Figure S2). Enzymes, immune-active proteins, and transport proteins were also the most abundant in Dutch human milk over the course of lactation (Figure S2). The BCA equivalent values for the groups enzymes, immune-active proteins, and transport proteins in Dutch human milk ranged over 4.5–9.0 g/L, 3.8–5.6 g/L, and 4.8–6.8 g/L, respectively. Although different patterns in Chinese and Dutch human milk can be observed, the difference was not significant between the same group of biological functions (data not shown), except for cell and signaling, where levels were higher in Chinese human milk.

The relations between the levels of different biological function groups of serum proteins within the Chinese and within the Dutch human milk populations were visualized in a correlation matrix plot (Figure 4).

3.3. Individual Milk Serum Proteins

Totals of 469 and 200 serum proteins were measured in Chinese and Dutch human milk, respectively. The milk serum proteomes of different Chinese and Dutch mothers were compared based on 166 common milk serum proteins. The overall 15 most abundant milk serum proteins can be found in Table 1.

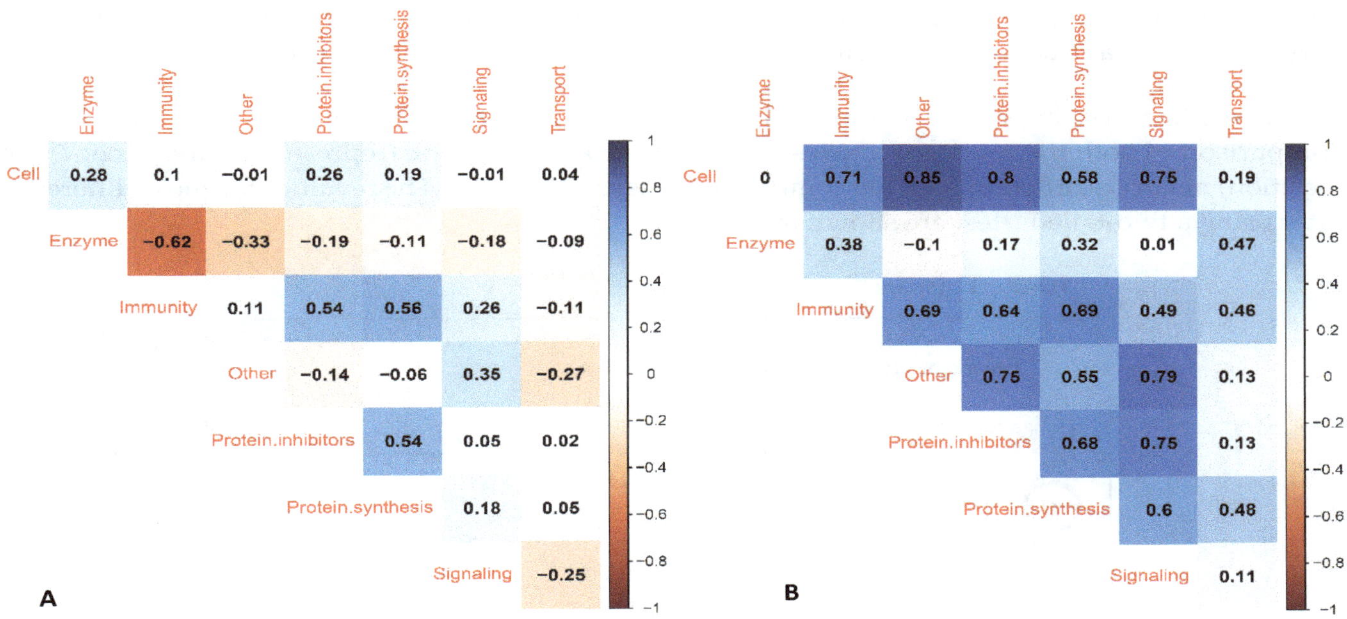

Figure 4. Calculated Pearson correlation coefficients between the different functional groups of serum proteins in Chinese and Dutch human milk, using the summed BCA equivalent values (g/L) over lactation. (**A**) Chinese human milk and (**B**) Dutch human milk.

Table 1. The 15 most abundant serum proteins categorized per function in both Chinese and Dutch human milk during lactation, with their corresponding BCA equivalent values (g/L) values at week 1.

Function	Protein Name	BCA Equivalent Values (g/L)	
		Chinese	Dutch
Enzyme	α-lactalbumin	6.98	8.73
	Bile salt-activated lipase	0.29	0.19
Immunity	Lactoferrin	3.74	2.10
	Ig α_1-chain c-region	0.91	0.71
	Ig λ_2-chain c-region	0.47	0.54
	Ig κ-chain c-region	0.39	0.90
	Polymeric immunoglobulin receptor	0.41	0.39
	Clusterin	0.23	0.17
	Osteopontin	0.17	0.19
	β_2-microglobulin	0.16	0.16
Protease inhibitors	α_1-antichymotrypsin	0.11	0.08
Transport	β-casein †	1.17	3.91
	α_{S1}-casein †	1.33	1.34
	Serum albumin	0.93	1.06
	κ-casein †	0.23	0.29
	Fatty acid-binding protein	0.07	0.13

† Micellar caseins were completely removed, while this was not the case for the free soluble part of the caseins.

In Dutch human milk, α_1-antichymotrypsin belongs to the top 15 serum proteins instead of the transport protein fatty acid-binding protein (Table 1). Within the group enzymes, the highly abundant α-lactalbumin and bile salt-activated lipase are mainly responsible for the changes in this group in human milk over the course of lactation (Table 1). Many immune-active proteins, like lactoferrin, osteopontin, different types of immunoglobulins, polymeric immunoglobulin receptor, and clusterin, belong to the most abundant serum proteins in human milk (Table 1). The changes within the group of transport proteins over the course of lactation can mainly be explained by the caseins (Table 1). The caseins in Table 1 probably refer to the free, non-micellar casein, as the micellar casein should have been removed during the sample preparation (Table 1). With the majority of the caseins in milk being part of the micellar fraction, the caseins in Table 1 therefore do not reflect the levels of total casein.

The differences in protein patterns between Chinese and Dutch human milk were examined by comparison of both the intercept (representing colostrum) and slope (representing the decline over lactation) of curves, fitted for the 166 common milk serum proteins. The *p*-values for these differences after using a two-tailed *t*-test are shown in Figure 5.

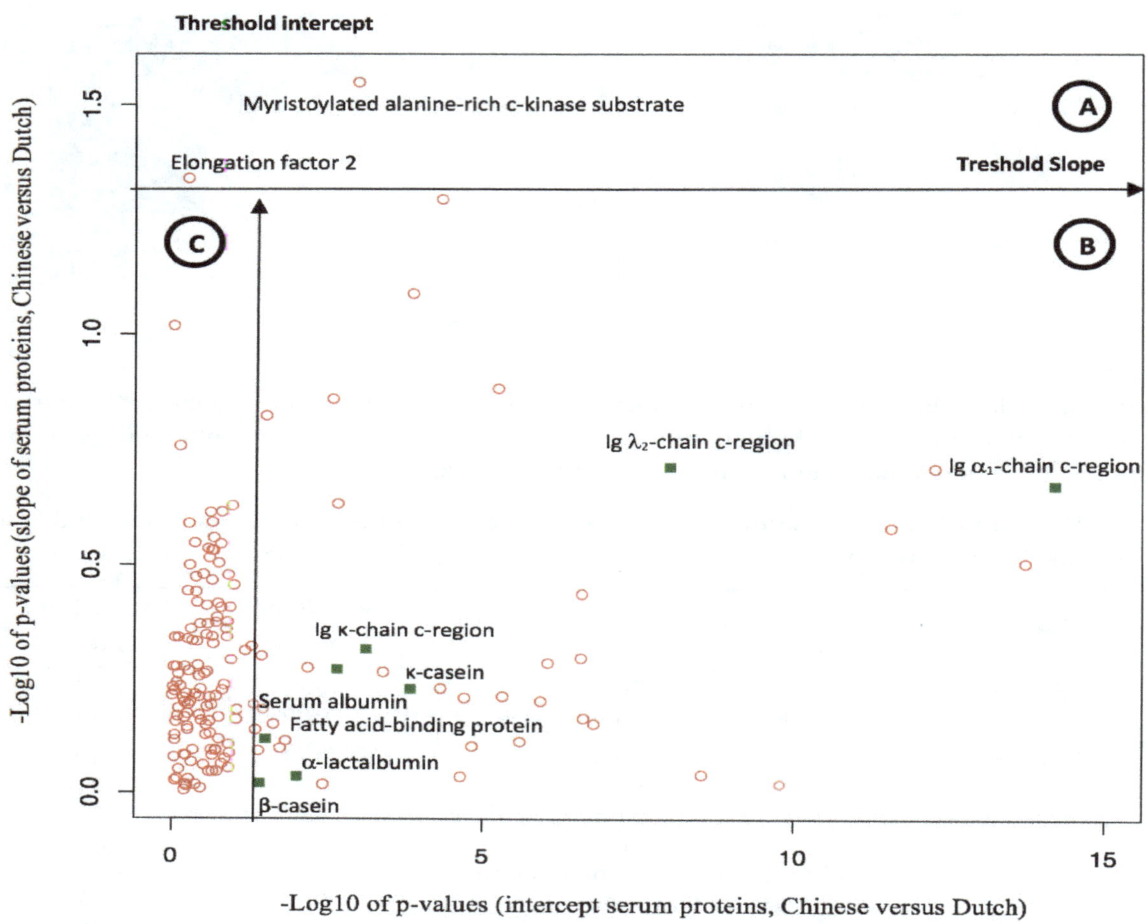

Figure 5. Comparison of the common serum proteins in Chinese and Dutch human milk during lactation. Green squares indicate the proteins displayed in Table 1. For each serum protein in Chinese and Dutch human milk over the course of lactation, a regression line was fitted, summarizing the profile for each protein into an intercept (representing week 1) and slope (representing rate of change over lactation). These profiles were used for comparison between Chinese and Dutch human milk, and the *p*-values for differences between them were plotted. (**A**) Significantly different proteins in Chinese and Dutch human milk over the course of lactation, based on difference in slope; (**B**) significantly different proteins in Chinese and Dutch human milk at week 1, based on intercept; and (**C**) no significant difference.

The levels of two serum proteins (elongation factor 2 and myristoylated alanine-rich c-kinase substrate) varied in the Chinese and Dutch human milk over the course of lactation, as shown by the significantly different slope (Figure 5, area A). Next to that, the levels of 35 serum proteins varied in intercept (Figure 5, area B), including several proteins from the top 15 (Table 1), as shown in green. The complete list of significantly different serum proteins in Chinese and Dutch human milk is shown in Table 2, grouped according to their biological function.

Table 2. Significantly different serum proteins in Chinese and Dutch human milk, with p-values for week 1 (intercept) and over the course of lactation (slope).

Function *	Protein Name	p-Values of Serum Proteins (Chinese Versus Dutch)	
		Intercept	Slope
Cell	Actin	0.002 *	0.540
	Calreticulin	0.000 *	0.620
	Follistatin-related protein 1	0.003 *	0.140
	MARCKS-like protein 1	0.004 *	0.959
	Protein deglycase DJ-1	0.000 *	0.051
	Peroxiredoxin 2	0.002 *	0.233
Enzyme	4-trimethylaminobutyraldehyde dehydrogenase	0.000 *	0.590
	α-lactalbumin	**0.010** *	**0.922**
	Fructose-bisphosphate aldolase A	0.000 *	0.710
	Isocitrate dehydrogenase 1	0.000 *	0.310
	L-lactate dehydrogenase A	0.000 *	0.772
	Nucleoside diphosphate kinase A	0.000 *	0.082
	Protein disulfide-isomerase	0.000 *	0.685
	Transketolase	0.023 *	0.707
	Triosephosphate isomerase	0.000 *	0.912
	Tryptophan-tRNA ligase	0.000 *	0.131
	UTP-glucose 1-phosphate uridylyltransferase	0.000 *	0.630
Immunity	Complement C4B	0.000 *	0.200
	Ig α_1-chain c-region	**0.000** *	**0.210**
	Ig γ_3 chain c-region	0.000 *	0.190
	Ig κ-chain c-region	**0.001** *	**0.490**
	Ig λ_2-chain c-region	**0.045** *	**0.640**
	Granulins	0.018 *	0.800
	Lysozyme C	0.000 *	0.937
	Monocyte differentiation antigen CD14	0.015 *	0.770
Protease inhibitors	Inter-α-trypsin inhibitor heavy chain H2	0.000 *	0.522
Protein synthesis	Elongation factor 2	0.547	0.050*
Signaling	14-3-3 protein β/α	0.000 *	0.372
Transport	Apolipoprotein E	0.036 *	0.500
	β-casein †	**0.000** *	**0.590**
	Fatty acid-binding protein	**0.000** *	**0.790**
	Heat shock protein HSP 90-beta	0.040 *	0.810
	κ-casein †	**0.038** *	**0.950**
	Selenium-binding protein 1	0.006 *	0.536
	Serum albumin	**0.031** *	**0.760**
	Transcobalamin 1	0.000 *	0.509
Other	Myristoylated alanine-rich c-kinase substrate	0.001	0.028 *

Bold type indicates the proteins also displayed in Table 1. † Micellar caseins were completely removed, while this was not the case for the free soluble part of the caseins. * Corresponding p-values (two-tailed t-test, $\alpha < 0.05$)

The levels of the 166 common milk serum proteins in the Chinese and Dutch populations that increased or decreased over the course of lactation, can be found as supporting information (Table S1). The levels of 17 (10%) and 21 (12%) of the 166 common milk serum proteins changed over the course of lactation in Chinese and Dutch human milk, respectively. In addition, the 166 common serum proteins were compared between Chinese and Dutch human milk for each week separately (Table S2). This showed that 16 of 17 proteins that significantly differed in week 1 were also significantly differing in one or more of the other weeks.

4. Discussion

4.1. The Level and Type of Serum Proteins in Chinese Human Milk

The total protein concentrations decrease significantly over a 20-week lactation period in each mother, although with individual variations (Figure 1). These milk serum protein concentrations match with those observed in earlier studies, ranging from 12 to 25 g/L [7,32–34], although other studies report lower values from 7 to 16 g/L over the course of lactation [3,24,35,36]. These differences may be explained by the BCA method [37,38], which generally overestimates the total protein in human milk by about 25–40% [37,38]. The serum protein levels in this study should thus be regarded as semi-quantitative, although this did not influence the comparisons reported here, as they are all based on the BCA method. Although the protein content seems high for milk serum, it should be taken into account that the samples with the highest protein content are actually those in early lactation. These samples are known to have higher protein and relatively lower casein contents [6], leading to higher milk serum protein contents. In addition, part of the casein remained in the sample after sample preparation and therefore also counted towards the BCA protein content.

As described previously [5], human milk becomes fully mature between 4 and 6 weeks postpartum, with the amounts of bioactive components decreasing relative to the nutrients. In early life, infants have an immature intestinal immune system, making them more vulnerable to infection by opportunistic pathogens [5]. The high levels of immune-related milk serum proteins in colostrum (Figure 3) may provide protection to the infant in this sensitive stage of development.

It was also observed that a large variability exists in the milk serum protein composition in colostrum among Chinese mothers (Figure 2). The results in this study comprising milk from seven mothers shows that immune-active proteins, enzymes, and transport proteins are highly abundant in Chinese human milk (Figure 3), which can also be observed from the individual data of mothers (Figure 2). Earlier studies had already shown that immune-active proteins, enzymes, and transport proteins were present in the largest quantities over the course of lactation [7,9,11].

4.2. The 15 Most Abundant Milk Serum Proteins

The large quantities of immune-active proteins are especially driven by the abundance of lactoferrin, immunoglobulins, polymeric immunoglobulin receptor, clusterin, osteopontin and β_2-microglobulin (Table 1), which may protect infants against pathogenic microorganisms, and confer passive immunity to the neonate until its own immune system has been developed [9–11]. As shown in Table 1, transport proteins, like free soluble caseins, serum albumin, and fatty acid binding protein were present in large quantities during lactation. Free soluble caseins could not be removed from the milk, unlike the micellar casein that can be pelleted by ultracentrifugation–a phenomenon that has also been reported by others [7,19,24]. Free soluble and micellar caseins belong to the most abundant proteins in human milk, and these proteins mainly supply infants with amino acids and minerals needed for their growth [23–25]. It can also be observed from Table 1 that enzymes are the largest group of proteins across lactation. The large quantities of enzymes in human milk can be explained by the presence of α-lactalbumin, which is known to be the most abundant milk serum protein (Table 1). This enzyme is required for the synthesis of lactose, the main macronutrient in milk [5,21]. It should be noticed that α-lactalbumin does not have enzymatic activity on its own. Besides α-lactalbumin, bile salt-activated lipase belongs to the 15 most important enzymes in Chinese and Dutch human milk during lactation (Table 1). Bile salt-activated lipase supports the digestion of fats in the immature infant digestive tract, and facilitates the absorption of cholesterol, vitamin A, and triacylglycerols [7]. The protease inhibitor α_1-antichymotrypsin is also among the 15 most abundant human milk serum proteins, and, like other protease inhibitors and proteases, might play a key role in the digestion of human milk [12–14]. Overall, the 15 most abundant proteins identified in this study were in levels dominating the entire milk composition, covering more than 95% of both the Chinese and Dutch milk serum proteomes.

4.3. Proteases and Protease Inhibitors

Proteases may play a key role in the digestion of human milk. Although trypsin was the most abundant protease in Chinese and Dutch human milk, many other proteases (e.g., cytosol aminopeptidase, elastase, kallikrein, plasmin, cathepsins) were found, albeit to a lesser extent (Supplementary Information, data file). As described by others, proteases might be present in human milk to hydrolyze proteins in the mammary gland to regulate casein micelle size [14,15]. Protein digestion in human milk by proteases target specific proteins (e.g., caseins, polymeric immunoglobulin receptor, osteopontin) that do not have an extensive tertiary structure and are thus more accessible to proteolytic cleavage [16,18]. These proteins were, in this study, part of the overall 15 most abundant proteins in Chinese and Dutch human milk during lactation (Table 1). In particular, the caseins are well digested [16–18], which indicates that proteases and bile salt-activated lipase in human milk aids overall in the digestion of two of its main macronutrients, fats and proteins [19].

Besides proteases, human milk also contains protease inhibitors. The ratio between protease inhibitors and proteases in colostrum is circa 10:1. The most abundant protease inhibitors were α_1-antichymotrypsin, α_1-antitrypsin, cystatin C, and phosphatidyletanolamine-binding protein (Supplementary Information, data file). As described by others, α_1-antichymotrypsin binds to chymotrypsin and other chymotrypsin-like serine proteases in human milk, while α_1-antitrypsin inhibits proteases, such as trypsin, elastase, plasmin, and thrombin, and irreversibly deactivates trypsin in vitro [12–15]. A correlation was found between protease inhibitors and immune-active proteins in Chinese and Dutch human milk (Figure 4). Previous literature focused specifically on the relation between serine protease inhibitors and immunoglobulins [7], which also in our data showed stronger correlations than for all protease inhibitors and all immune proteins (Figure S3). A correlation higher than 0.7 was also found in both Chinese and Dutch milk between proteases and protease inhibitors specifically (data not shown). A previous study presented an overview of the proteolytic system network in human milk [15], which consists of several proteases, protease inhibitors, and blood coagulation proteins, indicating that these protein groups share a common biochemical pathway; this may explain their correlations.

Where some of the major proteins are partially digested by milk proteases in human milk, most immune-active proteins are less sensitive to digestion by these proteases, due to their compact folded globular structure, that cannot be as easily digested [16]. For these immune-active proteins to have an immune-activating role in the small intestine, they must be protected against intestinal digestion, because they are sensitive to chymotrypsin and trypsin [17,18]. That might be the reason why protease inhibitors present in human milk seem to target intestinal enzymes, specifically blocking trypsin, chymotrypsin, and other proteases [17,18], especially through the relative abundant α_1-antichymotrypsin and α_1-antitrypsin. Overall, protease inhibitors may thus ensure that specific proteins stay intact in the infant's digestive tract. This may also explain previous findings that several immune-active proteins (e.g., lactoferrin, lysozyme, immunoglobulins) and protease inhibitors (e.g., α_1-antichymotrypsin, α_1-antitrypsin) can be found intact in the stool of breastfed infants [17,18]. The intact proteins in the infant's stool may also be related to the simultaneous decrease in the content of immune-active proteins and protease inhibitors over lactation. Protection is less necessary later in lactation due to the development of the infant's immune system and digestive tract over time, while digestion becomes important for the release of nutrients later in lactation.

4.4. Comparison of High- and Low- Abundance Serum Proteins in Chinese and Dutch Human Milk

It appears that the milk serum proteomes of Chinese and Dutch mothers are similar (Figure 3 and Figure S2). The main purpose of this study was to evaluate the common serum proteins in Chinese and Dutch human milk over the course of lactation. Totals of 469 and 200 serum proteins were found in Chinese and Dutch human milk, respectively. Although a lower number of serum proteins was identified in Dutch human milk, there was still an overlap of 166 serum proteins with Chinese human milk, which represents more than 95% of the milk serum proteome in term of concentrations. The reason for the higher number of serum proteins found in Chinese human milk might be due to the larger sample size (48 versus 24 human milk samples), which generally leads to more identified proteins [28].

In total, 22% (37 out of 166) of the common serum proteins in human milk differed between Chinese and Dutch mothers either at week 1 or over the course of lactation. The levels of 35 of the 166 (circa 21%) common serum proteins varied between Chinese and Dutch mothers in week 1 (Figure 5, area B). This, together with the results presented in Table 2 and Table S2, indicates that the differences between Chinese and Dutch human milk serum proteins were mainly in their level throughout lactation, and not in their changes over lactation, as the levels of only 2 of the 166 (circa 1%) common serum proteins identified in this study (myristoylated alanine-rich c-kinase substrate and elongation factor 2) differed over the course of lactation (Figure 5, area A, showing difference in slope). Overall, the main differences in the milk serum proteomes between Chinese and Dutch human milk were observed in the level of individual proteins, and not in rate of changes over lactation.

5. Conclusions

The milk serum proteome of Chinese and Dutch mothers were similar in term of relative the abundance of different functional groups as well as the most abundant proteins. Some quantitative differences were found, especially in absolute levels and not in rates of change over lactation. Human milk contains enzymes that can assist the digestion of milk proteins and lipids in the immature infant's digestive tract. Protease inhibitors, which are highly correlated to the immune-active proteins, are present in variable amounts in human milk; they could be relevant during digestion and might be involved in controlling protein breakdown in the infant's intestinal tract.

Supplementary Materials:
Figure S1: Total BCA serum protein concentrations (g/L) in Dutch human milk per mother over a 24-week lactation period. Raw data from Dutch human milk were re-used [7]; Figure S2: BCA equivalent values (g/L) of serum proteins in human milk of 4 Dutch mothers categorized per biological function over a 24-week lactation period. Raw data from Dutch human milk were re-used [7]; Figure S3: Correlations between the functional groups consisting of protease inhibitors (including serine and non-serine protease inhibitors) and immune-active proteins (including immunoglobulins and non-immunoglobulins) in Chinese human milk, using BCA equivalent values (g/L) over a 20-week lactation period; Table S1: Significantly different serum proteins in Chinese and Dutch human milk over the course of lactation, based on the BCA equivalent values (g/L) over lactation (slope); Table S2: Serum proteins that were significantly different in at least one of the lactation weeks. Numbers are the p-value for the difference between the Chinese human milk serum proteins and Dutch human milk serum proteins. To facilitate direct comparison between Chinese and Dutch data within this research, the time points 12 and 20 weeks postpartum were compared to week 16 and 24, respectively; Supporting Information, data file: Serum proteins in human milk of Chinese mothers over a 20-week lactation period. The columns described in the next tab are the individual proteins, their functions and their iBAQ values averaged for all mothers at weeks 1, 2, 4, 8, 12, and 20 postpartum.

Author Contributions: M.E., I.M.S., H.A.S., and K.A.H. conceived and planned the experiments. M.E. carried out the experiments. S.B. contributed to sample preparation and analysis. M.E. and J.H. calculated the statistics and all authors contributed to the interpretation of the results. M.E. worked on all the data and took the lead in writing the manuscript. All authors, especially H.A.S. and K.A.H. provided critical feedback and helped shape the research, analysis, and manuscript.

References

1. Kramer, M.; Kakuma, R. The optimal duration of exclusive breastfeeding: A systematic review. *Adv. Exp. Med. Biol.* **2004**, *554*, 63–77. [PubMed]
2. Liao, Y.; Alvarado, R.; Phinney, B.; Lönnerdal, B. Proteomic characterization of human milk whey proteins during a twelve-month lactation period. *J. Proteome Res.* **2011**, *10*, 1746–1756. [CrossRef] [PubMed]

3. Martin, C.; Ling, P.; Blackburn, G. Review of infant feeding: Key features of breastmilk and infant formula. *Nutrients* **2016**, *8*, 279. [CrossRef] [PubMed]
4. Gartner, L.; Morton, J.; Lawrence, R.; Naylor, A.; O'Hare, D.; Schanler, R.; Eidelman, A. Breastfeeding and the use of human milk. *Pediatrics* **2005**, *115*, 496–506. [PubMed]
5. Elwakiel, M.; Hageman, J.A.; Wang, W.; Szeto, I.M.; van Goudoever, J.B.; Hettinga, K.A.; Schols, H.A. Human milk oligosaccharides in colostrum and mature milk of Chinese mothers: Lewis positive secretor subgroups. *J. Agric. Food Chem.* **2018**, *66*, 7036–7043. [CrossRef] [PubMed]
6. Kunz, C.; Lönnerdal, B. Re-evaluation of the whey protein/casein ratio of human milk. *Acta Paediatr.* **1992**, *81*, 107–112. [CrossRef] [PubMed]
7. Zhang, L.; de Waard, M.; Verheijen, H.; Boeren, S.; Hageman, J.; van Hooijdonk, T.; Vervoort, J.; van Goudoever, J.; Hettinga, K. Changes over lactation in breast milk serum proteins involved in the maturation of immune and digestive system of the infant. *J. Proteomics* **2016**, *147*, 40–47. [CrossRef] [PubMed]
8. Zhang, L.; van Dijk, A.; Hettinga, K. An interactomics overview of the human and bovine proteome over lactation. *Proteome Sci.* **2016**, *15*, 1–14. [CrossRef] [PubMed]
9. Hettinga, K.; Van Valenberg, H.; De Vries, S.; Boeren, S.; Van Hooijdonk, T.; Van Arendonk, J.; Vervoort, J. The host defense proteome of human and bovine milk. *PLoS ONE* **2011**, *6*, 1–8. [CrossRef] [PubMed]
10. Hettinga, K.; Reina, F.; Boeren, S.; Zhang, L.; Koppelman, G. Difference in the breast milk proteome between allergic and non-allergic mothers. *PLoS ONE* **2015**, *10*, 1–11. [CrossRef] [PubMed]
11. Beck, K.; Weber, D.; Phinney, B.; Smilowitz, J.; Hinde, K.; Lönnerdal, B.; Korf, I.; Lemay, D. Comparative proteomics of human and macaque milk reveals species-specific nutrition during postnatal development. *J. Proteome Res.* **2015**, *14*, 2143–2157. [CrossRef] [PubMed]
12. Chowanadisai, W.; Lönnerdal, B. α_1-Antitrypsin and antichymotrypsin in human milk: Origin, concentrations, and stability. *Am. J. Clin. Nutr.* **2002**, *76*, 828–833. [CrossRef] [PubMed]
13. Lindberg, T. Protease inhibitors in human milk. *Pediatr. Res.* **1982**, *16*, 479–483. [CrossRef] [PubMed]
14. Dallas, D.; Murray, N.; Gan, J. Proteolytic systems in milk: Perspectives on the evolutionary function within the mammary gland and the infant. *J. Mammary Gland Biol. Neoplasia.* **2015**, *20*, 133–147. [CrossRef] [PubMed]
15. Kelly, A.; O'Flaherty, P.; Fox, P. Indigenous proteolytic enzymes in milk: A brief overview of the present state of knowledge. *Int. Dairy J.* **2006**, *16*, 563–572. [CrossRef]
16. Dingess, K.; de Waard, M.; Boeren, S.; Vervoort, J.; Lambers, T.; van Goudoever, J.; Hettinga, K. Human milk peptides differentiate between the preterm and term infant and across varying lactational stages. *Food Funct.* **2017**, *8*, 3769–3782. [CrossRef] [PubMed]
17. Dallas, D.; Guerrero, A.; Khaldi, N.; Borghese, R.; Bhandari, A.; Underwood, M. A peptidomic analysis of human milk digestion in the infant stomach reveals protein-specific degradation patterns. *J. Nutr.* **2014**, *144*, 815–820. [CrossRef] [PubMed]
18. Su, M.; Broadhurst, M.; Liu, C.; Gathercole, J.; Cheng, W.; Qi, X. Comparative analysis of human milk and infant formula derived peptides following in vitro digestion. *Food Chem.* **2017**, *221*, 1895–1903. [CrossRef] [PubMed]
19. Lönnerdal, B. Human milk proteins: Key components for the biological activity of human milk. *Adv. Exp. Med. Biol.* **2004**, *554*, 11–25.
20. Lönnerdal, B. Bioactive proteins in human milk: Mechanisms of action. *J. Pediatr.* **2010**, *156*, 26–30. [CrossRef] [PubMed]
21. Newburg, D. Bioactive components of human milk: Evolution, efficiency and protection. *Adv. Exp. Med. Biol.* **2001**, *501*, 3–10. [PubMed]
22. Spik, G.; Brunet, B.; Mazurier-Dehaine, C.; Fontaine, G.; Montreuil, J. Characterization and properties of the human and bovine lactotransferrins extracted from the faeces of newborn infants. *Acta Pædiatr. Scand.* **1982**, *71*, 979–985. [CrossRef] [PubMed]
23. Davidson, L.; Lönnerdal, B. Persistence of human milk proteins in the breastfed infant. *Acta Pædiatr.* **1987**, *76*, 733–740. [CrossRef]
24. Lönnerdal, B. Nutritional and physiologic significance of human milk proteins. *Am. J. Clin. Nutr.* **2003**, *77*, 1537–1543. [CrossRef] [PubMed]
25. Jakaitis, B.; Denning, P. Human breast milk and the gastrointestinal innate immune system. *Clin. Perinatol.* **2014**, *41*, 423–435. [CrossRef] [PubMed]

26. Jensen, H.; Poulsen, N.; Moller, H.; Stensballe, A.; Larsen, L. Comparative proteomic analysis of casein and whey as prepared by chymosin-induced separation, isoelectric precipitation or ultracentrifugation. *J. Dairy Res.* **2012**, *79*, 451–458. [CrossRef] [PubMed]
27. Lu, J.; Boeren, S.; de Vries, S.; van Valenberg, H.; Vervoort, J. Filter-aided sample preparation with dimethyl labeling to identify and quantify milk fat globule membrane proteins. *J. Proteomics* **2011**, *75*, 34–43. [CrossRef] [PubMed]
28. Cox, J.; Mann, M. MaxQuant enables high peptide identification rates, individualized ppb-range mass accuracies and proteome-wide protein quantification. *Nature* **2008**, *26*, 1367–1372.
29. Schwanhausser, B.; Busse, D.; Li, N.; Dittmar, G.; Schuchhardt, J.; Wolf, J.; Chen, W.; Selbach, M. Global quantification of mammalian gene expression control. *Nature* **2011**, 337–342. [CrossRef] [PubMed]
30. Huang, D.; Sherman, B.; Lempicki, R. Systematic and integrative analysis of large gene lists using DAVID Bioinformatics Resources. *Nat. Protoc.* **2009**, *4*, 44–57. [CrossRef] [PubMed]
31. Tyanova, S.; Temu, T.; Sinitcyn, P.; Carlson, A.; Hein, M.; Geiger, T.; Mann, M.; Cox, J. The Perseus computational platform for comprehensive analysis of proteomics data. *Nat. Methods* **2016**, *13*, 731–740. [CrossRef] [PubMed]
32. Breckwoldt, J.; Neulen, J.; Keck, C. Lactation. From cellular mechanisms to integration. In *Comprehensive Human Physiology*; Greger, R., Windhorst, U., Eds.; Springer: Berlin, Germany, 1996; Volume 1, pp. 2365–2373.
33. Monaco, M.; Donavan, S. Human milk: Nutritional properties. In *Nutrition in Pediatrics: Basic Science and Clinical Applications*; Walker, W., Watkins, J., Duggan, C., Eds.; BC Decker Inc.: Hamilton, ON, Canada, 2008; Volume 4, pp. 341–353.
34. Trend, S.; Strunk, T.; Hibbert, J.; Kok, C.; Zhang, G.; Doherty, D.; Richmond, P.; Burgner, D.; Simmer, K.; Davidson, D.; et al. Antimicrobial protein and peptide concentrations and activity in human breast milk consumed by preterm infants at risk of late-onset neonatal sepsis. *PLoS ONE* **2015**, *10*, 1–20. [CrossRef] [PubMed]
35. Liao, Y.; Weber, D.; Xu, W.; Durbin-Johnson, B.; Phinney, B.; Lönnerdal, B. Absolute quantification of human milk caseins and the whey/casein ratio during the first year of lactation. *J. Proteome Res.* **2017**, *16*, 4113–4121. [CrossRef] [PubMed]
36. Lönnerdal, B.; Erdmann, P.; Thakkar, S.; Sauser, J.; Destaillats, F. Longitudinal evolution of true protein, amino acids and bioactive proteins in breast milk: A developmental perspective. *J. Nutr. Biochem.* **2017**, *41*, 1–11. [CrossRef] [PubMed]
37. Wu, X.; Jackson, R.; Khan, S.; Ahuja, J.; Pehrsson, P. Human milk nutrient composition in the United States: Current knowledge, challenges, and research needs. *Curr. Dev. Nutr.* **2018**, *2*, 1–18. [CrossRef] [PubMed]
38. Perrin, M.; Fogleman, A.; Newburg, D.; Allen, J. A longitudinal study of human milk composition in the second year postpartum: Implications for human milk. *Matern. Child Nutr.* **2017**, *13*, 1–12. [CrossRef] [PubMed]

4

Breastfeeding Disparities between Multiples and Singletons by NICU Discharge

Roser Porta [1], Eva Capdevila [2], Francesc Botet [3], Gemma Ginovart [4], Elisenda Moliner [4], Marta Nicolàs [5], Antonio Gutiérrez [6,7], Jaume Ponce-Taylor [8] and Sergio Verd [9,*]

1 Neonatal Unit, Dexeus University Hospital, 5 Sabino Arana st, 08028 Barcelona, Spain; roser.porta@quiron.es
2 Pediatric Unit, Department of Primary Care, Catalonia Health Authority, Balmes st, 08007 Barcelona, Spain; e.capde@gmail.com
3 Neonatal Unit, University Maternity Hospital, 5 Sabino Arana st. 08028 Barcelona, Spain; fbotet@clinic.cat
4 Neonatal Unit, Santa Creu i Sant Pau University Hospital, 87 mSant Quinti st. 08041 Barcelona, Spain; gginovart@santpau.cat (G.G.); emoliner@santpau.cat (E.M.)
5 Neonatal Unit, Germans Trias i Pujol University Hospital, Canyet Road, 08916 Badalona, Spain; mnicolasl.germanstrias@gencat.cat
6 Department of Hematology, Son Espases University Hospital. IdISBa Balearic Medical Research Council, Valldemossa Road, 79, 07010 Palma de Mallorca, Spain; antoniom.gutierrez@ssib.es
7 COMIB Advisory, Passeig de Mallorca, 42, 07012 Palma de Mallorca, Spain
8 Urgent Care Centre, Department of Primary Care, Balearic Health Authority, 1 Illes Balears st. 07014 Palma de Mallorca, Spain; Jaume.ponce@gmail.com
9 Pediatric Unit, Department of Primary Care, Balearic Health Authority, Matamusinos st. 07013 Palma de Mallorca, Spain
* Correspondence: drsverd@gmail.com

Abstract: Multiple pregnancy increases the risk of a range of adverse perinatal outcomes, including breastfeeding failure. However, studies on predictive factors of breastfeeding duration in preterm twin infants have a conflicting result. The purpose of this observational study was to compare feeding practices, at hospital discharge, of twin and singleton very low birth weight infants. The study is part of a prospective survey of a national Spanish cohort of very low birth weight infants (SEN1500) that includes 62 neonatal units. The study population comprised all infants registered in the network from 2002 to 2013. They were grouped into singletons and multiples. The explanatory variables were first analyzed using univariate models; subsequently, significant variables were analyzed simultaneously in a multiple stepwise backward model. During the twelve-year period, 32,770 very low birth weight infants were included in the database, of which 26.957 were discharged alive and included in this analysis. Nine thousand seven hundred and fifty-eight neonates were multiples, and 17,199 were singletons. At discharge, 31% of singleton infants were being exclusively breastfed, 43% were bottle-fed, and 26% were fed a combination of both. In comparison, at discharge, only 24% of multiple infants were exclusively breastfed, 43% were bottle-fed, and 33% were fed a combination of both ($p < 0.001$). On multivariable analysis, twin pregnancy had a statistically significant, but small effect, on cessation of breastfeeding before discharge (OR 1.10; 95% CI: 1.02, 1.19). Risks of early in-hospital breastfeeding cessation were also independently associated with multiple mother-infant stress factors, such as sepsis, intraventricular hemorrhage, retinopathy, necrotizing enterocolitis, intubation, and use of inotropes. Instead, antibiotic treatment at delivery, In vitro fertilization and prenatal steroids were associated with a decreased risk for shorter in-hospital breastfeeding duration. Multiple pregnancy, even in the absence of pathological conditions associated to very low birth weight twin infants, may be an impeding factor for in-hospital breastfeeding.

Keywords: breastfeeding; multiple pregnancy; neonate; premature birth; milk bank; pregnancy outcomes

1. Introduction

Historically, formula was provided to very low birth weight (VLBW) infants to ensure rapid growth. However, recent studies show that feeding fortified human milk to preterm infants does not result in lower weight at discharge [1]. Achieving optimal development for preterm infants, whilst minimizing the risk for serious disease in the neonate, remains an important challenge for clinicians. Human milk is recommended for enteral feeding of preterm newborns [2], since it is associated with low rates of necrotizing enterocolitis (NEC) [3], sepsis, retinopathy of prematurity (ROP) [4], and a better neurocognitive development [5]. Despite efforts to offer human milk as the primary source of enteral nutrition during the stay in the neonatal intensive care unit (NICU), infant milk formulas are used in situations in which the mother's milk or donor's milk is not available.

Previous research has identified associations between the provision of breast milk in the NICU and maternal characteristics, infant characteristics, and environmental factors [6–8]. However, studies on predictive factors of breastfeeding duration in premature infants have conflicting results. Some studies have found that higher gestational age is associated with higher rates of breastfeeding [7,9], while others have found that mothers of VLBW infants acknowledge that human milk is a unique factor in improving outcomes for their infant [10] and, consequently, breastfeeding rates are higher among them.

The proportion of infants born preterm is higher for twins, when compared to singletons [11]. Breastfeeding poses unique challenges for the mothers of twins, but little attention has been paid to risk factors for early cessation of breastfeeding for these mothers. Only a few studies have focused on issues related to breastfeeding cessation for full term twins [12,13]. From a physiological standpoint, the World Health Organization (WHO) and other authorities state that mother's milk is sufficient for feeding multiple babies [14]. It provides optimal nutrition for full term or preterm twins. A study comparing singleton and multiple premature, under 30 weeks, gestations, found that the milk volume was higher in mothers of multiples compared with singletons (599 mL/day vs. 430 mL/day) [15]. It has also been reported that the milk yield of individual breasts of mothers of twins is 0.8–2.1 kg per 24 h at six months, whereas the total milk yield of mothers of triplets can reach 3.0 kg per 24 h at 2.5 months [16]. Previous research shows that preterm twin infants may be less likely to be breastfed compared to singleton infants, but the data on this subject remains contradictory [17]. When interpreting the results from these studies, it should be noted that the type of babies included is variable, and that most studies do not provide details on feeding maintenance and complications. One issue that further complicates efforts to address this question is the finding that most preterm complications (NEC, ROP, sepsis, etc.) may be a cause of breastfeeding cessation, and may also be a consequence of breastfeeding cessation. This makes it difficult to explain the relationship between feeding type and severe clinical complications. The aim of this study is to shed light on the influence of major neonatal morbidity, and multiple birth, on in-hospital breastfeeding success. Specifically, we hypothesize that twin birth exerts its own substantial influence on poor breastfeeding outcomes among VLBW infants, irrespective of the clinical situations of these patients.

To test this hypothesis, we have used a multicenter, electronic health record-derived database that represents roughly two-thirds of all Spanish VLBW infants. The objective is to compare breastfeeding rates at hospital discharge of singleton and twin VLBW infants, and to evaluate which neonatal conditions and diseases preclude the provision of breast milk at the time of hospital discharge.

2. Methods

2.1. Design

The study is part of a prospective survey of a national Spanish cohort of VLBW infants (SEN1500 database), based on questionnaires. The SEN1500 network prospectively collects maternal and neonatal data of live-born infants of ≤1500 g who were born in or admitted to the collaborating NICUs within the first 28 days of life. Data were collected using a pre-established form and were submitted electronically using common and specific software. The characteristics, quality control, and data confidentiality systems of this database have been described elsewhere [18]. For the purpose of the present study, data corresponding to all discharged alive newborns within the database over a period of twelve years were retrieved. The SEN1500 database includes 62 neonatal units, which encompasses about two-thirds of all Spanish VLBW infants. The study population comprises all infants registered in the database, during the period 2002–2013. They were grouped into singletons and multiples. The same cohort was used previously to analyze morbidity and mortality associated with multiple birth [19].

2.2. Data Collection

In this study, we assess clinical factors that are known to influence breastfeeding during the hospital stay of singletons and twins. The main variable of interest was any breastfeeding, i.e., not being completely weaned from breastmilk, on the day when hospital discharge was completed. Data on maternal and infant characteristics were obtained from medical records by local health care professionals, using a pretested standardized questionnaire. The study variables were defined according to the variables catalogue of the SEN1500 database. We collected demographic data (birth weight, gender), obstetrical data (fertilization, antenatal care, gestational age, type of delivery, twinning), procedures and treatment (intra partum antibiotics, inotropic therapy, intubation, surfactant administration, ventilation, oxygen therapy, ductus closure, retinopathy surgery), neonatal morbidity (necrotizing enterocolitis, intraventricular haemorrhage, sepsis), length of hospitalization and type of feeding at discharge.

2.3. Outcomes

Exclusive breast milk feeding was defined as the infant receiving no food or drink other than the mother's own milk. Any breast milk feeding was defined as the infant receiving mother's own milk, independent of the addition of formula or other food and/or drink. SEN1500 was set up by the Spanish Association of Neonatologists. It encompasses 62 neonatal units, about two-thirds of all national neonatal units. The operational definitions used to collect feeding data at discharge are: No breastfeeding, any breastfeeding, or exclusive breastfeeding. The database systems are locally controllable. Breastfeeding outcomes are recorded after discharge, in each neonatal unit by the neonatologist responsible for registering obstetric and neonatal information, routinely collected from the Perinatal Health files.

2.4. Statistical Analysis

Data analysis was performed using statistical package SPSS 14.0 for Windows (IBM Company, Chicago, IL, USA). p-Values below 0.05 were considered to be of statistical significance. Descriptive statistics were used to outline mother and infant characteristics. Variables following binomial distributions were expressed as frequencies and percentages; and quantitative variables as median and ranges. Comparisons between qualitative variables were made using the Fisher Exact Test or Chi-square. Comparisons between quantitative and qualitative variables were performed through non-parametric tests (U of Mann-Whitney or Kruskal-Wallis).

Logistic regression (both univariate and multivariate) was used to assess the relationship between potential predictor variables of breastfeeding at discharge, a broad range of explanatory variables with a p-value under 0.1 was chosen to appear in the final regression model, yet this less restrictive approach is accepted, as well as considering explanatory variables one at a time [20]. Out of the variables with a significant relation to breastfeeding at discharge after the univariate analysis, we excluded those that, from a clinical point of view, are a result rather than a cause of feeding practice (anthropometric data at discharge). Finally, the explanatory variables included in the stepwise backward regression model were birth weight, height at birth, birth head circumference, gender, In vitro fertilization, multiple birth, prenatal care, prenatal administration of corticosteroids or antibiotics, delivery type, NICU use of surfactant or inotropic drugs, intubation, ventilation duration, oxygen therapy duration, CRIB score, duct pharmacological closure, surgical management of ROP, NEC, late onset sepsis (LOS), intraventricular hemorrhage (IVH), and supplementary oxygen at 36 weeks PMA (bronchopulmonary dysplasia). The results are presented as odds ratio (OR) with a 95% confidence interval (CI).

2.5. Statement of Ethics

The study was conducted in accordance with the Declaration of Helsinki. The Local Health District Human Research Ethics Committees approved the collection of the data from the SEN1500 database and subsequent analysis. Data collection in SEN1500 is anonymous and has been previously approved by the Ethics and Investigation Committees of the Collaborative Centers. It is in compliance with the Spanish data protection law. Ethical approval code: IIBSP-LEC-2011-129. Informed consent was obtained a legally authorized person, such as a parent or guardian.

3. Results

3.1. Characteristics of the Study Population

The study included 26,957 VLBW infants, of which 9758 were multiples, and 17,199 were singletons—who were all alive when discharged from the NICU. The characteristics of the study sample are summarized in Table 1. The median gestational age was 29 weeks, with a median birth weight of 1190 g. Female infants made up 50% of the sample. Cesarean delivery was common (72%), and 6% of infants were outborn. Use of antenatal care was observed in 22,830 (88%) patients. Antenatal corticosteroid administration rate was 84%, and median length of hospital stay was 50 days. As we have reported elsewhere [18], most patient characteristics and major morbidities differed between multiples and singletons (see Table 2).

Table 1. Characteristics of 26,957 VLBW infants discharged alive from 62 Spanish neonatal units in 2002–2013.

Characteristic	Number (%)
Maternal Factors	
In vitro fertilization (%)	4747 (19)
Prenatal care (%)	22,830 (88)
Antenatal corticosteroid therapy (%)	22,059 (84)
Intrapartum antibiotic chemoprophylaxis (%)	11,502 (47)
Between hospital transfers	1651 (6)
Caesarean section (%)	19,503 (72)
Multiple birth (%)	9758 (36)
Median gestational age at birth, weeks (range)	29 (20–41)
Infant Factors	
Male sex (%)	13,374 (50)
Apgar score at 1 min (%)	7 (0–10)
Median birth weight, g. (range)	1190 (360–1499)
No breastfeeding at discharge (%)	11,592 (43)
Morbidities	
Early onset sepsis (%)	950 (4)
Late onset sepsis (%)	7672 (29)
Necrotising enterocolitis (any) (%)	1506 (6)
Bronchopulmonary dysplasia (%)	3127 (14)
Surgical management of ROP (%)	951 (4)
Median length of stay, days (range)	50 (1–238)

Data are presented as median (minimum–maximum) or number (percentile), unless specified. Abbreviations: ROP, retinopathy of prematurity; VLBW, very low birth weight; g, gram.

Table 2. Demographic and pathological characteristics of singletons versus multiples.

Variables	Singleton	Multiple	*p*-Value
	n = 17,199	*N* = 9758	
Maternal Factors			
Median gestational age (weeks) (range)	29 (20–41)	30 (20–39)	<0.001
In vitro fertilization	833 (5.2%)	3914 (44%)	<0.001
Outborn	1153 (6.7%)	498 (5.1%)	<0.001
Antenatal care	14,320 (86.3%)	8510 (90.8%)	<0.001
Antenatal steroids	13,741 (81.9%)	8318 (86.9%)	<0.001
Maternal *intra partum* antibiotics	7172 (46.3%)	4330 (49%)	<0.001
Vaginal delivery	5510 (32%)	1944 (19.9%)	<0.001
Infant Factors			
Median birthweight (g) (range)	1160 (360–1499)	1220 (395–1499)	<0.001
Male sex (%)	8728 (50.7)	4646 (47.6)	<0.001
Morbidities			
Days of ventilatory therapy	0 (0–835)	0 (0–672)	<0.001
Days of supplemental oxygen	4 (0–391)	3 (0–286)	<0.001
Surfactant at any time	7689 (45%)	4130 (42.6%)	<0.001
Inotropic therapy	3728 (22.7%)	1959 (21.1%)	0.003
Necrotizing enterocolitis (all grades)	1007 (5.9%)	499 (5.1%)	0.011
Early-onset sepsis	671 (3.9%)	279 (2.9%)	<0.001
Late-onset sepsis	5173 (30.5%)	2499 (26%)	<0.001
IVH (all grades)	3471 (21.7%)	1494 (16.5%)	<0.001
Supplementary Oxygen at discharge	1074 (6.3%)	507 (5.2%)	<0.001
NICU length of stay (days)	19 (0–187)	14 (0–238)	<0.001

Data are presented as mean (SD) or number (percentile), unless specified. Abbreviations: IVH, intraventricular hemorrhage; NICU, neonatal intensive care unit. Comparisons between qualitative variables were made using the Fisher Exact Test or Chi-square. Comparisons between quantitative and qualitative variables were performed through non-parametric tests (U of Mann-Whitney or Kruskal-Wallis).

3.2. *Breastfeeding Patterns by Study Factors*

At hospital discharge, 15,365 (57%) infants were being breastfed, 28% exclusively, and 29% non-exclusively. Out of the singleton infants, at hospital discharge, 31% were being exclusively breastfed, 43% exclusively bottle-fed, and 26% were being fed a combination of both. In comparison, at hospital discharge, only 24% of multiple infants were being exclusively breastfed, 43% exclusively bottle-fed, and 33% were being fed a combination of both. The distribution of the patients by feeding type at discharge differed in these two groups ($p < 0.001$).

3.3. *Determinants of Breastfeeding at Hospital Discharge*

The results of the univariate analysis are summarised in Table 3. With regards to mother and delivery characteristics, the unadjusted analysis shows that In vitro fertilization (IVF), prenatal care, administration of antenatal corticosteroids, intra partum antibiotics, and vaginal delivery, were all protective factors for being breastfed at discharge. Infant weight, height and head circumference at birth were also positively associated with breastfeeding rates at discharge. Additionally, infants that were being breastfed at discharge received less surfactant and were less often intubated or put on mechanical ventilation. They spent fewer days using supplemental oxygen, they received fewer inotropes and required less surgical treatment for ROP, and IVH (grades III and IV). NEC and LOS were more prevalent in infants not being breastfed at discharge.

Table 3. Univariate analysis of risk factors for no breastfeeding at NICU discharge.

Characteristics	Twins		Single	
	OR (95% CI)	p	OR (95% CI)	p
Birth weight	1 (1–1)	0.008	0.99 (0.99–0.99)	<0.001
Height at birth	0.99 (0.99–1)	0.011	0.99 (0.99–0.99)	<0.001
Birth head circumference	0.99 (0.99–1)	0.1	0.99 (0.99–0.99)	<0.001
Male gender	1.08 (0.99–1.17)	0.076	0.99 (0.93–1.05)	0.65
Twin birth		—		—
In vitro fertilization	0.93 (0.85–1.01)	0.099	0.59 (0.5–0.68)	<0.001
Prenatal care	0.84 (0.72–0.97)	0.022	1.46 (1.33–1.6)	<0.001
Prenatal steroids:		<0.001		<0.001
No				
Partial	0.66 (0.57–0.77)		0.84 (0.76–0.93)	
Complete	0.72 (0.63–0.82)		0.74 (0.68–0.8)	
Antibiotic treatment at delivery	0.72 (0.66–0.79)	<0.001	0.86 (0.81–0.92)	<0.001
Delivery type: C-section	1.12 (1.01–1.24)	0.038	0.87 (0.82–0.93)	<0.001
Intubation:	1.22 (1.1–1.35)	<0.001	1.58 (1.48–1.69)	<0.001
CRIB score	1.06 (1.04–1.08)	<0.001	1.11 (1.09–1.12)	<0.001
Conventional ventilation duration	1.01 (1.01–1.02)	<0.001	0.58 (0.55–0.62)	<0.001
Oxygen therapy duration	1 (1–1.01)	<0.001	0.62 (0.55–0.69)	<0.001
Surfactant administration	1.15 (1.06–1.25)	0.001	1.56 (1.46–1.66)	<0.001
Inotropic therapy	1.53 (1.38–1.7)	<0.001	1.96 (1.82–2.12)	<0.001
Ductus closure:		0.022		<0.001
None				
Indometacin	1.12 (0.98–1.28)		1.51 (1.36–1.67)	
Ibuprofen	0.88 (0.77–1)		1.2 (1.08–1.32)	
ROP surgery	1.42 (1.13–1.78)	0.002	2.43 (2.06–2.88)	<0.001
Necrotizing enterocolitis	1.65 (1.37–1.99)	<0.001	1.88 (1.65–2.15)	<0.001
Late onset sepsis	1.27 (1.15–1.39)	<0.001	1.59 (1.48–1.7)	<0.001
Intraventricular hemorrhage		0.001		<0.001
No				
Grade I–II	1.13 (0.99–1.28)		1.24 (1.14–1.36)	
Grade III–IV	1.48 (1.18–1.85)		1.94 (1.67–2.26)	
Supplemental oxygen *at* 36 weeks *PMA*	1.53 (1.33–1.76)	<0.001	2 (1.82–2.21)	<0.001

Data presented as median (range) or percentile. ABBREVIATIONS: NICU, neonatal intensive care unit; PMA, postmenstrual age; ROP, retinopathy of prematurity.

However, when these factors were put into a multivariable model to determine the effect of a factor, while holding all others constant (Table 4), multiple birth (OR 1.10), surfactant administration (OR 1.10), prenatal care (OR 1.11), intubation (OR 1.15), LOS (OR 1.23), surgical treatment for ROP (OR 1.33), use of inotropes (OR 1.38), IVH grades III or IV (OR 1.42), bronchopulmonary dysplasia (OR 1.43) and NEC (OR 1.47), were significantly associated with a lower chance of any breastfeeding at discharge. On the other hand, the primary findings of this study indicate that the odds of a VLBW infant of being breastfed at the time of hospital discharge correlate to (a) the use of ibuprofen for ductus closure, (b) prenatal steroid treatment, (c) In vitro fertilization, and (d) intrapartum antibiotics.

Table 4. Logistical regression analysis of no breastfeeding at discharge as a function of selected predictor variables.

Variables	Odds Ratio (95% CI)	*p*-Value
	Maternal Factors	
Prenatal care	1.11 (1.01–1.22)	0.036
Partial prenatal steroids	0.79 (0.71–0.88)	<0.001
Complete prenatal steroids	0.82 (0.75–0.89)	<0.001
In vitro fertilization	0.84 (0.77–0.92)	<0.001
Antibiotic treatment at delivery	0.86 (0.81–0.92)	<0.001
Multiple birth	1.10 (1.02–1.19)	0.009
	Infant Factors	
Surfactant administration	1.10 (1.01–1.19)	0.023
Endotracheal intubation	1.15 (1.06–1.25)	0.001
	Morbidities	
Ibuprofen treatment for ductus closure	0.73 (0.66–0.81)	<0.001
Late onset sepsis	1.27 (1.18–1.36)	<0.001
Surgical management of ROP	1.33 (1.13–1.57)	0.001
Inotrope support	1.38 (1.26–1.50)	<0.001
Grade III–IV intraventricular hemorrhage	1.42 (1.21–1.67)	<0.001
Supplemental oxygen at 36 weeks PMA	1.43 (1.3–1.59)	<0.001
Necrotizing enterocolitis	1.47 (1.29–1.69)	<0.001

−2 log likelihood: 23234; DF: 17. Abbreviations: ROP, retinopathy of prematurity.

4. Discussion

The incidence of multiple births has risen since the 1970s [21]. Within this group, the proportion of infants born preterm is higher compared to singletons [22]. There is strong evidence that not being fed breastmilk carries greater risks, with preterm babies having specific additional risks. However, mothers of preterm infants may terminate lactation earlier than mothers of full term infants [23]. Researching the obstacles for breastfeeding in preterm babies is a central issue in perinatology [8]. The low prevalence of breastfeeding among preterm infants may be explained by several factors. First, by difficulties inherent to their higher neonatal morbidity [24,25]. Also, maternal socio-demographic factors, and health-care services related factors may play an important role in the initiation and duration of breastfeeding. Although previous studies have examined a wide range of factors related to breastfeeding during a hospital stay for preterm infants, only a few have focused on the effects of multiple births on breastfeeding rates in this population.

Moreover, the few studies that have taken into account this variable have produced controversial results. The results on this issue are quite diverse depending on the study population and on the time of investigation of the nutritional method. To the best of our knowledge, from 1997 to 2017, four papers have found that the combination of prematurity and twin birth results in lower rates and shorter duration of breastfeeding among preterm multiples. On the other hand, six papers have found no breastfeeding differences between singleton and twin preterm infants. A 2004 study assessed exclusive and non-exclusive breastfeeding at day 1, day 3, week 2, month 1, and month 6 postpartum, among 346 mothers of full term and preterm singleton and multiple babies. They found that at any time point, except week 2 and month 1, the proportion of preterm multiples who fed at least some breast milk was less than in other groups [26]. A 2007 telephone survey on 94 VLBW infants reported that mothers of preterm multiples were 16 times more likely to provide formula before week 12 postpartum than mothers who delivered a singleton [27]. A 2014 Danish cohort of preterm infants (24–36 weeks of gestation) has found that multiple birth is significantly associated with the later establishment of exclusive breastfeeding [28]. A 2016 study on a very large sample of very preterm infants shows that the odds for exclusive breastfeeding at discharge for singletons was significantly higher than for twins [29]. Similarly, we found that singleton preterm infants were more likely to be exclusively breastfed at discharge than multiple preterm infants (31% versus 24%). Our results are in line with the previous research on the prevalence of exclusive breastfeeding for VLBW infants at NICU discharge, ranging from 11.4 to 30.5% in various countries [10,17,30]. All studies on this topic report that rates of breastfeeding (exclusive or non-exclusive) decrease with time. Exclusive breastfeeding at NICU discharge is essential to help women in continuing breastfeeding for durations recommended by the WHO. Accordingly, Kaneko et al. reported that the prevalence of exclusive breastfeeding was 22.6% at NICU discharge, and it had dropped only to 15.7% by the start of complementary feeding. These values are slightly higher or lower than those of recent large Japanese or Italian cohorts, respectively [17,31].

On the other hand, six authors have reported that preterm twins can breastfeed as successfully as preterm singleton infants. A 1997 paper on 15 singleton and 18 twin preterm infants showed no differences in feeding method from birth to discharge [32]. More recently, a Danish paper has reported no differences in exclusive breastfeeding rates at discharge [33], an Israeli paper has reported no differences in breastfeeding beyond six months of age [34], and three other papers from Western countries have shown no differences in any breastfeeding rates at discharge from the NICU [6,35,36].

For the majority of mothers, breastfeeding evolves naturally. However, it is not so when mothers experience the unique stress associated with the NICU environment [37]. Most maternal and NICU characteristics that challenge the success of breastfeeding have been extensively studied. Conversely, scarce attention has been devoted to the influence on breastfeeding of a variety of stress factors that preterm and fragile infants face. These include aggressive procedures, life-threatening and damaging conditions, such as IVH or ROP, without forgetting expected feeding difficulties related to the infant's clinical status at feeding time. Therefore, in this study, we chose to examine the link of common neonatal medical complications with the infant continuing to receive breastmilk upon discharge.

VLBW infants are at risk for a variety of medical complications, any of which further limits the mother-infant dyad progression to breastfeeding competence. However, according to our multivariable analysis, only intubation, NEC, LOS, IVH grades III or IV, surgical ROP, the use of inotropes and twin pregnancy were risk factors for breastfeeding cessation before NICU discharge.

Our findings cannot substantiate previous research in this field, yet we have found only one article that identified absence of history of NEC or LOS as significant predictors of continued provision of mother's milk in VLBW infants through to day of life 30 [38], and we have found no published research that reports that lower rates of breastfeeding among multiple preterm infants may reflect their distinct neonatal morbidity.

Our analysis of a very large sample of babies has reduced the number of variables linked to in-hospital breastfeeding cessation to fifteen independent risk factors. Twin pregnancy is one such risk factor, but its magnitude (OR = 1.10) is small enough to explain contradictory results in previous research on this topic. It is expected that small samples with bigger margins of error cannot detect this effect.

Finally, our research confirms that surgical NEC, ROP, bronchopulmonary dysplasia and LOS are linked to no breastfeeding at discharge. It is likely that this is a matter of reverse causation, since it is well established that lack of breastfeeding is a risk factor for such conditions in preterm infants. Likewise, it is reasonable to speculate that prenatal care, including prenatal steroid treatment, boost successful breastfeeding rates. Conversely, surfactant administration, intubation, inotropes, and IVH have not been previously linked to breastfeeding difficulties, and are, therefore, worth further investigation. On the other hand, the same applies to *ductus* closure, In vitro fertilization or *intra partum* antibiotics.

Limitations

The large sample study, the exclusion of recall bias concerning breastfeeding duration and the diverse patient population, are strengths of our study. We were able to show some variation in maternal breast milk provision between multiple and singleton preterm infants. While these findings are important in broadening our knowledge, they are not without limitations.

Breastfeeding was not the focus of the primary study. Consequently, the questions concerning breastfeeding were less detailed than those that would be used in a prospective study. An additional limitation of this study is the use of maternal breast milk feedings at discharge to represent mothers continued provision of breast milk. We were also unable to quantify the volume of maternal breast milk received.

5. Conclusions

Our study of a very large sample of VLBW infants, shows that singleton pregnancy predicts a discrete increase of in-hospital breastfeeding rates, when compared to twin pregnancy. This study encourages a closer look at breastfeeding in the NICU. We support that breastfeeding among VLBW twin infants at NICU discharge is feasible; however, identification of multiple risk factors for the cessation of breastfeeding reflects the complexity of this process. By understanding predictive maternal or infant factors associated with poor breastfeeding outcomes, mothers at risk can be identified for more successful interventions. In addition, we can work to come up with adequate interventions for twin VLBW infants so that, when compared with singleton VLBW infants, neonatal morbidities will no longer be factors associated with failed breastfeeding. It is possible that early interventions for a few serious complications linked to breastfeeding cessation could have minimized the other problems and made it possible for the women to continue. Interventions in the NICU should enable mothers to transition to breastfeeding as soon as possible to promote success until discharge and beyond.

Going forward, for NICUS to excel at feeding human milk, in-depth work remains to determine barriers to a mother's ability to provide breast milk and to establish evidence-based lactation care.

Author Contributions: All authors contributed extensively to the work presented in this paper. S.V. and R.P. conceived the study; E.C. and F.B. developed the methodology; E.M. and M.N. monitored data collection; A.G. analyzed the data; R.P., G.G., F.B. and J.P.-T. critically reviewed the manuscript for important intellectual content; S.V. and J.P.-T. wrote the paper.

Acknowledgments: We want to thank all children, mothers and caregivers who participated in this study, as well as the nursing staff participating in the research for their cooperation. This project would not have been possible without the generous support from the Library of the Balearic Health Authority and from SEN1500 network.

Abbreviations

CI, 95% confidence interval; IVH, intraventricular hemorrhage; LOS, late onset sepsis; NEC, necrotizing enterocolitis; NICU, neonatal unit; OR, odds ratio; ROP, retinopathy of prematurity; SEN1500, Spanish cohort of very low birth weight; VLBW, very low birth weight; WHO, World Health Organization.

References

1. Lewis, E.D.; Richard, C.; Larsen, B.M.; Field, C.J. The importance of human milk for immunity in preterm infants. *Clin. Perinatol.* **2017**, *44*, 23–47. [CrossRef] [PubMed]
2. Lechner, B.E.; Vohr, B.R. Neurodevelopmental outcomes of preterm infants fed human milk: A Systematic Review. *Clin. Perinatol.* **2017**, *44*, 69–83. [CrossRef] [PubMed]
3. Lloyd, M.L.; Malacova, E.; Hartmann, B.; Simmer, K. A clinical audit of the growth of preterm infants fed predominantly pasteurised donor human milk v. those fed mother's own milk in the neonatal intensive care unit. *Br. J. Nutr.* **2019**, *121*, 1018–1025. [CrossRef] [PubMed]
4. Kumar, R.K.; Singhal, A.; Vaidya, U.; Banerjee, S.; Anwar, F.; Rao, S. Optimizing nutrition in preterm low birth weight infants-Consensus Summary. *Front. Nutr.* **2017**′ *4*, 20. [CrossRef] [PubMed]

5. Maffei, D.; Schanler, R.J. Human milk is the feeding strategy to prevent necrotizing enterocolitis! *Semin. Perinatol.* **2017**, *41*, 36–40. [CrossRef] [PubMed]
6. Pineda, R.G. Predictors of breastfeeding and breastmilk feeding among very low birth weight infants. *Breastfeed. Med.* **2011**, *6*, 15–19. [CrossRef] [PubMed]
7. Powers, N.G.; Bloom, B.; Peabody, J.; Clark, R.; Md, N.G.P.; Md, B.B.; Md, J.P.; Md, R.C. Site of care influences breastmilk feedings at NICU discharge. *J. Perinatol.* **2003**, *23*, 10–13. [CrossRef] [PubMed]
8. Sisk, P.; Quandt, S.; Parson, N.; Tucker, J. Breast milk expression and maintenance in mothers of very low birth weight infants: Supports and barriers. *J. Hum. Lact.* **2010**, *26*, 368–375. [CrossRef]
9. Espy, K.A.; Senn, T.E. Incidence and correlates of breast milk feeding in hospitalized preterm infants. *Soc. Sci. Med.* **2003**, *57*, 1421–1428. [CrossRef]
10. Lee, H.C.; Gould, J.B. Factors influencing breast milk versus formula feeding at discharge for very low birth weight infants in California. *J. Pediatr.* **2009**, *155*, 657–662.e2. [CrossRef]
11. Branum, A.M.; Schoendorf, K.C. Changing patterns of low birthweight and preterm birth in the United States, 1981–1998. *Paediatr. Perinat. Epidemiol.* **2002**, *16*, 8–15. [CrossRef] [PubMed]
12. Damato, E.G.; Dowling, D.A.; Standing, T.S.; Schuster, S.D. Explanation for cessation of breastfeeding in mothers of twins. *J. Hum. Lact.* **2005**, *21*, 296–304. [CrossRef]
13. Östlund, Å.; Nordström, M.; Dykes, F.; Flacking, R. Breastfeeding in preterm and term twins–maternal factors associated with early cessation: A population-based study. *J. Hum. Lact.* **2010**, *26*, 235–241. [CrossRef] [PubMed]
14. Royal College of Paediatrics and Child Health. *Guidance for Health Professionals on Feeding Twins, Triplets and Higher Order Multiples*; RCPCH: London, UK, 2011.
15. Lau, C.; Hurst, N.; Burns, P.; Schanler, R.J. Interaction of stress and lactation differs between mothers of premature singletons and multiples. *Adv. Exp. Med. Biol.* **2004**, *554*, 313–316. [PubMed]
16. Leonard, L.G. Breastfeeding rights of multiple birth families and guidelines for health professionals. *Twin. Res.* **2003**, *6*, 34–45. [CrossRef] [PubMed]
17. Davanzo, R.; Monasta, L.; Ronfani, L.; Brovedani, P.; Demarini, S.; Breastfeeding in Neonatal Intensive Care Unit Study Group. Breastfeeding at NICU discharge: A multicenter Italian study. *J. Hum. Lact.* **2013**, *29*, 374–380. [CrossRef] [PubMed]
18. Moro, M.S.; Fernández, C.P.; Figueras, J.A.; Pérez, J.R.; Coll, E.; Doménech, E.M.; Jiménez, R.; Pérez, V.S.; Quero, J.J.; Roques, V.S. Sen1500: Design and implementation of a registry of infants weighing less than 1500 g. at birth in Spain. *An. Pediatr.* **2008**, *68*, 181–188.
19. Porta, R.; Capdevila, E.; Botet, F.; Verd, S.; Ginovart, G.; Moliner, E.; Nicolàs, M.; Rios, J.; SEN1500 Network. Morbidity and mortality of very low birth weight multiples compared with singletons. *J. Matern. Fetal. Neonatal. Med.* **2019**, *32*, 389–397. [CrossRef] [PubMed]
20. Lang, T. Documenting research in scientific articles: Guidelines for Authors: 3. Reporting multivariate analysis. *Chest* **2007**, *131*, 628–632. [CrossRef]
21. Wallis, S.K.; Dowswell, T.; West, H.M.; Renfrew, M.J.; Whitford, H.M. Breastfeeding education and support for women with twins or higher order multiples. *Cochrane Database Syst. Rev.* **2017**, CD012003. [CrossRef]
22. NICE. Multiple Pregnancy: Twin and Triplet Pregnancies. NICE Quality Standard [QS46]. Available online: http://www.nice.org.uk/guidance/qs46/resources/guidance-multiple-pregnancy-pdf2013 (accessed on 24 January 2019).
23. Killersreiter, B.; Grimmer, I.; Bührer, C.; Dudenhausen, J.W.; Obladen, M. Early cessation of breastmilk feeding in very low birthweight infants. *Early Hum. Dev.* **2001**, *60*, 193–205. [CrossRef]
24. Morag, I.; Harel, T.; Leibovitch, L.; Simchen, M.J.; Maayan-Metzger, A.; Strauss, T. Factos associated with breast milk feeding of very preterm infants from birth to 6 months corrected age. *Breastfeed. Med.* **2016**, *11*, 138–143. [CrossRef] [PubMed]
25. Kirchner, L.; Jeitler, V.; Waldhör, T.; Pollak, A.; Wald, M. Long hospitalization is the most important risk factor for early weaning from breast milk in premature babies. *Acta Paediatr.* **2009**, *98*, 981–984. [CrossRef] [PubMed]
26. Geraghty, S.R.; Pinney, S.M.; Sethuraman, G.; Roy-Chaudhury, A.; Kalkwarf, H.J. Breast milk feeding rates of mothers of multiples compared to mothers of singletons. *Ambul. Pediatr.* **2004**, *4*, 226–231. [CrossRef] [PubMed]

27. Hill, P.D.; Aldag, J.C.; Zinaman, M.; Chatterton, R.T. Predictors of preterm infant feeding methods and perceived insufficient milk supply at week 12 postpartum. *J. Hum. Lact.* **2007**, *23*, 32–38. [CrossRef] [PubMed]
28. Maastrup, R.; Hansen, B.M.; Kronborg, H.; Bojesen, S.N.; Hallum, K.; Frandsen, A.; Kyhnaeb, A.; Svarer, I.; Hallström, I.K. Breastfeeding progression in preterm infants is influenced by factors in infants, mothers and clinical practice: The results of a national cohort study with high breastfeeding initiation rates. *PLoS ONE* **2014**, *9*, e108208. [CrossRef]
29. Ericson, J.; Flacking, R.; Hellström-Westas, L.; Eriksson, M. Changes in the prevalence of breast feeding in preterm infants discharged from neonatal units: A register study over 10 years. *BMJ Open* **2016**, *6*, e012900. [CrossRef]
30. Maia, C.; Brandão, R.; Roncalli, A.; Maranhão, H. Length of stay in a neonatal intensive care unit and its association with low rates of exclusive breastfeeding in very low birth weight infants. *J. Matern. Fetal. Neonatal Med.* **2011**, *24*, 774–777. [CrossRef]
31. Kaneko, A.; Kaneita, Y.; Yokoyama, E.; Miyake, T.; Harano, S.; Suzuki, K.; Ibuka, E.; Tsutsui, T.; Yamamoto, Y.; Ohida, T. Factors associated with exclusive breast- feeding in Japan: For activities to support child-rearing with breast-feeding. *J. Epidemiol.* **2006**, *16*, 57–63. [CrossRef]
32. Liang, R.; Gunn, A.J.; Gunn, T.R. Can preterm twins breast feed successfully? *N. Z. Med. J.* **1997**, *110*, 209–212.
33. Zachariassen, G.; Faerk, J.; Grytter, C.; Esberg, B.; Juvonen, P.; Halken, S. Factors associated with successful establishment of breastfeeding in very preterm infants. *Acta Paediatr.* **2010**, *99*, 1000–1004. [CrossRef]
34. Pinchevski-Kadir, S.; Shust-Barequet, S.; Zajicek, M.; Leibovich, M.; Strauss, T.; Leibovitch, L.; Morag, I. Direct feeding at the breast Is associated with breast milk feeding duration among preterm infants. *Nutrients* **2017**, *9*, 1202. [CrossRef]
35. Rodrigues, C.; Teixeira, R.; Fonseca, M.J.; Zeitlin, J.; Barros, H.; Couto, A.S.; Lopes, A.; Almeida, A.; Portela, A.; Portuguese EPICE (Effective Perinatal Intensive Care in Europe) Network; et al. Prevalence and duration of breast milk feeding in very preterm infants: A 3-year follow-up study and a systematic literature review. *Paediatr. Perinat. Epidemiol.* **2018**, *32*, 237–246. [CrossRef]
36. Mamemoto, K.; Kubota, M.; Nagai, A.; Takahashi, Y.; Kamamoto, T.; Minowa, H.; Yasuhara, H. Factors associated with exclusive breastfeeding in low birth weight infants at NICU discharge and the start of complementary feeding. *Asia Pac. J. Clin. Nutr.* **2013**, *22*, 270–275. [CrossRef]
37. Lau, C. Breastfeeding challenges and the preterm mother-infant dyad: A conceptual model. *Breastfeed. Med.* **2018**, *13*, 8–17. [CrossRef]
38. Romaine, A.; Clark, R.H.; Davis, B.R.; Hendershot, K.; Kite, V.; Laughon, M.; Updike, I.; Miranda, M.L.; Meier, P.P.; Patel, A.L.; et al. Predictors of prolonged breast milk provision to very low birth weight infants. *J. Pediatr.* **2018**, *202*, 23–30. [CrossRef]

5

Human Milk Casein and Whey Protein and Infant Body Composition over the First 12 Months of Lactation

Zoya Gridneva [1,*], Wan J. Tie [1], Alethea Rea [2], Ching Tat Lai [1], Leigh C. Ward [3], Kevin Murray [4], Peter E. Hartmann [1] and Donna T. Geddes [1]

1 School of Molecular Sciences, M310, The University of Western Australia, Crawley, Perth, WA 6009, Australia; ash.tie@uwa.edu.au (W.J.T.); ching-tat.lai@uwa.edu.au (C.T.L.); peter.hartmann@uwa edu.au (P.E.H.); donna.geddes@uwa.edu.au (D.T.G.)

2 Centre for Applied Statistics, The University of Western Australia, Crawley, Perth, WA 6009, Australia; alethea.rea@uwa.edu.au

3 School of Chemistry and Molecular Biosciences, The University of Queensland, St. Lucia, Brisbane, QLD 4072, Australia; l.ward@uq.edu.au

4 School of Population and Global Health, The University of Western Australia, Crawley, Perth, WA 6009, Australia; kevin.murray@uwa.edu.au

* Correspondence: zoya.gridneva@uwa.edu.au

Abstract: Human milk (HM) influences infant feeding patterns and body composition (BC). This small proof-of concept longitudinal study investigated relationships between infant/maternal BC and HM casein, whey and total protein during the first 12 months of lactation. BC of breastfeeding dyads (n = 20) was measured at 2 (n = 15), 5 (n = 20), 9 (n = 19), and/or 12 (n = 18) months postpartum with ultrasound skinfolds (infants) and bioimpedance spectroscopy (infants/mothers). Proteins concentrations and 24-h milk intake were measured and calculated daily intakes (CDI) determined. Higher maternal weight, body mass index, fat-free mass, fat-free mass index, and fat mass index were associated with higher concentration of whey protein ($p \leq 0.034$, $n = 20$). There were no associations between infant BC and concentrations of all proteins, and CDI of whey and total protein. Higher CDI of casein were associated with lower infant fat-free mass ($p = 0.003$, $n = 18$) and higher fat mass ($p < 0.001$), fat mass index ($p = 0.001$, $n = 18$), and % fat mass ($p < 0.001$, $n = 18$) measured with ultrasound skinfolds. These results show a differential effect of HM casein on development of infant BC during the first year of life, suggesting that there is a potential to improve outcome for the infant through interventions, such as continuation of breastfeeding during the first 12 months of life and beyond, which may facilitate favourable developmental programming that could reduce risk of non-communicable diseases later in life.

Keywords: casein; whey; protein; breastfeeding; infant; body composition; bioelectrical impedance spectroscopy; ultrasound skinfolds; human milk; calculated daily intakes; lactation

---

1. Introduction

An epidemic of childhood obesity and the associated non-communicable diseases (NCD), such as diabetes and cardiovascular disease are of increasing international concern [1]. Increasingly, data suggests the lifelong risk of NCD could be modified through early programming effects on obesity and adiposity [2,3]. It is evident that breastfed infants are at 15–20% reduced risk of obesity and obesity related disease later in life [4,5]. Whilst the protective mechanisms of breastfeeding are not fully understood [6], the development of body composition (BC) in early life [7], composition of human milk (HM) [8–10], and infant breastfeeding patterns and behavior [11–13] are all known to play an important role in the programming of these health outcomes.

An increased risk of obesity has been associated with both rapid weight gain [14] and the elevated protein content in infant formulas [9,15]. Compared with 9 g/L in term HM (6–12 g/L, week 10/12) [16], protein content ranged from 12 to 19 g/L in infant formulas and from 16 to 27 g/L in follow-up formulas [15]. Thus, limiting protein intake from infant foods could be an effective strategy in reduction of childhood obesity, leading to the development of lower protein formulas to mimic growth rates of HM fed infants [15]. HM is recognized as the best form of nutrition for optimal growth and development of the human infant and as such is species specific in composition. The stark compositional differences between HM and formula have been implicated in the differences in weight and BC between breastfed and formula-fed infants and decreased risk of later obesity for breastfed infants [8,9].

The protein content of HM, which is low yet highly bioavailable, appears to play a key role in infant growth [9] and might provide a rationale for the reduced risk of being in rapid-growth trajectory [17] and for the lower fat-free mass (FFM) and higher fat mass (FM) and percentage FM (%FM) of breastfed infants compared with formula-fed [18] during early infancy. In term infants, the protein intakes from HM (three months, boys: 6.4 ± 1.2 g/day; girls: 5.8 ± 1.0 g/day) were found to be almost half that of formula (boys: 11.4 ± 2.0 g/day; girls: 10.5 ± 1.8 g/day), and at three and six months differences in protein intake and weight gain were associated with disproportionate gain in FM and FFM, resulting in %FM difference between the groups [8]. These variations suggest a self-regulatory mechanism of milk intake (MI), which may be in part driven by HM components [10] that are associated with feeding frequency (FFQ) [19].

Despite MI and protein intakes being associated with breastfed infants' weight and FFM gain [8] very few comprehensive longitudinal HM protein intake studies are available through the exclusive breastfeeding and weaning periods. Also, there has been no investigation of the effect of either concentrations or daily intakes of specific HM fractions—such as casein and whey—on infant BC, yet these are highly variable between breastfeeding dyads. Daily intakes of HM components are the true reflection on what infant receives, unlike the concentrations, which can be misleading, especially if the milk intake is inadequate or if mixed feeding is present.

The protective role of HM and breastfeeding may be attributable to the effect of specific protein fractions on development of infant BC. Thus, the aim of this longitudinal study was to investigate relationships of concentrations and daily intakes of HM casein, whey and total protein with anthropometrics and BC of healthy term breastfed infants and their mothers during first 12 months postpartum. Further exploration of relationships of infant 24-h MI and FFQ with HM proteins was carried out.

2. Materials and Methods

2.1. Study Participants

Breastfed infants ($n = 20$; 10 males, 10 females) of English-speaking, predominantly Caucasian, mothers of higher social-economic status from a developed country were recruited from the community, primarily from the West Australian branch of the Australian Breastfeeding Association. Inclusion criteria were: healthy singletons, gestational age ≥37 weeks, exclusively breastfed [20] at 2 and 5 months, and maternal intention to breastfeed until 12 months. Exclusion criteria were: infant factors that could potentially influence growth and development of BC, maternal smoking, and low milk supply. All mothers provided written informed consent to participate in the study, which was approved by The University of Western Australia Human Research Ethics Committee (RA/1/4253, RA/4/1/2639) and registered with the Australian New Zealand Clinical Trials Registry (ACTRN12616000368437).

2.2. Study Session

Measurements were made when the infants were 2 and/or 5, 9, and 12 months of age. Participants visited our laboratory at King Edward Memorial Hospital for Women (Subiaco, Perth, WA, Australia) for up to four monitored breastfeeding sessions between March 2013 and September 2015. At each study session, the infant was weighed pre-feed, and then the mother breastfed her infant. Infant bioelectrical impedance spectroscopy (BIS) measurements were made pre-feed, unless impractical, then they were taken post-feed [21]. Ultrasound skinfold and anthropometric measurements were made post-feed. Clothing was removed for the measurements except for a dry diaper and a sleeveless shirt.

Maternal weight, height, and BIS measurements were recorded. Small (1−2 mL) pre- and post-feed milk samples were collected into 5 mL polypropylene vials (Disposable Products, Adelaide, SA, Australia) from the breast/s that infant was fed from and samples were frozen at −20 °C for biochemical analysis. Current feeding frequency (FFQ) of the infants was self-reported by mothers.

2.3. Anthropometric Measurements

Infants weight was determined before breastfeeding using Medela Electronic Baby Weigh Scales (±2.0 g; Medela Inc., McHenry, IL, USA). Infant crown-heel length was measured once to the nearest 0.1 cm using non-stretch tape and a headpiece and a footpiece, both applied perpendicularly to the hard surface. Infant head circumference was measured with a non-stretch tape to the nearest 0.1 cm.

Maternal weight was measured using Seca electronic scales (±0.1 kg; Seca, Chino, CA, USA). Height was self-reported by participants or measured against a calibrated marked wall (accuracy ±0.1 cm).

Infant and maternal body mass index (BMI) were calculated as kg/m^2.

2.4. Body Composition with Bioelectrical Impedance Spectroscopy

The methods for measuring maternal and infant BC with BIS using Impedimed SFB7 bioelectrical impedance analyser (ImpediMed, Brisbane, QLD, Australia) as well as age-specific equations used for calculations of infant BC parameters during this study have been published previously [22]. The within participant coefficient of variation (CV) for maternal %FM was 0.21% [23]. Within participant CV for infant resistance measurements at 50 kHz (R_{50}) was 1.5% [21].

2.5. Ultrasound Skinfold Measurements

The method for measuring infant skinfolds using the Aplio XG ultrasound machine (Toshiba, Tokyo, Japan) with a 14-8 MHz transducer (PLT-1204BX) and sterile water-based ultrasonic gel (Parker Laboratories Inc., Fairfield, NJ, USA) as well as the equations for calculations of infant BC parameters during this study have been published previously [22,24]. Briefly, single ultrasound scans of four anatomical sites (biceps, subscapular, suprailiac and triceps) were performed on the left side of the body with minimal compression. At all tome points, infant BC was calculated with both, 2-skinfolds (US 2SF: triceps, subscapular) and 4-skinfolds (US 4SF: biceps, subscapular, suprailiac and triceps).

2.6. Body Composition Indices

The indices of height-normalized BC were calculated for mothers and infants: FM index (FMI) was calculated as $FM/length^2$, and FFM index (FFMI) was calculated as $FFM/length^2$; both expressed as kg/m^2 [25].

2.7. 24-h Milk Intake and Feeding Frequency

Infant 24-h MI was measured by mothers using the 24-h milk production (MP) protocol, weighing infants at home with the Medela Electronic Baby Weigh Scales pre- and post each breastfeed during a 24-h period plus one breastfeeding, and recording amounts of HM (g) consumed by the infant (including expressed HM if any) [26]. 24-h MI was determined as previously described with potential underestimation of 3–10% [26] and FFQ (meals per 24-h) was recorded [27]. 24-h MI was measured at three time points: between 2 and 5 (4.0 ± 1.3) months, when MI is shown to be stable [27], and within 2 weeks of 9 (9.4 ± 0.3) and 12 (12.2 ± 0.4) months. Given that measuring 24-h MI is not always practical, particularly at the later stages of lactation, mothers were also asked to estimate how frequently the infant fed, and self-reported (SR) the typical time between the meals (e.g., each 2 h) during the week prior to the study session as a proxy measure of FFQ.

2.8. Calculated Daily Intakes of Human Milk Proteins

24-h MI values from the 24-h MP, and casein, whey and total protein concentrations (pooled pre-/post-feed) from samples taken at the study sessions were used for determination of calculated daily intakes (CDI). These CDI were considered representative of a typical daily intake due to the absence of significant short-term (weekly) [28] and circadian [29,30] variations in HM protein concentrations during the established lactation.

2.9. Sample Preparation

Prior to further analysis, HM samples were thawed for 2 h at room temperature, mixed on Intelli-Mixer RM-2M (ELMI, Riga, Latvia) at 50 revolutions per min in "UU" mode for 15 s, then, after gentle inversion (three times), aliquoted into 1.5 mL tubes (Sarstedt, Numbrecht, Germany). Pre- and post-feed samples were pooled for measuring casein and whey and total protein. Milk samples were defatted by centrifugation at room temperature in a Beckman Microfuge 11 (Aberdon Enterprise Inc., Elk Grove Village, IL, USA) at 10,000× g for 10 min and removing the fat layer by clipping it off together with the top of the tube [31]. Skim HM was used for measuring protein concentrations. Standard assays were adapted for and carried out using a JANUS workstation (PerkinElmer, Inc., Waltham, MA, USA) and measured on EnSpire (PerkinElmer, Inc., Waltham, MA, USA).

2.10. Human Milk Fractions

Casein and whey proteins were separated by the method described by Kunz and Lonnerdal [32] and Khan et al. [30]. Protein concentrations (total protein, casein, and whey proteins) were measured using the Bradford Protein Assay adapted from Mitoulas et al. [29]. Recovery of protein was 100.6 ± 5.2% (n = 5) with a detection limit of 0.031 g/L and an inter-assay CV of 7.8% (n = 18). Casein-whey ratio was calculated as follows:

$$Casein - whey\ ratio = \text{casein concentration/whey protein concentration.} \quad (1)$$

2.11. Statistical Analyses

Data for this analysis came from the longitudinal study, the details of which have been described previously [22]. Descriptive statistics are reported as mean ± standard deviation (SD) (range); model parameters as estimate ± SE (standard error).

During this longitudinal study infants were measured at four time points (2 and/or 5, 9 and 12 months). An approximate sample size was calculated using the 'F tests–Linear multiple regression: Fixed model: R^2 increase' option in G*Power [33] as if this was a cross-sectional study with equal numbers at each time. Allowing four predictors (three for age comparisons), $\alpha = 0.05$ and 14 participants (56 sample points = 14 participants × 4 time points) would give the study power of 0.80 to detect an effect size of 0.15. This approach was selected, as there is no closed form expression suitable for the calculation of sample sizes for this research design [34], with the consideration that longitudinal study design is more powerful. Recruitment of participants at the 5-months point was introduced, as many mothers would not commit to a study that required breastfeeding to 12 months, when approached at 2 months. As a result, required number of participants was increased to 20 in order to maintain predicted power; this also addressed issues relating to missed visits. Missing data was dealt with using available case analysis.

The analyses for systematic differences in concentrations and CDI of adipokines at different months after birth used linear mixed model with age as effect factor and participant as a random factor. Differences between each month were analysed using general linear hypothesis tests (Tukey's all pair comparisons).

Relationships between: (a) maternal BC and protein concentrations/CDI, and (b) protein concentrations/CDI and infant BC, (c) protein concentrations and breastfeeding parameters (24-h MI/FFQ), and (d) FFQ and CDI of proteins were analysed using linear mixed effects models. Each protein concentration/CDI or infant BC measure/index was considered separately as the response variable, and each model contained fixed effects of infant age (months), a predictor (maternal BC measure/index, protein concentration/CDI and breastfeeding parameters (24-h MI/FFQ)) and an interaction between infant age and predictor, as well as a random intercept per participant. If the interaction was not significant results were reported for the same model fitted without the interaction to assist in understanding the nature of the relationship between the predictor and outcome.

To investigate if there were differences by sex, relationships between infant characteristics and protein concentrations were also analysed using linear mixed effects models accounting for age and sex and an interaction between infant age and predictor, as well as a random intercept per participant.

Relationships between CDI of proteins measured between 2 and 5, and at 9 and 12 months after birth and changes (Δ) in infant BC and anthropometric parameters between the time points were analysed using linear regression models.

Owing to the large number of comparisons, a false discovery rate adjustment [35] was performed on associated subgroupings of results to the interaction p-value if it was less than 0.05 or to the main effect p-value. The adjusted significance levels are reported in Results and Tables and set at the 5% level otherwise. Statistical analysis was performed in R 3.1.2 [36]. Additional packages were used for linear mixed effects models (nlme, lme4, and car) [37–39], intra-class correlations (irr) [40], Tukey's all pair comparisons (multcomp) [41] and graphics (ggplot2) [42].

3. Results

3.1. Subjects

Twenty-two infants were recruited; two infants (one male, one female) were excluded from the study after the 2-months visit (commenced weaning; personal circumstances). One female infant weaned after the 5-months visit and was not followed up further; 19 remaining infants were breastfed at 9 months; 17 infants continued to breastfeed at 12 months. Out of 18 infants measured at 12 months, 16 infants (89%) still continued to breastfeed; one male infant ceased breastfeeding 2 weeks before the 12-month appointment and one female infant stopped at 10 months after birth.

Therefore, overall six infants missed one study session and one infant missed two study sessions. Five of these infants were not recruited until 5 months, one infant did not attend the study session at 9 months and two did not attend the study session at 12 months.

Overall, 80 measures were expected however some were missing, specifically: infant weight (n = 9); infant BC parameters measured with US 2SF, and maternal age, weight, height, BMI and BC parameters measured with BIS (n = 10); infant head circumference (n = 11); infant length, BMI and BC parameters measured with US 4SF, concentrations of casein, whey and total protein (n = 12); infant BC parameters measured with BIS (n = 13); self-reported FFQ (n = 20). Missing data also occurred due to difficulties with conducting 24-h MI measurements at later stages of lactation. The following measurements from the 60 expected were missing: FFQ from 24-h MP (n = 26), 24-h MI and CDI of casein, whey and total protein (n = 27). Missing data were spread across the time points (Table 1).

Participant demographic characteristics collected at the start of the study are presented in Table 2, anthropometric and breastfeeding characteristics measured at the four study sessions are presented in Table 1. The more detailed determinants of maternal and infant BC as well as description of longitudinal changes in infant and maternal BC and breastfeeding parameters, and the associations between them have been reported previously [22].

Table 1. Participant anthropometric and breastfeeding characteristics throughout 12 months of lactation.

Characteristics	2 Months Mean ± SD (Range)	5 Months Mean ± SD (Range)	9 Months Mean ± SD (Range)	12 Months Mean ± SD (Range)
Mothers				
	$n = 14$	$n = 20$	$n = 18$	$n = 18$
Weight (kg)	78.8 ± 19.3 [a] (57.5–116.2)	70.1 ± 17.8 (53.7–115.3)	63.0 ± 10.0 (50.4–121.9)	64.2 ± 17.3 (51.4–121.9)
BMI (kg/m^2)	27.2 ± 5.5 (20.4–35.5)	24.8 ± 5.0 (19.0–35.2)	22.7 ± 3.9 (17.9–37.2)	23.9 ± 5.9 (18.2–37.2)
Infants				
	$n = 14$	$n = 20$	$n = 19$	$n = 18$
Sex (M/F) Age (months)	9 M/6 F 2.04 ± 0.14 (1.87–2.33)	10 M/10 F 5.16 ± 0.22 (4.77–5.47)	10 M/9 F 9.22 ± 0.27 (8.83–9.77)	9 M/9 F 12.26 ± 0.28 (11.63–12.67)
Length (cm)	58.1 ± 1.9 (54.2–60.0)	64.8 ± 2.3 (60.5–69.5)	71.7 ± 1.9 (66.0–74.0)	73.6 ± 3.2 (69.0–78.5)
Weight (kg)	5.630 ± 0.660 (4.420–7.400)	7.431 ± 1.134 (5.808–9.510)	8.836 ± 0.975 (6.675–10.095)	9.650 ± 0.618 (7.165–11.085)
BMI (kg/m^2)	16.6 ± 1.2 (14.5–18.1)	17.6 ± 1.9 (14.9–20.4)	17.7 ± 1.7 (14.2–20.2)	17.8 ± 0.9 (13.7–19.2)
Head circumference (cm)	39.7 ± 1.6 (37.0–42.0)	42.1 ± 1.5 (40.0–45.9)	45.6 ± 1.7 (43.0–48.5)	46.6 ± 1.7 (44.2–49.5)
Breastfeeding Characteristics				
		$n = 17$	$n = 8$	$n = 8$
24-h milk intake (g)	n/a [b]	818.8 ± 204.9 (498–1185)	478.3 ± 154.0 (300–775)	451.1 ± 215.7 (255–795)
		$n = 17$	$n = 8$	$n = 9$
24-h feeding frequency (MP)	n/a [b]	8.1 ± 1.4 (6–11)	5.4 ± 1.3 (4–7)	4.4 ± 2.1 (2–8)
	$n = 11$	$n = 19$	$n = 17$	$n = 13$
Feeding frequency (SR)	2.3 ± 0.4 [c] (1.5–3.0)	2.8 ± 0.8 (1.5–4.0)	3.7 ± 1.2 (2.0–6.0)	5.4 ± 2.9 (2.2–12.0)

[a] Data are mean ± SD and ranges. [b] Milk intake and feeding frequency as meals per 24-h was determined from 24-h milk production (MP) measured between 2 and 5 months (presented at 5 months here) and within 2 weeks of 9 and 12 months; n/a, not applicable. [c] Maternal self-report (SR) of feeding frequency at the time of the visit as a typical time between meals (e.g., each 2 h). BMI, body mass index. M/F, male/female.

Table 2. Participant demographic characteristics at the start of the study.

Characteristics $n = 20$	Mean ± SD (Range)
Maternal age (years)	33.3 ± 4.7 (24–44) [a]
Maternal height (cm)	167.4 ± 7.4 (150–181)
Parity	2.3 ± 0.9 (1–4)
Infant sex (Male/Female)	10/10
Infant birth weight (kg)	3.486 ± 0.498 (2.660–4.455)
Infant gestational age (weeks)	39.4 ± 1.3 (37.6–43.0)

[a] Data are mean ± standard deviation (SD) and ranges.

3.2. Breastfeeding Parameters and Human Milk Proteins

HM protein concentrations and CDI at 4 time points are detailed in Table 3. CDI of casein, whey and total protein, 24-h MI, and both SR and MP FFQ decreased across the lactation (see Table 4 for estimates and significances).

Table 3. Human milk proteins presented as concentrations and 24-h intakes at months after birth [a].

	2 Months	**5 Months**	**9 Months**	**12 Months**
Components	**Mean ± SD**	**Mean ± SD**	**Mean ± SD**	**Mean ± SD**
	(Range)	**(Range)**	**(Range)**	**(Range)**
	Concentrations [b]			
	***n* = 15**	***n* = 20**	***n* = 19**	***n* = 15**
Total protein (g/L)	11.03 ± 1.40 [c] (7.60–12.32)	11.90 ± 4.31 (7.93–24.16)	9.69 ± 1.12 (7.25–14.96)	10.72 ± 2.84 (5.89–16.80)
Casein (g/L)	1.24 ± 0.24 (0.69–1.57)	1.51 ± 0.44 (0.78–3.45)	1.11 ± 0.38 (0.49–2.00)	1.07 ± 0.35 (0.65–1.87)
Whey protein (g/L)	6.44 ± 1.62 (4.12–9.08)	5.43 ± 0.90 (3.82–7.38)	5.43 ± 0.93 (3.94–9.40)	7.61 ± 1.85 (4.49–9.76)
Casein-whey ratio	0.21 ± 0.07 (0.10–0.31)	0.28 ± 0.05 (0.13–0.73)	0.21 ± 0.08 (0.07–0.38)	0.16 ± 0.09 (0.09–0.36)
	CDI [d]			
		***n* = 17**	***n* = 8**	***n* = 8**
Total protein (g)	n/a [e]	9.19 ± 3.82 [d] (4.51–20.34)	5.24 ± 1.84 (2.18–7.48)	4.18 ± 2.11 (1.93–7.23)
Casein (g)	n/a	1.45 ± 0.82 (0.56–3.63)	0.60 ± 0.23 (0.17–0.95)	0.54 ± 0.34 (0.24–1.19)
Whey protein (g)	n/a	4.23 ± 1.14 (2.65–6.76)	3.02 ± 1.11 (1.70–4.64)	2.78 ± 1.34 (1.15–4.40)

[a] Milk components' concentrations and 24-h components' intakes are presented grouped by the month after birth. [b] Concentrations as measured at 2, 5, 9, and 12 months. [c] Data are mean ± SD and ranges. [d] Calculated daily intakes (CDI) of proteins were calculated between 2 and 5 months (presented at 5 months here) and within 2 weeks of 9 and 12 months. [e] n/a, not applicable.

Table 4. Differences by infant age/lactation duration (between time points) within measured human milk proteins and breastfeeding parameters [a].

Changes in Characteristics between Time Points	Months after Birth						
	5 and 2 Months	9 and 2 Months	12 and 2 Months	9 and 5 Months	12 and 5 Months	12 and 9 Months	*p* Overall
	Milk Components						
	n = 15	*n* = 13	*n* = 10	*n* = 18	*n* = 14	*n* = 15	*n* = 20
ΔTotal protein (g/L)	0.57 (0.80) [b] 0.89	−0.52 (0.81) 0.92	0.08 (0.86) 1.00	−1.08 (0.75) 0.46	−0.49(0.80) 0.93	0.60 (0.81) 0.88	0.59 [c]
ΔCasein (g/L)	**0.38 (0.15)** [d] **0.047**	0.87 −0.11 (0.15)	1.00 −0.01 (0.16)	**0.002** **−0.50 (0.14)**	**0.043** **−0.39(0.15)**	0.89 0.11 (0.15)	**0.010**
ΔWhey protein (g/L)	**−1.06 (0.36)** **0.016**	−0.36 (0.36) 0.75	0.13 (0.39) 0.099	0.69 (0.33) 0.15	**1.19(0.36)** **0.005**	0.49 (0.36) 0.52	**0.006**
ΔCasein-whey ratio	**0.11 (0.03)** **0.004**	−0.01 (0.03) 1.00	0.01 (0.03) 1.00	**−0.11 (0.03)** **<0.001**	**−0.10 (0.03)** **0.006**	0.01 (0.03) 0.98	**0.002**
	Breastfeeding Characteristics						
	n = 11	*n* = 11	*n* = 7	*n* = 17	*n* = 13	*n* = 13	*n* = 19
ΔFeeding frequency (SR) [e]	0.46 (0.53) 0.82	**1.40 (0.54)** **0.045**	**3.14 (0.58)** **<0.001**	0.94 (0.46) 0.17	**2.69 (0.50)** **<0.001**	**1.75 (0.51)** **0.003**	**<0.001**
				n = 7	*n* = 7	*n* = 7	*n* = 10
ΔFeeding frequency (MP) [f]	n/a [g]	n/a [g]	n/a [g]	**−2.81 (0.49)** **<0.001**	**−3.71 (0.46)** **<0.001**	−0.90 (0.52) 0.19	**<0.001**
				n = 7	*n* = 7	*n* = 7	*n* = 9
Δ24-h milk intake (g) [f]	n/a	n/a	n/a	**−325 (64)** **<0.001**	**−376 (64)** **<0.001**	−52 (69) 0.73	**<0.001**
	CDI of Milk Components						
				n = 7	*n* = 7	*n* = 7	*n* = 9
ΔTotal protein (g) [f]	n/a	n/a	n/a	**−3.81 (0.83)** **<0.001**	**−4.09 (0.83)** **<0.001**	−0.28 (0.86) 0.94	**<0.001**
ΔCasein (g) [f]	n/a	n/a	n/a	**−0.91 (0.26)** **0.005**	**−0.91 (0.26)** **0.005**	−0.002 (0.31) 1.00	**<0.001**
ΔWhey protein (g) [f]	n/a	n/a	n/a	**−1.52 (0.37)** **<0.001**	**−1.49 (0.37)** **<0.001**	0.03 (0.39) 1.00	**0.002**

[a] Systematic differences in the measured variables between different months after birth were calculated using general linear hypothesis test (Tukey's all pair comparisons). [b] Data are parameter estimate and standard error of estimate and *p*-value. [c] Overall *p*-value is associated with age as reported in linear mixed model. [d] Bold text indicates significant difference ($p < 0.05$) between two time points or overall. [e] Feeding frequency was self-reported (SR) by mothers at the time of the visit as an average time between meals (e.g., each 2 h). [f] 24-h milk intake and feeding frequency as meals per 24-h was measured at 24-h milk production (MP) and daily intakes (CDI) calculated between 2 and 5 months (presented at 5 months here) and within 2 weeks of 9 and 12 months. [g] Results are not presented for impractical combinations; n/a, not applicable.

3.3. Maternal Body Composition and Human Milk Proteins

Higher maternal characteristics and BC measures (weight, BMI, FFM, FFMI, and FMI) were associated with higher whey protein concentrations (Figure 1).

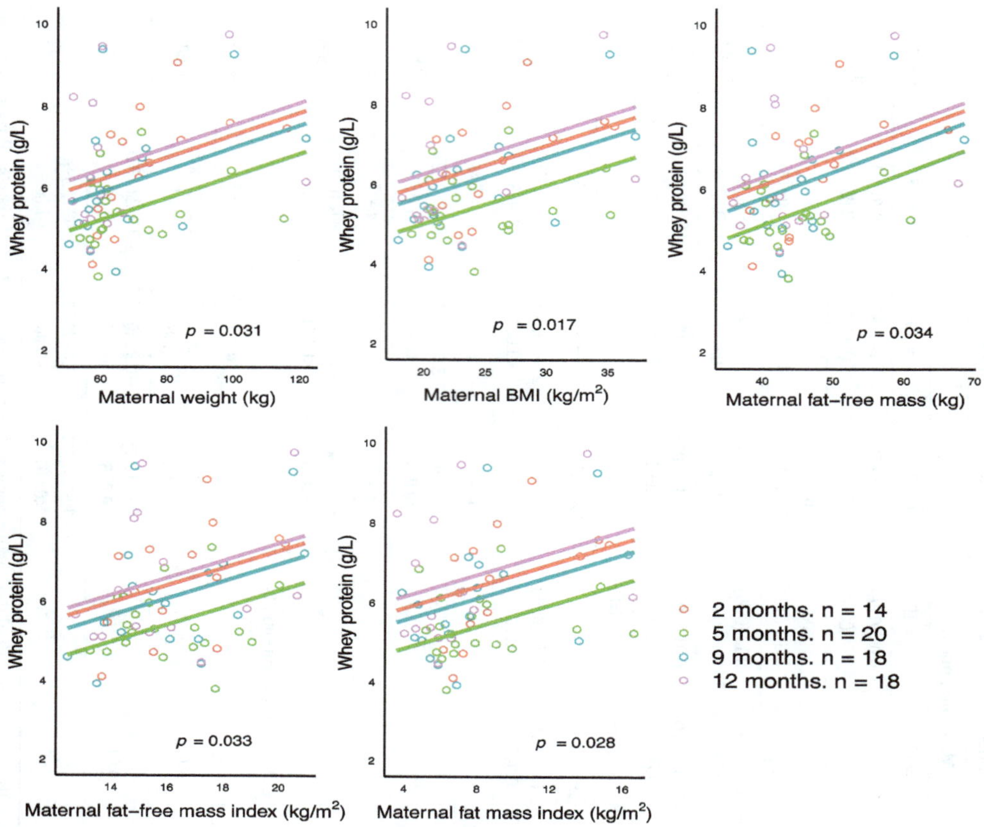

Figure 1. Significant positive associations between concentrations of human milk whey protein and maternal anthropometrics and body composition parameters measured with bioelectrical impedance spectroscopy. Lines represent linear regression and grouped by the month of lactation.

No associations were seen between maternal characteristics and casein–whey ratio, total protein and casein concentrations, and CDI of all proteins after adjusting for the false discovery rate (see Table A1 for estimates and significances).

3.4. Infant Body Composition and Concentrations of Proteins

No significant associations between concentrations of proteins and infant characteristics were seen after adjusting for the false discovery rate (see Table A2 for estimates and significances).

When infant sex was included in the models, significant differences were found for infant head circumference, weight, FFM (US 2SF, 4SF, and BIS) and FFMI (US 4SF and BIS), but none of the models reported an effect of either total protein, whey protein and casein concentrations or whey-to-casein ratio (details are not reported).

3.5. Infant Body Composition and Calculated Daily Intakes of Proteins

Higher CDI of casein were associated with lower infant FFM (US 4SF) and increased FM (US 4SF), %FM (US 4SF), and FMI (US 4SF) after adjusting for the false discovery rate (Figure 2).

No associations were seen between infant characteristics and both CDI of total protein and whey protein (see Table A3 for estimates and significances).

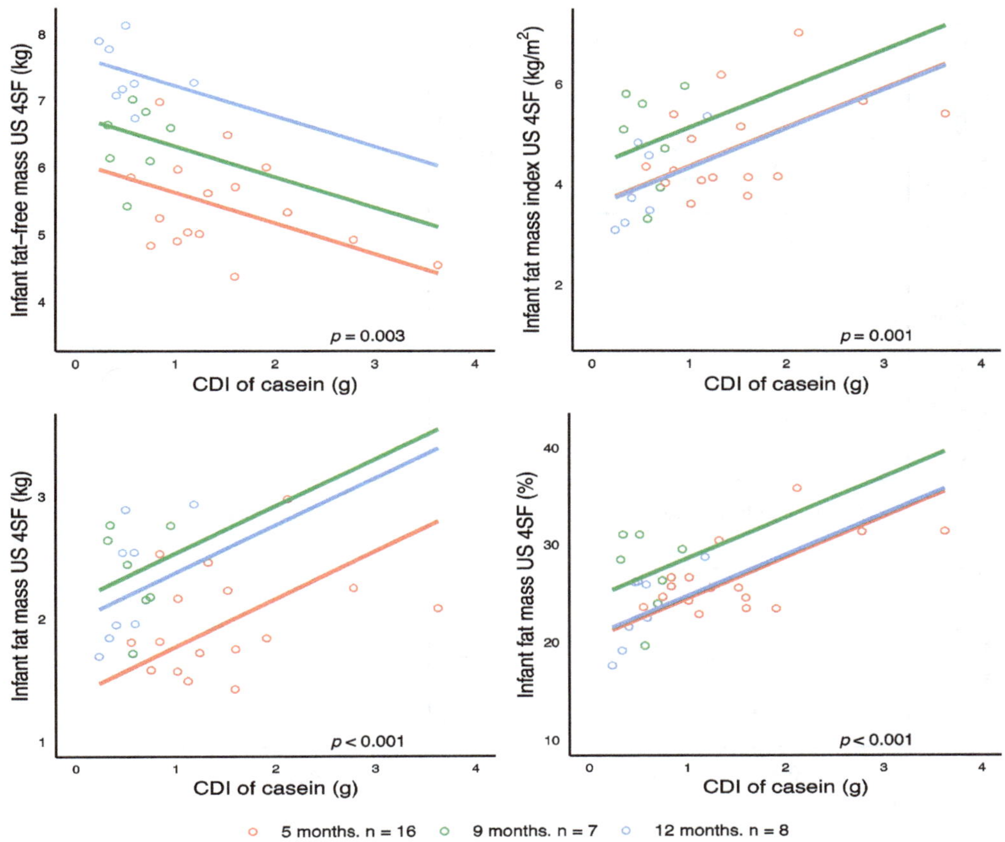

Figure 2. Significant associations between calculated daily intakes (CDI) of human milk casein and infant body composition parameters measured with ultrasound four-skinfolds. Lines represent linear regression and grouped by the month of lactation.

3.6. Breastfeeding Parameters and Human Milk Proteins

No significant associations were seen between concentrations of proteins and 24-h MI, 24-h MP FFQ, and SR FFQ after adjusting for the false discovery rate (see Table A4 for estimates and significances).

Higher FFQ (both, SR and 24-h MP) were associated with higher CDI of all, casein, whey and total protein (Figure 3) after adjusting for the false discovery rate (see Table A4 for estimates and significances).

3.7. Changes in Infant Characteristics and Calculated Daily Intakes of Human Milk Proteins

After adjusting for the false discovery rate, no significant associations were seen at any time points between changes in infant BC (Δ) between the time points and CDI of either total protein, casein or whey protein (see Tables A5–A7 for estimates and significances).

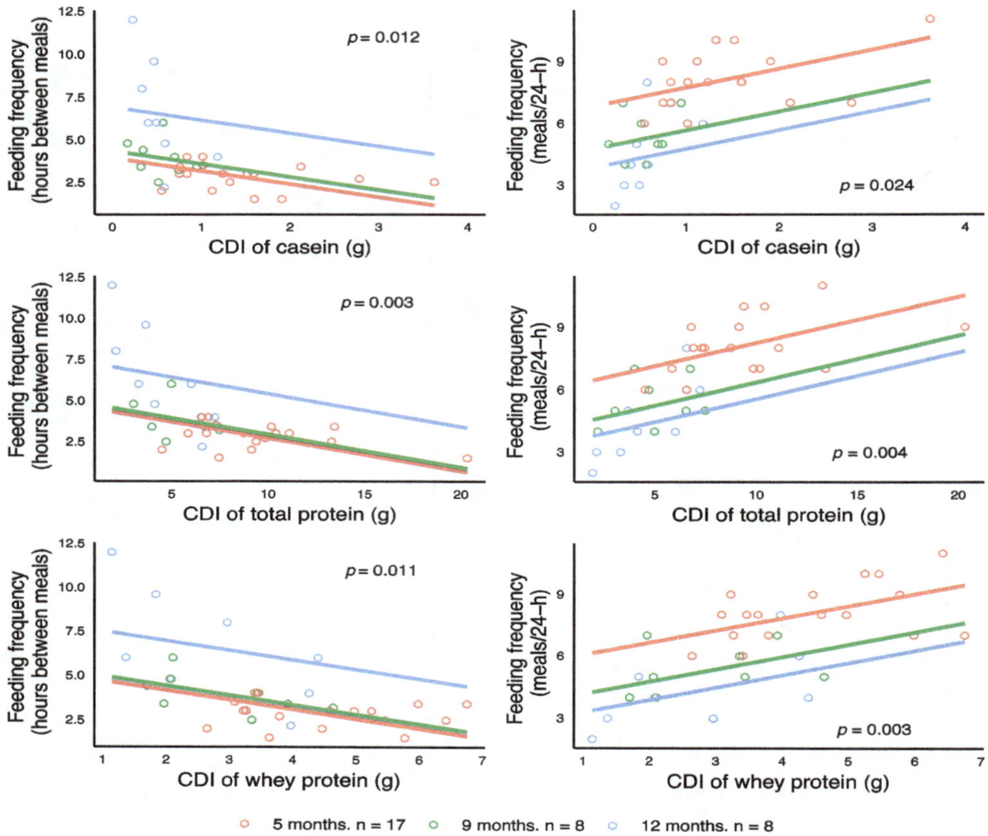

Figure 3. Significant associations between infant feeding frequency (self-reported feeding frequency (hours between meals) or 24-h milk production feeding frequency (meals per 24-h)) and calculated daily intakes (CDI) of casein and total and whey protein. Lines represent linear regression and grouped by the month of lactation.

4. Discussion

A dose–response relationship between breastfeeding duration and childhood obesity has been previously confirmed [43] and this longitudinal study provides more knowledge on the complex mechanisms by which breastfeeding and HM may influence infant BC and confer some degree of protection from obesity. In this small proof-of-concept study, calculated daily intakes of HM casein have been associated with the development of infant BC and are differentially related to infant FM and FFM (Figure 4). Furthermore, infant FFQ was associated with higher CDI of casein, whey and total protein, emphasizing the critical role of HM and breastfeeding in programming of infant appetite control and growth in the first year of life.

Within the normal developmental context of breastfeeding we found that concentrations of total protein (approximately 11 g/L) were not associated with infant anthropometrics or BC during first 12 months of lactation (Section 3.4; Table A2). However, in formula-fed infants high protein formulas (15–19 g/L) are related to accelerated growth trajectory with greater weight gain [15], while breastfed infants display reduced lean body mass and increased adiposity during the early infancy compared to formula-fed [18]. Also in contrast to our results, higher HM protein concentrations at four to eight weeks postpartum were related to higher infant BMI at 12 months but not weight gain or BC [44]. These contrasting results are likely due to the differences in protein composition of formulas and shorter breastfeeding durations. Our study focused on women who breastfed for 12 months and therefore is more reflective of normative development of BC of the breastfed infant.

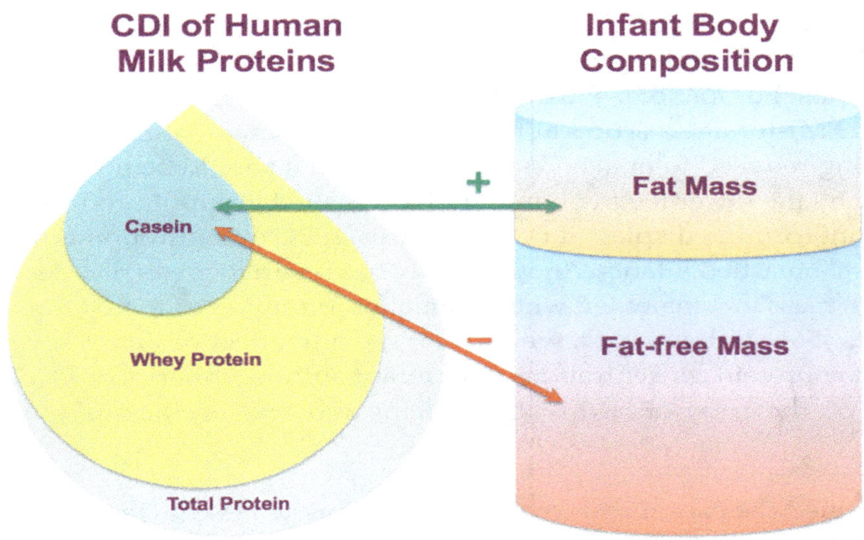

Figure 4. Possible lactocrine programming of the infant body composition during the first year of life as researched. Green arrow indicates positive associations of calculated daily intakes (CDI) of casein with measured body composition parameters and red arrow—negative associations.

To account for variation in infant MI we calculated the CDI of total protein and found no association with infant anthropometrics or BC during first 12 months of lactation (Section 3.5; Table A3). Whilst volume of HM is known to be related to infant growth rate [29,45,46], it has been shown that infants consuming higher daily intakes of protein at various times during first 12 months have higher weight and FFM [8,47,48]. These studies however included formula-fed infants and concentrated on differences between breastfeeding and formula feeding by calculating combined protein intakes from HM/formula and solids. Our study showed multiple positive associations between CDI of total protein between two and five months and changes in infant BC, but statistical significance did not remain after correction for multiple comparisons (Table A5). One recent study measured protein intakes from HM during the first three months in two groups of breastfed infants, with higher and lower weight gain [10] and found protein intakes were not different between the groups. It therefore remains to be elucidated if total protein intake in breastfed infants does impact BC development and larger longitudinal trials are required to do this.

Notwithstanding the absence of infant dietary data, we found that higher CDI of HM casein are associated with both lower infant lean body mass and higher adiposity (Section 3.5; Table A3), with associations strengthening at the later months of lactation. Casein is present in HM at a very low concentrations, compared with other species [49] and is not only a source of amino acids and trace elements (calcium and phosphorus) for the infant [50] but also breaks down to the bioactive peptides that have an array of functions including antimicrobial, gastrointestinal, immuno-modulating and opioid effects [51]. Indeed, increased CDI of casein was also related to increased FFQ. Previously we have shown that higher FFQ was related to lower FFM and higher 24-h MI and adiposity [22]. Furthermore, we have also found higher casein-whey ratios of HM are associated with shorter gastric emptying time in a cross-sectional cohort of exclusively breastfed infants [52]. Casein-whey ratios also interacted with feed volumes, with higher casein-whey ratios associating with faster gastric emptying of smaller feed volumes and slower gastric emptying of larger feed volumes [52]. Thus, HM casein may be modulating the development of infant BC via gastric emptying and breastfeeding frequency that in turn influences infant MI.

CDI of HM whey protein produced similar associations with infant BC to CDI of casein; negative with lean mass and positive with adiposity (Table A3) however, correction for multiple comparisons eliminated significance. We have found previously that higher HM whey protein concentrations are associated with larger post-feed stomach volumes in exclusively breastfed infants [52], and may therefore have an effect on infant BC, in combination with casein, via modulation of breastfeeding patterns. Studies in animal models indicate that whey from bovine milk may promote the growth of the soft (and adipose) tissue [53]. Furthermore, infants fed whey-dominant formula had higher weight-for-age and BMI-for-age z-scores at four months compared with breastfed infants despite the protein content being reduced to match HM [54], although it should be noted that these differences could be explained by the lower feed volumes in the breastfed group. In contrast infants fed a whey- and casein-dominant formula displayed no differences in BC or anthropometrics at four months of age [55], compared to breastfed infants. Another study has reported greater fat deposition in males and greater gains in lean mass in females fed whey-dominant formula during first three months compared to breastfed infants [56]. In this study, we did not see any effect of infant sex on relationships of either casein or whey protein concentrations with infant anthropometrics or BC. Larger longitudinal studies that focus on the array of HM whey proteins and sex-specific analysis may resolve these conflicting results.

We have examined the casein and total whey proteins of HM however, the HM whey fraction contains proteins that remain soluble in the liquid portion after precipitation of caseins—such as α-lactalbumin, lactoferrin, lysozyme, and secretory IgA [57]—as well as various hormones, enzymes, and binding proteins [49]. Many of these proteins have not been studied in relation to infant growth and BC and may either act synergistically or in an antagonistic manner. Administered bovine and HM lysozyme [58,59] have been linked to increased weight gain in preterm infants. Furthermore, high levels of lactoferrin in bovine formula was associated with lower weight gain rate in healthy term female infants during first two months after birth compared with control [60]. Interestingly, α-lactalbumin-enriched formula did not result in any differences in weight gain, weight-for-age and weight-for-length z-scores compared with breastfed infants or infants fed standard formula at four months of age [61]. This suggests that α-lactalbumin, a rich source of essential amino acids, may play optimal nutritive but not necessarily programming role in infant growth. It is yet to be determined whether the proportions of the most abundant whey proteins impact growth and BC development, in particular lysozyme, which may act via promotion of the colonization of infant gut by the infant-type human-residential bifidobacteria [62] and via change in gut microbiome composition through both, detrimental microbe reduction and beneficial microbe enrichment as shown in porcine model [63].

The number of studies showing associations between maternal characteristics and HM components is increasing. We found that higher whey protein concentrations are related to higher maternal weight, BMI, and both fat and lean body mass throughout the first 12 months of lactation (Section 3.3, Table A1). This represents a potential pathway by which the protein composition of HM may be altered and potentially improved via optimal maternal BC which may impact infant development. The absence of an association with HM casein concentration suggests it is not modifiable, and reflects the intrinsic synthesis of casein in the breast [64] as opposed to movement of whey components from the maternal circulation into the milk [65]. Whilst we did not find any associations between maternal characteristics and total protein concentrations, total protein has previously been positively related to maternal %FM [23] and BMI [66–69]. Other studies have shown no associations [70] or a negative association [71]. Larger longitudinal studies would help to clarify these associations.

Breastfeeding frequency is likely a reflection of appetite regulation of the infant [72] and is highly variable between breastfeeding dyads [27]. Recently we have shown increased FFQ was associated with increased 24-h MI, and both of these breastfeeding parameters were related to higher infant adiposity [22]. Both methods that we used to measure infant FFQ have some limitations, especially self-reported FFQ which has been shown to be biased towards reporting higher numbers of feeds in infants that feed more frequently in comparison with 24-h MP FFQ [22], which is again limited to one measure at the time point of data collection. Nevertheless, positive relationships between FFQ (which were also associated with higher FM accretion) and CDI of HM proteins casein in particular (Section 3.6; Table A4) help us to assemble the possible pathways of the mechanisms of infant BC regulation. These results emphasize the importance of including these measures in order to elucidate the mechanisms by which HM components affect infant growth and BC and the degree by which the mother influences HM composition and volumes.

Daily intakes may be a more relevant factor than concentrations of HM components for examining the nutritional physiology of the breastfed infant. In this study, daily intakes were calculated and are considered representative of a typical daily intake due to the absence of significant within-feed [23], short-term (weekly) [28], and circadian [29] variations in HM protein concentrations, including casein and whey [30], during the established lactation. Furthermore, measurement of 24-h milk intake by test-weighing is an accurate [73] and reproducible procedure from within two to four days to within one to two weeks between measurements [45,74–76]. Although no dietary data was collected in this study, the evidence is emerging that protein from dairy/milk sources may have different and/or more potent effects on infant growth and adiposity than the vegetable and meat proteins probably due to the bioactive factors present in milks [77,78]. The major source of milk protein in this study was HM, as no formula was used by mothers. Furthermore, differences in protein intake between breastfed and formula-fed infants during first 12 months are mainly attributed to a lower intake of protein from HM, not to a difference in protein intake from solid foods [48].

The strength of this proof-of-concept study is that infants were breastfed on demand up to 12 months and the broad range of adiposity levels among the mothers. The limitations are the small number of participants, the small number of 24-h MP at 9 and 12 months and the absence of infant dietary data between 5 and 12 months of age. Our population was term healthy fully-breastfed singletons from predominantly Caucasian mothers of higher social-economic status therefore, our results may not be applicable to dyads from other backgrounds.

5. Conclusions

The results of this small proof-of-concept study provide more evidence that HM impacts infant developmental programming and show differential associations between HM casein intakes and development of infant fat and fat-free mass during the first 12 months of life. Thus, the continuation of breastfeeding past the exclusive breastfeeding period may facilitate developmental programming that could potentially reduce risk of obesity and NCD later in life.

Author Contributions: All authors critically reviewed and approved the final manuscript. Conceptualization, Z.G., L.C.W., K.M., P.E.H., and D.T.G.; Data curation, Z.G.; Formal analysis, Z.G., A.R., and K.M.; Funding acquisition, D.T.G.; Investigation, Z.G., W.J.T., C.T.L., and D.T.G.; Methodology, C.T.L. and D.T.G.; Resources, D.T.G.; Supervision, C.T.L., L.C.W., K.M., P.E.H., and D.T.G.; Visualization, Z.G., A.R., and K.M.; Writing—Original draft, Z.G., A.R., and D.T.G.; Writing—Review & editing, W.J.T., C.T.L., L.C.W., K.M., and P.E.H.

Acknowledgments: Authors wish to thank Anna R. Hepworth for consultation on research design and assistance with data analyses. Many thanks are extended to all mothers and infants who participated in this study.

Appendix A

Table A1. Associations between maternal characteristics and human milk proteins.

	2 Months		5 Months		9 Months		12 Months		p-Value		
Maternal Predictor	Intercept (SE)	Slope (SE)	Intercept (SE)	Slope (SE)	Intercept (SE)	Slope (SE)	Intercept (SE)	Slope (SE)	Predictor	Infant Age (Months)	Interaction
	$n = 14$		$n = 20$		$n = 18$		$n = 15$			$n = 20$	
Concentration of Whey Protein (g/L)											
Weight (kg)	4.58 (0.96) [a]	0.027 (0.013)	3.58 (0.91)	0.027 (0.013)	4.27 (0.90)	0.027 (0.013)	4.82 (0.89)	0.027 (0.013)	**0.031** [b]	0.003	0.26 [c]
BMI [d] (kg/m^2)	4.05 (1.09)	0.098 (0.041)	3.06 (1.04)	0.098 (0.041)	3.76 (1.03)	0.098 (0.041)	4.32 (1.01)	0.098 (0.041)	**0.017**	0.002	0.25
FFM [d] (kg)	3.55 (1.44)	0.064 (0.030)	2.56 (1.39)	0.064 (0.030)	3.23 (1.39)	0.064 (0.030)	3.74 (1.40)	0.064 (0.030)	**0.034**	0.004	0.39
FFMI [d] (kg)	2.97 (1.71)	0.216 (0.102)	1.98 (1.66)	0.216 (0.102)	2.64 (1.66)	0.216 (0.102)	3.16 (1.66)	0.216 (0.102)	**0.033**	0.004	0.43
FM [d] (kg/m^2)	5.53 (0.60)	0.040 (0.020)	4.51 (0.55)	0.040 (0.020)	5.21 (0.54)	0.040 (0.020)	5.79 (0.53)	0.040 (0.020)	0.048	0.002	0.24
FMI [d] (kg/m^2)	5.32 (0.64)	0.138 (0.063)	4.31 (0.59)	0.138 (0.063)	5.02 (0.58)	0.138 (0.063)	5.61 (0.56)	0.138 (0.063)	**0.028**	0.002	0.25
	n/a [e]		$n = 17$		$n = 7$		$n = 8$			$n = 18$	
CDI of Total Protein (g)											
FM (%)	n/a [e]	n/a [e]	12.40 (4.28)	−0.090 (0.128)	5.30 (4.54)	0.019 (0.145)	−3.27 (4.47)	0.325 (0.153)	0.59	<0.001	0.046
CDI of Whey Protein (g)											
FFM (kg)	n/a	n/a	5.45 (2.24)	−0.002 (0.050)	−0.90 (2.54)	0.091 (0.057)	9.37 (4.76)	−0.155 (0.152)	0.82	<0.001	0.030

[a] Parameter estimate ± SE; effects of predictors taken from linear mixed effects models that accounted for month after birth and an interaction between month after birth and predictor with a random effect per participant; if the interaction is not significant parameter estimates are taken from a model with no interaction. [b,c] Results are presented only for interactions or predictors with raw p-values < 0.05; after the false discovery rate adjustment, the interaction/predictor p-values were considered to be significant at <0.048 for concentration of whey protein (indicated by the bold text), at <0.05 for concentrations of total protein and casein, casein-whey ratio and CDI of casein (none are significant, data not shown), at <0.046 for CDI of total protein and at <0.030 for CDI of whey protein (none are significant). [d] BMI, body mass index; FFM, fat-free mass; FFMI, fat-free mass index; FM, fat mass; FMI, fat mass index. [e] CDI were measured between 2 and 5 months (presented at 5 months here) and within 2 weeks of 9 and 12 months; n/a, not applicable.

Table A2. Associations between concentrations of human milk proteins and infant characteristics.

	2 Months		5 Months		9 Months		12 Months		*p*-Value		
Predictor (Concentration, g/L)	Intercept (SE)	Slope (SE)	Intercept (SE)	Slope (SE)	Intercept (SE)	Slope (SE)	Intercept (SE)	Slope (SE)	Predictor	Infant Age (Months)	Interaction
	$n = 13$		$n = 20$		$n = 18$		$n = 13$			$n = 20$	
Infant Fat-Free Mass Index with Bioelectrical Impedance Spectroscopy (kg/m^2)											
Total protein	4.67 (0.29) [a]	−0.034 (0.022)	5.66 (0.30)	−0.034 (0.022)	6.82 (0.28)	−0.034 (0.022)	7.48 (0.28)	−0.034 (0.022)	0.032 [b]	0.070	0.55 [c]
	$n = 13$		$n = 19$		$n = 18$		$n = 15$			$n = 20$	
Infant Fat Mass with Ultrasound 4 Skinfolds (%)											
Casein-whey ratio	23.70 (1.36)	9.09 (4.62)	23.40 (1.70)	9.09 (4.62)	24.00 (1.28)	9.09 (4.62)	21.90 (1.33)	9.09 (4.62)	0.046	0.21	0.23

[a] Parameter estimate ± SE; effects of predictors taken from linear mixed effects models that accounted for month after birth and an interaction between month after birth and predictor with a random effect per participant; if the interaction is not significant parameter estimates are taken from a model with no interaction. [b,c] Results are presented only for interactions or predictors with raw p-values < 0.05; after the false discovery rate adjustment, the interaction/predictor p-values were considered to be significant at <0.032 for total protein concentration (none are significant), at <0.046 for casein-whey ratio (none are significant), and at <0.05 for casein and whey protein concentrations (none are significant, data not shown).

Table A3. Associations between calculated daily intakes of casein and whey protein and infant characteristics.

Predictor (CDI [d], g)	5 Months		9 Months		12 Months		*p*-Value		
	Intercept (SE)	Slope (SE)	Intercept (SE)	Slope (SE)	Intercept (SE)	Slope (SE)	Predictor	Infant Age (months)	Interaction
	$n = 17$		$n = 7$		$n = 8$			$n = 18$	
Infant Fat Mass with Ultrasound 2 Skinfolds (kg)									
Whey protein	1.31 (0.30) [a]	0.148 (0.062)	1.98 (0.23)	0.148 (0.062)	2.03 (0.24)	0.148 (0.062)	0.024 [b]	<0.001	0.56 [c]
Infant fat mass with ultrasound 2 skinfolds (%)									
Whey protein1	20.60 (2.65)	1.330 (0.554)	22.90 (2.12)	1.330 (0.554)	21.60 (2.03)	1.330 (0.554)	0.033	0.62	0.53
	$n = 17$		$n = 7$		$n = 7$			$n = 18$	
Infant Head Circumference (cm)									
Casein	43.10 (0.45)	−0.243 (0.194)	44.70 (0.55)	1.330 (0.680)	46.80 (0.46)	−0.334 (0.490)	0.23	<0.001	0.046
Infant Body Mass Index (kg/m^2)									
Casein	16.70 (0.65)	0.676 (0.358)	18.30 (0.98)	−0.788 (1.430)	18.80 (0.74)	−2.10 (1.040)	0.33	0.59	0.047
Infant Fat-Free Mass Index with Bioelectrical Impedance Spectroscopy (kg/m^2)									
Whey protein	14.10 (0.61)	−0.319 (0.121)	14.70 (0.48)	−0.319 (0.121)	14.30 (0.50)	−0.319 (0.121)	0.004	0.075	0.20
Infant Fat Mass Index with Ultrasound 2 Skinfolds (kg/m^2)									
Casein	3.99 (0.42)	0.517 (0.248)	4.55 (0.36)	0.517 (0.248)	4.15 (0.35)	0.517 (0.248)	0.048	0.32	0.77
Whey protein	3.22 (0.65)	0.336 (0.135)	3.88 (0.51)	0.336 (0.135)	3.42 (0.52)	0.336 (0.135)	0.016	0.20	0.73
	$n = 16$		$n = 7$		$n = 8$			$n = 18$	
Infant Fat-Free Mass with Ultrasound 4 Skinfolds (kg)									
Casein	6.08 (0.26)	−0.456 (0.144)	6.77 (0.21)	−0.456 (0.144)	7.68 (0.21)	−0.456 (0.144)	**0.003**	<0.001	0.79

Table A3. *Cont.*

Predictor (CDI [d], g)	5 Months		9 Months		12 Months		*p*-Value		
	Intercept (SE)	Slope (SE)	Intercept (SE)	Slope (SE)	Intercept (SE)	Slope (SE)	Predictor	Infant Age (months)	Interaction
Infant Fat Mass with Ultrasound 4 Skinfolds (kg)									
Casein	1.38 (0.18)	0.390 (0.100)	2.14 (0.15)	0.390 (0.100)	1.99 (0.14)	0.390 (0.100)	**<0.001**	<0.001	0.28
Infant Fat Mass with Ultrasound 4 Skinfolds (%)									
Casein	20.30 (1.62)	4.220 (0.932)	24.40 (1.31)	4.220 (0.932)	20.60 (1.26)	4.220 (0.932)	**<0.001**	0.002	0.31
Whey protein	21.30 (2.65)	1.190 (0.565)	23.60 (2.18)	1.190 (0.565)	20.10 (2.05)	1.190 (0.565)	0.038	0.16	0.62
	n = 16		*n* = 7		*n* = 7		*n* = 18		
Infant Fat-Free Mass Index with Ultrasound 4 Skinfolds (kg/m²)									
Casein	13.70 (0.43)	−0.484 (0.235)	13.20 (0.61)	−0.119 (0.901)	14.90 (0.47)	−2.28 (0.662)	0.001	0.021	0.022
Infant Fat Mass Index with Ultrasound 4 Skinfolds (kg/m²)									
Casein	3.57 (0.42)	0.789 (0.240)	4.35 (0.34)	0.789 (0.240)	3.55 (0.34)	0.789 (0.240)	**0.001**	0.013	0.55
Whey protein	3.39 (0.67)	0.309 (0.143)	3.94 (0.55)	0.309 (0.143)	3.07 (0.55)	0.309 (0.143)	0.034	0.12	0.74

[a] Parameter estimate ± SE; effects of predictors taken from linear mixed effects models that accounted for month after birth and an interaction between month after birth and predictor with a random effect for participant; if the interaction is not significant parameter estimates are taken from a model with no interaction. [b,c] Results are presented only for interactions or predictors with raw *p*-values < 0.05; after the false discovery rate adjustment interaction/predictor *p*-values were considered to be significant at <0.022 for calculated daily intakes (CDI) of casein (indicated by the bold text), at <0.004 for CDI of whey protein (none are significant) and at <0.05 for CDI of total protein (none are significant, data not shown). [d] CDI were measured between 2 and 5 months and within 2 weeks of 9 and 12 months.

Table A4. Associations between feeding frequency and human milk proteins.

Predictor (Concentration of Proteins or Breastfeeding Parameter)	2 Months		5 Months		9 Months		12 Months		*p*-Value		
	Intercept (SE)	Slope (SE)	Intercept (SE)	Slope (SE)	Intercept (SE)	Slope (SE)	Intercept (SE)	Slope (SE)	Predictor	Infant Age (Months)	Interaction
	n = 11		*n* = 19		*n* = 17		*n* = 11		*n* = 19		
Infant Feeding Frequency (Self-Reported as Hours between Feeds) [e]											
Total protein (g/L)	3.97 (0.94) [a]	−0.158 (0.078)	4.56 (0.95)	−0.158 (0.078)	5.29 (0.87)	−0.158 (0.078)	7.16 (0.94)	−0.158 (0.078)	0.039 [b]	<0.001	0.30 [c]
	n/a [d]		*n* = 17		*n* = 8		*n* = 8		*n* = 18		
CDI of Total Protein (g)											
Feeding frequency (24-h MP) [d]	n/a [d]	n/a [d]	2.15 (2.68)	0.317 (0.004)	0.87 (1.92)	0.317 (0.004)	1.34 (1.69)	0.317 (0.004)	**0.004**	0.41	0.22
Feeding frequency (SR) [e]	n/a	n/a	11.10 (0.97)	0.19 (0.002)	7.93 (1.17)	0.19 (0.002)	9.15 (1.51)	0.19 (0.002)	**0.003**	<0.001	0.90

Table A4. *Cont.*

Predictor (Concentration of Proteins or Breastfeeding Parameter)	2 Months		5 Months		9 Months			12 Months	*p*-Value		
	Intercept (SE)	Slope (SE)	Intercept (SE)	Slope (SE)	Intercept (SE)	Slope (SE)	Intercept (SE)	Slope (SE)	Predictor	Infant Age (Months)	Interaction
CDI of Casein (g) [d]											
Feeding frequency (24-h MP)	n/a	n/a	0.01 (0.62)	0.074 (0.017)	−0.34 (0.44)	0.074 (0.017)	−0.18 (0.02)	0.074 (0.017)	**0.024**	0.36	0.54
Feeding frequency (SR)	n/a	n/a	1.81 (0.22)	0.054 (0.014)	1.19 (0.29)	0.054 (0.014)	1.54 (0.40)	0.054 (0.014)	**0.012**	0.005	0.57
CDI of Whey Protein (g) [d]											
Feeding frequency (24-h MP)	n/a	n/a	1.39 (1.10)	0.131 (0.003)	0.95 (0.78)	0.131 (0.003)	1.30 (0.68)	0.131 (0.003)	**0.003**	0.36	0.084
Feeding frequency (SR)	n/a	n/a	5.16 (0.39)	0.095 (0.017)	3.88 (0.52)	0.095 (0.017)	4.50 (0.71)	0.095 (0.017)	**0.011**	<0.001	0.25

[a] Parameter estimate ± SE; effects of predictors taken from linear mixed effects models that accounted for month after birth and an interaction between month after birth and predictor with a random effect for participant; if the interaction is not significant parameter estimates are taken from a model with no interaction. [b,c] Results are presented only for interactions or predictors with raw *p*-values < 0.05; after the false discovery rate adjustment interaction/predictor *p*-values were considered to be significant at <0.039 for self-reported feeding frequency and concentrations of the proteins, at <0.05 for 24-h milk production (MP) feeding frequency and concentrations of the proteins (none are significant, data not shown), at <0.05 for calculated daily intakes (CDI) of total protein, casein and whey protein and both FFQ (indicated by the bold text). [d] CDI, 24-h milk intake and 24-h milk production (24-h MP) feeding frequency were measured between 2 and 5 months (presented at 5 months here) and within 2 weeks of 9 and 12 months; n/a–not applicable. [e] Feeding frequency was self-reported (SR) by mothers at the time of the visit as an average time between meals (e.g., each 2 h).

Table A5. Associations between calculated daily intakes of human milk total protein at given time points and changes in infant body composition between the time points.

Changes in Infant Characteristics between Time Points	Months after Birth					
	5 and 2 Months	9 and 2 Months	12 and 2 Months	9 and 5 Months	12 and 5 Months	12 and 9 Months
CDI of Total Protein (g) between 2 and 5 Months (n = 17) [e]						
ΔHead circumference (cm)	−0.14 (0.14) [a] 0.35 [b,c]	0.03 (0.17) 0.88	0.14 (0.16) 0.43	−0.04 (0.05) 0.44	0.03 (0.03) 0.33	**0.09 (0.04)** **0.046**
ΔLength (cm)	−0.08 (0.17) 0.62	**0.40 (0.15)** **0.025**	**0.57 (0.17)** **0.011**	−0.01 (0.11) 0.91	0.15 (0.13) 0.29	0.21 (0.12) 0.12
ΔWeight (kg)	0.09 (0.05) 0.11	**0.18 (0.07)** **0.030**	0.17 (0.09) 0.096	0.03 (0.03) 0.36	0.03 (0.04) 0.42	0.01 (0.01) 0.50
ΔBMI [d] (kg/m^2)	**0.29 (0.09)** **0.013**	0.13 (0.16) 0.42	0.06 (0.21) 0.79	0.03 (0.08) 0.67	−0.05 (0.10) 0.62	−0.09 (0.05) 0.13
ΔFat-free mass US 4SF [d] (kg)	0.04 (0.07) 0.55	**0.19 (0.07)** **0.037**	0.18 (0.12) 0.19	0.004 (0.03) 0.89	0.03 (0.04) 0.46	0.03 (0.02) 0.13
ΔFat-free mass BIS [d] (kg)	0.05 (0.03) 0.13	0.13 (0.09) 0.15	**0.18 (0.07)** **0.041**	0.02 (0.03) 0.60	0.08 (0.04) 0.065	**0.08 (0.03)** **0.041**

Table A5. *Cont.*

Changes in Infant Characteristics between Time Points	Months after Birth					
	5 and 2 Months	9 and 2 Months	12 and 2 Months	9 and 5 Months	12 and 5 Months	12 and 9 Months
ΔFat-free mass index US 4SF (kg/m^2)	**0.27 (0.09)** **0.023**	0.18 (0.14) 0.25	0.39 (0.22) 0.12	0.01 (0.05) 0.86	−0.02 (0.07) 0.81	−0.02 (0.06) 0.71
ΔFat-free mass index BIS (kg/m^2)	**0.14 (0.06)** **0.042**	0.11 (0.15) 0.46	0.11 (0.15) 0.49	0.04 (0.06) 0.51	0.04 (0.07) 0.59	0.03 (0.06) 0.59
ΔFat mass US 2SF (kg/m^2)	**0.13 (0.06)** **0.049**	0.07 (0.05) 0.22	0.12 (0.08) 0.16	0.03 (0.03) 0.43	0.004 (0.03) 0.91	−0.02 (0.01) 0.25
ΔFat mass index US 2SF (kg/m^2)	0.26 (0.13) 0.081	0.07 (0.12) 0.58	0.09 (0.19) 0.64	0.04 (0.08) 0.58	−0.03 (0.08) 0.70	**−0.07 (0.03)** **0.029**
ΔFat mass index BIS (kg/m^2)	**0.17 (0.07)** **0.044**	0.04 (0.15) 0.82	−0.03 (0.14) 0.84	−0.003 (0.07) 0.97	−0.13 (0.08) 0.12	−0.14 (0.07) 0.075
CDI of Total Protein (g) at 9 Months (n = 8) [e]						
ΔHead circumference (cm)	n/a [f]	−0.54 (0.22) 0.14	0.04 (0.33) 0.91	0.13 (0.09) 0.21	−0.17 (0.10) 0.14	**−0.30 (0.09)** **0.021**
ΔFat-free mass index BIS (kg/m^2)	n/a	**−0.36 (0.02)** **0.004**	0.07 (0.43) 0.89	−0.20 (0.12) 0.14	−0.12 (0.16) 0.47	0.08 (0.20) 0.70
CDI of Total Protein (g) at 12 Months (n = 8) [e]						
ΔBMI [d] (kg/m^2)	n/a [f]	n/a [f]	0.08 (0.32) 0.84	n/a [f]	−0.24 (0.25) 0.40	**−0.30 (0.09)** **0.021**
ΔFat-free mass index US 2SF (kg/m^2)	n/a	n/a	−0.32 (0.30) 0.39	n/a	**−0.48 (0.18)** **0.045**	−0.20 (0.12) 0.17
ΔFat-free mass index US 4SF (kg/m^2)	n/a	n/a	−0.30 (0.38) 0.51	n/a	**−0.50 (0.09)** **0.006**	−0.21 (0.17) 0.26
ΔFat mass US 2SF (kg)	n/a	n/a	**0.21 (0.05)** **0.024**	n/a	**0.14 (0.06)** **0.043**	−0.001 (0.04) 0.99
ΔFat mass US 2SF (%)	n/a	n/a	2.66 (0.93) 0.064	n/a	**1.60 (0.59)** **0.036**	−0.17 (0.55) 0.77
ΔFat mass index US 2SF (kg/m^2)	n/a	n/a	**0.38 (0.08)** **0.045**	n/a	0.25 (0.14) 0.13	−0.11 (0.10) 0.33

[a] Parameter estimates ± SE and [b] p-values for associations between calculated daily intakes (CDI) of casein at given time points and the changes (Δ) in measured variables between different months after birth. [c] Results are presented only for variables with at least one significant raw p-value ($p < 0.05$, indicated by the bold text); after the false discovery rate adjustment, the predictor p-values were considered to be significant at <0.011 for CDI of total protein between 2 and 5 months, at <0.004 for CDI at 9 months and at <0.006 for CDI at 12 months (none are significant). [d] BIS—bioelectrical impedance spectroscopy; BMI—body mass index; US 2SF—ultrasound 2-skinfolds; US 4SF—ultrasound 4-skinfolds. [e] CDI were measured between 2 and 5 months and within 2 weeks of 9 and 12 months. [f] Results are not presented for impractical time combinations, n/a–not applicable.

Table A6. Associations between calculated daily intakes of human milk casein at given time points and changes in infant body composition between the time points.

Changes in Infant Characteristic	Months after Birth					
	5 and 2	9 and 2	12 and 2	9 and 5	12 and 5	12 and 9
CDI of Casein (g) between 2 and 5 Months (n = 17) [e]						
ΔHead circumference (cm)	**−1.17 (0.39)** [a] **0.016** [b,c]	−0.79 (0.60) 0.23	−0.68 (0.58) 0.28	0.01 (0.22) 0.97	0.17 (0.15) 0.29	0.23 (0.22) 0.31
ΔFat mass US 4SF (kg)	0.02 (0.10) 0.83	**−0.47 (0.17)** **0.031**	**−0.49 (0.20)** **0.040**	−0.07 (0.15) 0.67	−0.17 (0.13) 0.21	−0.06 (0.07) 0.40
ΔFat mass US 2SF (%)	2.94 (3.17) 0.38	**−3.62 (1.50)** **0.042**	−2.02 (3.41) 0.57	−0.05 (1.76) 0.98	−1.37 (1.66) 0.42	−1.01 (0.68) 0.16
ΔFat mass US 4SF (%)	0.35 (1.53) 0.83	**−6.67 (1.36)** **0.002**	**−6.27 (2.42)** **0.036**	−1.18 (1.60) 0.47	−2.51 (1.31) 0.078	−0.92 (0.79) 0.27
ΔFat mass BIS (%)	0.94 (1.36) 0.51	−4.12 (2.78) 0.18	**−4.48 (1.61)** **0.027**	0.24 (1.51) 0.88	−0.77 (1.63) 0.64	−1.48 (1.73) 0.41
ΔFat mass index US 4SF (kg/m^2)	0.001 (0.27) 1.00	**−1.29 (0.32)** **0.005**	**−1.44 (0.50)** **0.028**	−0.23 (0.36) 0.53	−0.48 (0.33) 0.18	−0.20 (0.15) 0.19
CDI of Casein (g) at 9 Months (n = 8) [e]						
ΔHead circumference (cm)	n/a [f]	3.33 (3.00) 0.38	−1.04 (2.72) 0.74	0.62 (0.79) 0.47	**−1.78 (0.62)** **0.036**	**−2.40 (0.74)** **0.023**
CDI of Casein (g) at 12 Months (n = 8) [e]						
ΔHead circumference (cm)	n/a [f]	n/a [f]	**4.01 (0.60)** **0.022**	n/a [f]	−0.97 (0.55) 0.14	−0.66 (1.11) 0.58
ΔBMI [d] (kg/m^2)	n/a	n/a	−1.36 (3.92) 0.76	n/a	−2.33 (1.57) 0.20	**−2.09 (0.61)** **0.019**
ΔFat−free mass US 4SF [d] (kg)	n/a	n/a	**−3.77 (0.73)** **0.014**	n/a	−1.05 (0.83) 0.26	−0.51 (0.53) 0.38
ΔFat−free mass index US 2SF (kg/m^2)	n/a	n/a	−5.39 (2.60) 0.17	n/a	−2.99 (1.40) 0.086	**−2.13 (0.45)** **0.005**
ΔFat−free mass index US 4SF (kg/m^2)	n/a	n/a	−7.12 (1.69) 0.052	n/a	**−2.84 (0.87)** **0.031**	**−2.40 (0.78)** **0.028**
ΔFat mass US 4SF (%)	n/a	n/a	**33.56 (8.59)** **0.030**	n/a	6.08 (7.30) 0.44	4.85 (4.71) 0.35

[a] Parameter estimates ± SE and [b] p-values for associations between calculated daily intakes (CDI) of whey protein at given time points and the changes (Δ) in measured variables between different months after birth. [c] Results are presented only for variables with at least one significant raw p-value ($p < 0.05$, indicated by the bold text); after the false discovery rate adjustment, the predictor p-values were considered to be significant at <0.002 for CDI of casein between 2 and 5 months, at <0.023 for CDI at 9 months and at <0.005 for CDI at 12 months (none are significant). [d] BIS—bioielctrical impedance spectroscopy; BMI—body mass index; US 2SF—ultrasound 2-skinfolds; US 4SF—ultrasound 4-skinfolds. [e] CDI were measured between 2 and 5 months and within 2 weeks of 9 and 12 months. [f] Results are not presented for impractical time combinations, n/a, not applicable.

Table A7. Associations between calculated daily intakes of total human milk whey protein at given time points and changes in infant body composition between the time points.

Changes in Infant Characteristic	Months after Birth					
	5 and 2	9 and 2	12 and 2	9 and 5	12 and 5	12 and 9
CDI of Whey Protein (g) between 2 and 5 Months (n = 17) [e]						
ΔLength (cm)	−0.24 (0.33) [a] 0.49 [b,c]	0.44 (0.39) 0.29	**1.01 (0.35)** **0.024**	−0.06 (0.31) 0.85	0.17 (0.40) 0.67	0.37 (0.38) 0.35
ΔBMI [d] (kg/m^2)	**0.58 (0.19)** **0.017**	0.31 (0.31) 0.35	−0.02 (0.40) 0.97	−0.02 (0.22) 0.94	−0.23 (0.28) 0.42	−0.21 (0.16) 0.20
ΔFat-free mass index US 4SF (kg/m^2)	**0.65 (0.21)** **0.016**	0.20 (0.35) 0.58	0.12 (0.55) 0.83	0.003 (0.16) 0.99	−0.15 (0.21) 0.50	−0.05 (0.17) 0.77
ΔFat mass US 2SF (kg)	**0.29 (0.12)** **0.032**	0.15 (0.10) 0.18	0.26 (0.15) 0.12	0.01 (0.10) 0.96	−0.01 (0.10) 0.89	0.01 (0.04) 0.89
ΔFat mass index US 2SF (kg/m^2)	**0.61 (0.25)** **0.042**	0.21 (0.23) 0.38	0.25 (0.36) 0.51	−0.03 (0.22) 0.88	−0.15 (0.24) 0.54	−0.09 (0.10) 0.38
CDI of Whey Protein (g) at 12 Months (n = 8) [e]						
ΔFat-free mass index US 4SF (kg/m^2)	n/a [f]	n/a [f]	−0.18 (0.57) 0.78	n/a [f]	**−0.62 (0.22)** **0.049**	−0.10 (0.31) 0.76
ΔFat mass US 2SF (kg)	n/a	n/a	**0.26 (0.06)** **0.025**	n/a	0.13 (0.11) 0.27	−0.01 (0.06) 0.92

[a] Parameter estimates ± SE and [b] p-values for associations between calculated daily intakes (CDI) of total protein at given time points and the changes (Δ) in measured variables between different months after birth. [c] Results are presented only for variables with at least one significant raw p-value ($p < 0.05$, indicated by the bold text); after the false discovery rate adjustment, the predictor p-values were considered to be significant at < 0.016 for CDI of casein between 2 and 5 months, at < 0.05 for CDI at 9 months and at <0.025 for CDI at 12 months (none are significant). [d] BIS—bioielectrical impedance spectroscopy; BMI—body mass index; US 2SF—ultrasound 2-skinfolds; US 4SF—ultrasound 4-skinfolds. [e] CDI were measured between 2 and 5 and within 2 weeks of 9 (none are significant, data not shown) and 12 months. [f] Results are not presented for impractical time combinations, n/a–not applicable.

References

1. Wells, J.C.K.; Shirley, M.K. Body composition and the monitoring of non-communicable chronic disease risk. *Glob. Health Epidemiol. Genom.* **2016**, *1*, e18. [CrossRef] [PubMed]
2. Koletzko, B.; Brands, B.; Chourdakis, M.; Cramer, S.; Grote, V.; Hellmuth, C.; Kirchberg, F.; Prell, C.; Rzehak, P.; Uhl, O.; et al. The power of programming and the EarlyNutrition project: Opportunities for health promotion by nutrition during the first thousand days of life and beyond. *Ann. Nutr. Metab.* **2014**, *64*, 187–196. [CrossRef] [PubMed]
3. Ratnasingham, A.; Eiby, Y.; Dekker Nitert, M.; Donovan, T.; Lingwood, B.E. Review: Is rapid fat accumulation in early life associated with adverse later health outcomes? *Placenta* **2017**, *54*, 125–130. [CrossRef] [PubMed]
4. Weng, S.F.; Redsell, S.A.; Swift, J.A.; Yang, M.; Glazebrook, C.P. Systematic review and meta-analyses of risk factors for childhood overweight identifiable during infancy. *Arch. Dis. Child.* **2012**, *97*, 1019–1026. [CrossRef] [PubMed]
5. Koletzko, B.; von Kries, R.; Monasterolo, R.C.; Subias, J.E.; Scaglioni, S.; Giovannini, M.; Beyer, J.; Demmelmair, H.; Gruszfeld, D. Infant feeding and later obesity risk. *Adv. Exp. Med. Biol.* **2009**, *646*, 15–29. [PubMed]
6. Thompson, A.L. Developmental origins of obesity: Early feeding environments, infant growth, and the intestinal microbiome. *Am. J. Hum. Biol.* **2012**, *24*, 350–360. [CrossRef] [PubMed]
7. Wells, J.C.; Chomoto, S.; Fewtrell, M.S. Programming of body composition by early growth and nutrition. *Proc. Nutr. Soc.* **2007**, *66*, 423–434. [CrossRef] [PubMed]
8. Butte, N.; Wong, W.; Hopkinson, J.; Smith, E.; Ellis, K. Infant feeding mode affects early growth and body composition. *Pediatrics* **2000**, *16*, 1355–1366. [CrossRef]
9. Luque, V.; Closa-Monasterolo, R.; Escribano, J.; Ferre, N. Early programming by protein intake: The effect of protein on adiposity development and the growth and functionality of vital organs. *Nutr. Metab. Insights* **2015**, *8*, 49–56. [CrossRef] [PubMed]
10. Kon, I.Y.; Shilina, N.M.; Gmoshinskaya, M.V.; Ivanushkina, T.A. The study of breast milk IGF-1, leptin, ghrelin and adiponectin levels as possible reasons of high weight gain in breast-fed infants. *Ann. Nutr. Metab.* **2014**, *65*, 317–323. [CrossRef] [PubMed]
11. Sievers, E.; Oldigs, H.D.; Santer, R.; Schaub, J. Feeding patterns in breast-fed and formula-fed infants. *Ann. Nutr. Metab.* **2002**, *46*, 243–248. [CrossRef] [PubMed]
12. Savino, F.; Liguori, S.A.; Fissore, M.F.; Oggero, R. Breast milk hormones and their protective effect on obesity. *Int. J. Pediatr. Endocrinol.* **2009**, *2009*, 327505. [CrossRef] [PubMed]
13. Bartok, C. Babies fed breastmilk by breast versus by bottle: A pilot study evaluating early growth patterns. *Breastfeed. Med.* **2011**, *6*, 117–124. [CrossRef] [PubMed]
14. Druet, C.; Stettler, N.; Sharp, S.; Simmons, R.K.; Cooper, C.; Smith, G.D.; Ekelund, U.; Levy-Marchal, C.; Jarvelin, M.R.; Kuh, D.; et al. Prediction of childhood obesity by infancy weight gain: An individual-level meta-analysis. *Paediatr. Perinat. Epidemiol.* **2011**, *26*, 19–26. [CrossRef] [PubMed]
15. Koletzko, B.; von Kries, R.; Closa, R.; Escribano, J.; Scaglioni, S.; Giovannini, M.; Beyer, J.; Demmelmair, H.; Gruszfeld, D.; Dobrzanska, A.; et al. Lower protein in infant formula is associated with lower weight up to age 2 y: A randomized clinical trial. *Am. J. Clin. Nutr.* **2009**, *89*, 1836–1845. [PubMed]
16. Gidrewicz, D.A.; Fenton, T.R. A systematic review and meta-analysis of the nutrient content of preterm and term breast milk. *BMC Pediatr.* **2014**, *14*, 216. [CrossRef] [PubMed]
17. Rzehak, P.; Oddy, W.H.; Mearin, M.L.; Grote, V.; Mori, T.A.; Szajewska, H.; Shamir, R.; Koletzko, S.; Weber, M.; Beilin, L.J.; et al. Infant feeding and growth trajectory patterns in childhood and body composition in young adulthood. *Am. J. Clin. Nutr.* **2017**, *102*, 568–580. [CrossRef] [PubMed]
18. Gale, C.; Logan, K.; Santhakumaran, S.; Parkinson, J.; Hyde, M.; Modi, N. Effect of breastfeeding compared with formula feeding on infant body composition: A systematic review and meta-analysis. *Am. J. Clin. Nutr.* **2012**, *95*, 656–669. [CrossRef] [PubMed]
19. Khan, S.; Hepworth, A.R.; Prime, D.K.; Lai, C.T.; Trengove, N.J.; Hartmann, P.E. Variation in fat, lactose, and protein composition in breast milk over 24 hours: Associations with infant feeding patterns. *J. Hum. Lact.* **2013**, *29*, 81–89. [CrossRef] [PubMed]
20. Binns, C.W.; Fraser, M.L.; Lee, A.H.; Scott, J. Defining exclusive breastfeeding in Australia. *J. Paediatr. Child Health* **2009**, *45*, 174–180. [CrossRef] [PubMed]

21. Gridneva, Z.; Hepworth, A.; Ward, L.; Lai, C.T.; Hartmann, P.; Geddes, D.T. Bioimpedance spectroscopy in the infant: Effect of milk intake and extracellular fluid reservoirs on resistance measurements in term breastfed infants. *Eur. J. Clin. Nutr.* **2016**, *70*, 843–851. [CrossRef] [PubMed]
22. Gridneva, Z.; Rea, A.; Hepworth, A.R.; Ward, L.C.; Lai, C.T.; Hartmann, P.E.; Geddes, D.T. Relationships between breastfeeding patterns and maternal and infant body composition over the first 12 months of lactation. *Nutrients* **2018**, *10*, 45. [CrossRef] [PubMed]
23. Kugananthan, S.; Gridneva, Z.; Lai, C.T.; Hepworth, A.R.; Mark, P.J.; Kakulas, F.; Geddes, D.T. Associations between maternal body composition and appetite hormones and macronutrients in human milk. *Nutrients* **2017**, *9*, 252. [CrossRef] [PubMed]
24. Gridneva, Z.; Hepworth, A.R.; Ward, L.C.; Lai, C.T.; Hartmann, P.E.; Geddes, D.T. Determinants of body composition in breastfed infants using bioimpedance spectroscopy and ultrasound skinfolds—Methods comparison. *Pediatr. Res.* **2016**, *81*, 423–433. [CrossRef] [PubMed]
25. Van Itallie, T.B.; Yang, M.U.; Heymsfield, S.B.; Funk, R.C.; Boileau, R.A. Height-normalized indices of the body's fat-free mass and fat mass: Potentially useful indicators of nutritional status. *Am. J. Clin. Nutr.* **1990**, *52*, 953–959. [CrossRef] [PubMed]
26. Arthur, P.; Hartmann, P.; Smith, M. Measurement of the milk intake of breast-fed infants. *J. Pediatr. Gastroenterol. Nutr.* **1987**, *6*, 758–763. [CrossRef] [PubMed]
27. Kent, J.C.; Mitoulas, L.R.; Cregan, M.D.; Ramsay, D.T.; Doherty, D.A.; Hartmann, P.E. Volume and frequency of breastfeedings and fat content of breast milk throughout the day. *Pediatrics* **2006**, *117*, e387–e395. [CrossRef] [PubMed]
28. Khan, S.; Prime, D.K.; Hepworth, A.R.; Lai, C.T.; Trengove, N.J.; Hartmann, P.E. Investigation of short-term variations in term breast milk composition during repeated breast expression sessions. *J. Hum. Lact.* **2013**, *29*, 196–204. [CrossRef] [PubMed]
29. Mitoulas, L.R.; Kent, J.C.; Cox, D.B.; Owens, R.A.; Sherriff, J.L.; Hartmann, P.E. Variation in fat, lactose and protein in human milk over 24 h and throughout the first year of lactation. *Br. J. Nutr.* **2002**, *88*, 29–37. [CrossRef] [PubMed]
30. Khan, S.; Casadio, Y.; Lai, C.; Prime, D.; Hepworth, A.; Trengove, N.; Hartmann, P. Investigation of short-term variations in casein and whey proteins in breast milk of term mothers. *Hepatol. Nutr.* **2012**, *55*, 136–141. [CrossRef] [PubMed]
31. Keller, R.; Neville, M. Determination of total protein in human milk: Comparison of methods. *Clin. Chem.* **1986**, *32*, 120–123. [PubMed]
32. Kunz, C.; Lonnerdal, B. Human milk proteins: Separation of whey proteins and their analysis by polyacrylamide gel electrophoresis, fast protein liquid chromatography (FPLC) gel filtration, and anion-exchange chromatography. *Am. J. Clin. Nutr.* **1989**, *49*, 464–470. [CrossRef] [PubMed]
33. Faul, F.; Erdfelder, E.; Buchner, A.; Lang, A.-G. Statistical power analyses using G*power 3.1: Tests for correlation and regression analyses. *Behav. Res. Methods* **2009**, *41*, 1149–1160. [CrossRef] [PubMed]
34. Diggle, P.J.; Heagerty, P.J.; Liang, K.-Y.; Zeger, S.L. *Analysis of Longitudinal Data*; Oxford University Press Inc.: New York, NY, USA, 2002.
35. Curran-Everett, D. Multiple comparisons: Philosophies and illustrations. *Am. J. Physiol. Regul. Integr. Comp. Physiol.* **2000**, *279*, R1–R8. [CrossRef] [PubMed]
36. R Core Team. *R: A Language and Environment for Statistical Computing*; R Foundation for Statistical Computing: Vienna, Austria, 2017.
37. Pinheiro, J.B.; Bates, D.; DebRoy, S.; Sarkar, D.; R Core Team. *nlme: Linear and Nonlinear Mixed Effects Models*; R Package Version 3.1-131; R Foundation for Statistical Computing: Vienna, Austria, 2017.
38. Bates, D.; Maechler, M.; Bolker, B.; Walker, S. *lme4: Linear Mixed-Efects Models Using Eigen and s4*; R package Version 1.1-7; R Foundation for Statistical Computing: Vienna, Austria, 2014.
39. Fox, J.; Weisberg, S. *An R Companion to Applied Regression*; Sage: Thousand Oaks, CA, USA, 2011.
40. Gamer, M.; Lemon, J.; Fellows, I.; Singh, P. *Various Coefficients of Interrater Reliability and Agreement*; R package Version 0.84; R Foundation for Statistical Computing: Vienna, Austria, 2012.
41. Hothorn, T.; Bretz, F.; Westfall, P. Simultaneous inference in general parametric models. *Biom. J.* **2008**, *50*, 346–363. [CrossRef] [PubMed]
42. Wickham, H. *Ggplot2: Elegant Graphics for Data Analysis*; Springer: New York, NY, USA, 2009.

43. Yan, J.; Liu, L.; Zhu, Y.; Huang, G.; Wang, P.P. The association between breastfeeding and childhood obesity: A meta-analysis. *BMC Public Health* **2014**, *14*, 1267. [CrossRef] [PubMed]
44. Prentice, P.; Ong, K.K.; Schoemaker, M.H.; van Tol, E.A.F.; Vervoort, J.; Hughes, I.A.; Acerini, C.L. Breast milk nutrient content and infancy growth. *Acta Paediatr.* **2016**, *105*, 641–647. [CrossRef] [PubMed]
45. Dewey, K.; Heinig, M.; Nommsen, L.; Lonnerdal, B. Maternal versus infant factors related to breast milk intake and residual milk volume: The Darling study. *Pediatrics* **1991**, *87*, 829–837. [PubMed]
46. Kent, J.; Mitoulas, L.; Cox, D.B.; Owens, R.; Hartmann, P. Breast volume and milk production during extended lactation in women. *Exp. Physiol.* **1999**, *84*, 435–447. [CrossRef] [PubMed]
47. De Bruin, N.C.; Degenhart, H.J.; Gal, S.; Westerterp, K.R.; Stijen, T.; Visser, H.K.A. Energy utilization and growth in breast-fed and formula-fed infants measured prospectively during the first year of life. *Am. J. Clin. Nutr.* **1998**, *67*, 885–896. [CrossRef] [PubMed]
48. Heinig, M.J.; Nommsen, L.A.; Peerson, J.M.; Lonnerdal, B.; Dewey, K.G. Energy and protein intakes of breast-fed and formula-fed infants during the first year of life and their association with growth velocity: The Darling study. *Am. J. Clin. Nutr.* **1993**, *58*, 152–161. [CrossRef] [PubMed]
49. Artym, J.; Zimecki, M. Milk-derived proteins and peptides in clinical trials. *Postepy Hig. Med. Dosw.* **2013**, *67*, 800–816. [CrossRef]
50. Czank, C.; Mitoulas, L.R.; Hartmann, P.E. Human milk composition: Nitrogen and energy content. In *Hale and Hartmann's Text Book of Human Lactation*; Hartmann, P.E., Hale, T.W., Eds.; Hale Publishing, L.P.: Dallas, TX, USA, 2007; pp. 89–102.
51. Clare, D.A.; Swaisgood, H.E. Bioactive milk peptides: A prospectus. *J. Dairy Sci.* **2000**, *83*, 1187–1195. [CrossRef]
52. Gridneva, Z.; Kugananthan, S.; Hepworth, A.R.; Tie, W.J.; Lai, C.T.; Ward, L.C.; Hartmann, P.E.; Geddes, D.T. Effect of human milk appetite hormones, macronutrients, and infant characteristics on gastric emptying and breastfeeding patterns of term fully breastfed infants. *Nutrients* **2017**, *9*, 15. [CrossRef] [PubMed]
53. Budek, A.Z.; Bjornvad, C.R.; Molgaard, C.; Bugel, S.; Vestergaard, M.; Pulkkinen, P.; Michaelsen, K.F.; Sangild, P.T. Effects of casein, whey and soy proteins on volumetric bone density and bone strength in immunocompromised piglets. *Eur. J. Clin. Nutr. Metab.* **2007**, *2*, 57–62. [CrossRef]
54. Alexander, D.D.; Yan, J.; Bylsma, L.C.; Northigton, R.S.; Grathwohl, D.; Steenhout, P.; Erdmann, P.; Spivey-Krobath, E.; Haschke, F. Growth of infants consuming whey-predominant term infant formulas with a protein content of 1.8 g/100 kcal: A multicenter pooled analysis of individual participant data. *Am. J. Clin. Nutr.* **2016**, *104*, 1083–1092. [CrossRef] [PubMed]
55. Harrison, G.G.; Graver, E.J.; Vargas, M.; Churella, H.R.; Paule, C.L. Growth and adiposity of term infants fed whey-predominant or casein-predominant formulas or human milk. *J. Pediatr. Gastroenterol. Nutr.* **1987**, *6*, 739–747. [CrossRef] [PubMed]
56. Shepherd, R.W.; Oxborough, D.B.; Holt, T.L.; Thomas, B.J.; Thong, Y.H. Longitudinal study of the body composition of weight gain in exclusively breast-fed and intake-measured whey-based formula-fed infants to age 3 months. *J. Pediatr. Gastroenterol. Nutr.* **1988**, *7*, 732–739. [CrossRef] [PubMed]
57. Ballard, O.; Morrow, A.L. Human milk composition: Nutrients and bioactive factors. *Pediatr. Clin. N. Am.* **2013**, *60*, 49–74. [CrossRef] [PubMed]
58. Bol'shakova, A.M.; Shcherbakova, E.G.; Ivanova, S.D.; Medvedeva, M.M.; Zhuravleva, T.P. Lysozyme in the feeding of premature infants with mixed pathology. *Antibiotiki* **1984**, *29*, 784–790. [PubMed]
59. Braun, O.H.; Sandkuhler, H. Relationships between lysozyme concentration of human milk, bacteriologic content, and weight gain of premature infants. *J. Pediatr. Gastroenterol. Nutr.* **1985**, *4*, 583–586. [CrossRef] [PubMed]
60. Johnston, W.H.; Ashley, C.; Yeiser, M.; Harris, C.L.; Stolz, S.I.; Wampler, J.L.; Wittke, A.; Cooper, T.R. Growth and tolerance of formula with lactoferrin in infants through one year of age: Double-blind, randomized, controlled trial. *BMC Pediatr.* **2015**, *15*, 173. [CrossRef] [PubMed]
61. Trabulsi, J.; Capeding, R.; Lebumfacil, J.; Ramanujam, K.; Feng, P.; McSweeney, S.; Harris, B.; DeRusso, P. Effect of an α-lactalbumin-enriched infant formula with lower protein on growth. *Eur. J. Clin. Nutr.* **2011**, *65*, 167–174. [CrossRef] [PubMed]
62. Wong, C.B.; Xiao, J. Breast milk on the infant faecal microbiome: Components of breast milk orchestrating the establishment of bifidobacteria species. *J. Hum. Nutr. Food Sci.* **2018**, *6*, 1123.

63. Maga, E.A.; Desai, P.T.; Weimer, B.C.; Dao, N.; Kultz, D.; Murray, J.D. Consumption of lysozyme-rich milk can alter microbial fecal populations. *Appl. Environ. Microbiol.* **2012**, *78*, 6153–6160. [CrossRef] [PubMed]
64. Neville, M.C.; Allen, J.C.; Watters, C. The mechanisms of milk secretion. In *Lactation: Physiology, Nutrition, and Breast-Feedin*; Neville, M.C., Neifert, M.R., Eds.; Plenum Press: New York, NY, USA, 1983; pp. 49–102.
65. Mather, I.H.; Keenan, T.W. Function of endomembranes and the cell surface in the secretion of organic milk constituents. In *Biochemistry of Lactation*; Mepham, T.B., Ed.; Elsevier: Amsterdam, The Netherlands, 1983; pp. 231–283.
66. Chang, N.; Jung, J.A.; Kim, H.; Jo, A.; Kang, S.; Lee, S.-W.; Yi, H.; Kim, J.; Yim, J.-G.; Jung, B.-M. Macronutrient composition of human milk from Korean mothers of full term infants born at 37–42 gestational weeks. *Nutr. Res. Pract.* **2015**, *9*, 433–438. [CrossRef] [PubMed]
67. Grote, V.; Verduci, E.; Scaglioni, S.; Vecchi, F.; Contarini, G.; Giovannini, M.; Koletzko, B.; Agostoni, C. Breast milk composition and infant nutrient intakes during the first 12 months of life. *Eur. J. Clin. Nutr.* **2016**, *70*, 250–256. [CrossRef] [PubMed]
68. Innis, S.M. Impact of maternal diet on human milk composition and neurological development of infants. *Am. J. Clin. Nutr.* **2014**, *99*, S734–S741. [CrossRef] [PubMed]
69. Nommsen, L.A.; Lovelady, C.A.; Heinig, M.; Lonnerdal, B.; Dewey, K.G. Determinants of energy, protein, lipid, and lactose concentrations in human milk during the first 12 mo of lactation: The Darling study. *Am. J. Clin. Nutr.* **1991**, *53*, 457–465. [CrossRef] [PubMed]
70. De Luca, A.; Frasquet-Darrieux, M.; Gaud, M.A.; Christin, P.; Boquien, C.-Y.; Millet, C.; Herviou, M.; Darmaun, D.; Robins, R.J.; Ingrand, P.; et al. Higher leptin but not human milk macronutrient concentration distinguishes normal-weight from obese mothers at 1-month postpartum. *PLoS ONE* **2016**, *11*, e0168568. [CrossRef] [PubMed]
71. Bachour, P.; Yafawi, R.; Jaber, F.; Choueiri, E.; Abdel-Razzak, Z. Effects of smoking, mother's age, body mass index, and parity number on lipid, protein, and secretory immunoglobulin a concentrations of human milk. *Breastfeed. Med.* **2012**, *7*, 179–188. [CrossRef] [PubMed]
72. Hassiotou, F.; Geddes, D.T. Programming of appetite control during breastfeeding as a preventative strategy against the obesity epidemic. *J. Hum. Lact.* **2014**, *30*, 136–142. [CrossRef] [PubMed]
73. Meier, P.P.; Engstrom, J.L. Test weighing for term and premature infants is an accurate procedure. *Arch. Dis. Child. Fetal Neonatal Ed.* **2007**, *92*, F155–F156. [CrossRef] [PubMed]
74. Butte, N.; Garza, C.; Smith, E.; Nichols, B. Human milk intake and growth in exclusively breast-fed infants. *J. Pediatr.* **1984**, *104*, 187–195. [CrossRef]
75. Rattigan, S.; Ghisalberti, A.V.; Hartmann, P.E. Breast-milk production in Australian women. *Br. J. Nutr.* **1981**, *45*, 243–249. [CrossRef] [PubMed]
76. Kent, J.; Hepworth, A.; Sherriff, J.; Cox, D.; Mitoulas, L.; Hartmann, P. Longitudinal changes in breastfeeding patterns from 1 to 6 months of lactation. *Breastfeed. Med.* **2013**, *8*, 401–407. [CrossRef] [PubMed]
77. Hoppe, C.; Udam, T.R.; Lauritzen, L.; Molgaard, C.; Juul, A.; Michaelsen, K.F. Animal protein intake, serum insulin-like growth factor I, and growth in healthy 2.5-yold danish children. *Am. J. Clin. Nutr.* **2004**, *80*, 447–452. [CrossRef] [PubMed]
78. Gunther, A.L.B.; Remer, T.; Kroke, A.; Buyken, A.E. Early protein intake and later obesity risk: Which protein sources at which time points throughout infancy and childhood are important for body mass index and body fat percentage at 7 y of age? *Am. J. Clin. Nutr.* **2007**, *86*, 1765–1772. [CrossRef] [PubMed]

6

Online Video Instruction on Hand Expression of Colostrum in Pregnancy is an Effective Educational Tool

Therese A. O'Sullivan [1,*], Joy Cooke [2], Chris McCafferty [3] and Roslyn Giglia [4]

1 School of Medical and Health Sciences, Edith Cowan University, 270 Joondalup Drive, Joondalup, WA 6027, Australia
2 Maternity Unit, Glengarry Private Hospital, Duncraig, WA 6023, Australia; joy.cooke@westnet.com.au
3 School of Nursing and Midwifery, Edith Cowan University, Joondalup, WA 6027, Australia; c.mccafferty@ecu.edu.au
4 Telethon Kids Institute, University of Western Australia, Subiaco, WA 6008, Australia; roslyn.giglia@telethonkids.org.au
* Correspondence: t.osullivan@ecu.edu.au

Abstract: The use of antenatal colostrum expression in the weeks prior to birth may help improve long-term breastfeeding, but few large-scale studies exist. Typically, antenatal colostrum expression instruction relies on face-to-face education, making large interventions costly. We aimed to determine whether an expert online instructional video can improve knowledge and confidence around antenatal colostrum expressing. Pregnant women were asked to complete a questionnaire pre- and post-watching the instructional video online. Ninety five pregnant women completed both pre- and post-questionnaires. Total antenatal colostrum expression knowledge scores improved after watching the video, from a mean of 3.05 ± 1.70 correct out of a maximum of 7, to 6.32 ± 0.76 ($p < 0.001$). Self-reported confidence around hand expressing in pregnancy also improved from an average ranking of not confident (2.56 ± 1.17, out of a possible 5) to confident (4.32 ± 0.80, $p < 0.001$). Almost all women (98%) reported that they would recommend the video to a friend or family member if antenatal colostrum expression was suggested by their healthcare provider. Findings suggest that the use of an online expert video is an acceptable and effective way to educate pregnant women in antenatal colostrum expression.

Keywords: antenatal; expressing; pregnancy; video instruction; colostrum; breastfeeding; online

1. Introduction

During pregnancy, breasts begin to produce the first milk, colostrum. Historically, antenatal colostrum expression (ACE) was performed as a means of preparing the breasts for breastfeeding after birth. More recently, ACE is performed to collect a supply of colostrum. Colostrum can be collected using a syringe, and safely stored in a freezer. The colostrum can then be defrosted and given to the baby. The stored colostrum can be used to treat hypoglycaemia in the infant after birth, or if breastfeeding issues occur. The collection and storage of colostrum can ensure that an infant receives its own mother's milk as the first feed after birth, instead of reliance on formula during this time. In women intending to exclusively breastfeed, formula supplementation while in hospital has been associated with a two- to three-fold risk of early breastfeeding cessation [1]. Some have proposed that ACE can also promote the onset of Lactogenesis II, the "coming in" of breastmilk, however there is no evidence to support this effect, and the efficacy of the ACE practice is yet to be established in this regard [2].

In addition, there has been some concern that antenatal nipple stimulation while teaching hand expression will act as a precursor for the release of oxytocin, and may induce premature labour [3]. In a Cochrane review of the literature [4], breast stimulation was shown to reduce the number of women in labour after 72 h (i.e., had given birth), along with reduced postpartum haemorrhage rates. However, the authors went on to recommend not promoting this practice in high-risk women and noted that more information on maternal satisfaction was required. More recently, evidence suggests a role for nipple stimulation at term as a non-pharmacological method of labour induction [5,6]. In 2017, results of the Diabetes and Antenatal Milk Expressing (DAME) trial of 635 pregnant women with low-risk diabetes demonstrated that antenatal expressing did not result in a lower gestational age or increased admissions to the Neonatal Intensive Care Unit [7]. The authors concluded that there is no harm in advising women with diabetes in pregnancy at low risk of complications to express colostrum for the last few weeks of gestation. Other results from the DAME trial show a non-significant trend toward improvements in breastfeeding outcomes for women in the antenatal expressing intervention group, although the study was not powered for breastfeeding outcomes, and indicators for collecting infant feeding methods differed from standardised national indicators [8].

The question remains as to the effectiveness of ACE in promoting positive breastfeeding outcomes, and the safety of its practice as part of regular antenatal education at 37 weeks gestation in healthy, low-risk pregnant women. In our own medical record audit of a secondary, general hospital in Greater Perth, Western Australia, we compared the inclusion of ACE in antenatal education in relation to birthing outcomes in a hospital which had previously not included ACE in this education, using a retrospective control group. Results showed that inclusion of ACE in antenatal care was not associated with an increased risk of premature birth or admission to special care nursery [9].

Very few randomised controlled trials have been published in the area of ACE, with none in healthy women, and most using a small sample size (<100). Due to a lack of research investigating the safety and efficacy of antenatal colostrum expression in the general population, ACE is therefore not uniformly encouraged across Australian maternity health services. One major barrier to large scale trials in Australia is the cost of high-quality ACE instruction. A one-on-one session with a midwife (or lactation consultant) provides optimal ACE instruction, however it is not routinely taught as part of antenatal education. In our experience, detailed instruction and assistance with hand expressing is most often provided postnatally, commonly when women are experiencing breastfeeding difficulties (e.g., to relieve engorgement), are sleep deprived, and are potentially anxious about their ability to feed their babies.

Online videos can be an effective and cheap tool for instruction, in areas where the internet is easily accessible. The expert expressing instructional videos that are currently available demonstrate breastmilk expressing in women who have already given birth. Given that expressing in postnatal women is conceptually different, this type of video is not well suited to an antenatal setting. Colostrum has a different look and consistency to mature milk, and the presence of the baby often stimulates milk "let down". Feedback from West Australian midwives and lactation consultants, along with our local consumer reference group, indicated that a video of a lactation consultant-led demonstration of ACE using pregnant women would be very valuable. We have therefore developed an online instructional video on ACE specifically for pregnant women. To our knowledge, no such expert-informed video exists nationally or internationally that provides specific enough detail to suit requirements for use in a large-scale trial or in our health setting. The 20 min video featured a real-life situation, with two pregnant women in a session with a lactation consultant. The lactation consultant explained how to use ACE and how to collect and store the colostrum, and guided both women through the process in a practical demonstration (Appendix A, Figures A1–A3). The women had differing prior breastfeeding experience (one was primiparous, the other had previously breastfed multiple children), and differing breast sizes and nipples. The women also asked questions as they went through the process.

The aim of this study was to investigate whether the instruction on antenatal expression of colostrum via this instructional online video is an effective way to increase knowledge around ACE and confidence in using it, in pregnant women. If so, the use of an instructional video for ACE will provide an economical and feasible education option for future research.

2. Materials and Methods

2.1. Study Setting

This was a pre- and post-test study, using online questionnaires and video. Data collection for the study was completed online between August 2017 and April 2018.

2.2. Study Sample

Pregnant women were recruited through social media via local university and research institutions, and infant and mother organizations, along with personal contacts. The only inclusion criteria were being currently pregnant (any stage) and having access to the internet. Potential participants were provided with an online information letter and were requested to provide online consent prior to the start of the questionnaires. Ethics approval was granted from the Edith Cowan University Human Research Ethics Committee (17501).

2.3. Measurement

Two linked online questionnaires were developed using Qualtrics survey software (Provo, UT, USA). The first was a pre-video questionnaire which contained the ACE video at the end, followed by a second questionnaire which participants completed after viewing the video (post-video questionnaire). The pre-video questionnaire asked about age, gestation of current pregnancy, previous children and previous breastfeeding experience. The post-video questionnaire asked for feedback on the video, including aspects that were liked and disliked (free text response), the length of the video (too long, too short or appropriate), use of real pregnant women in the video (free text), and satisfaction on the depth of information covered, clarity of voices, image quality and overall satisfaction (assessed on a continuous 1–5 scale) from very unsatisfied to very satisfied. Respondents were also asked whether they would recommend the video to pregnant family and friends if ACE was suggested by their healthcare provider, and whether they had any suggestions for improvement of the video. Knowledge and confidence were assessed in both the pre- and post-questionnaires. Knowledge was assessed over seven areas and also as a total knowledge score (one point for each correct answer). To assess confidence about hand expressing in pregnancy, respondents were asked to move a sliding scale which ranged from 1–5, representing very unconfident to very confident.

2.4. Data Analysis

Descriptive statistics were used to report on subject characteristics, with means and standard deviations used for normally distributed results, and medians and interquartile ranges used to report results that were not normally distributed. The related samples McNemar statistical test was used to compare the number of correct answers in knowledge questions in the pre-video and post-video questionnaires, and the paired samples *t*-test was used to compare total knowledge scores and confidence around using ACE. Significance was set at $p < 0.05$.

For free text responses, information was grouped into themes and quotes that were identified as appropriate.

3. Results

A total of 171 pregnant women completed at least one aspect of the survey. Of these, 112 completed the full pre-questionnaire, with 95 going on to also complete the post-questionnaire after watching the video. Subject characteristics for the women who completed both questionnaires are shown in Table 1.

Knowledge of ACE improved significantly for all areas after watching the video (Table 2), as did the total knowledge score (for all $p < 0.001$, Figure 1). Confidence in hand expressing during pregnancy also significantly increased from a mean score of 2.56 ± 1.17 to 4.32 ± 0.80 ($n = 93$, $p < 0.001$) (Figure 2). IQR: Inter quartile range.

Table 1. Characteristics of the pregnant women participating in the video evaluation ($n = 95$).

Characteristic/Response	Mean (SD) or Median (IQR)/n (%)
Age (years)	30.8 (4.7)
Gestation of current pregnancy (weeks)	31.0 (23.0–37.0)
Number of previous children:	
0	103 (60.2)
1	40 (23.4)
2	2 (12.3)
3+	7 (4.1)
Have previously breastfed an infant (yes)	56 (32.7%)

Table 2. Knowledge questions asked in pre- and post-questionnaires, with responses ($n = 95$). The related samples McNemar statistical test was used to compare the number of correct answers pre- and post-questionnaire for each question, and the paired t-test was used to compare the total knowledge scores.

Knowledge Questions and Responses * Indicates Correct Response to the Question	Pre n (%)	Post n (%)	p
If you wanted to do hand expressing in pregnancy, approximately when should you start? (with healthcare provider permission)			
After 28 weeks gestation	5 (5.3)	1 (1.1)	
After 32 weeks gestation	2 (2.1)	0	<0.001
After 35 weeks gestation	16 (16.8)	0	
After 37 weeks gestation *	40 (42.1)	94 (98.9)	
Not sure	32 (33.7)	0	
Click on the picture below that shows the correct finger placement for hand expressing (set of three photos displayed)			
Photo showing narrow finger placement	3 (3.2)	0	
Photo showing correct placement *	48 (50.5)	78 (82.1)	<0.001
Photo showing wide finger placement	16 (16.8)	17 (17.9)	
Not sure	28 (29.5)	0	
If you were doing hand expressing in pregnancy, how often should you express?			
Once per day	16 (16.8)	1 (1.1)	
Two or three times per day *	25 (26.3)	90 (94.7)	<0.001
Four times a day	2 (2.1)	2 (2.1)	
Not sure	52 (54.7)	2 (2.1)	
Can you reuse the same syringe for collecting colostrum over the day?			
Yes, can be left at room temperature	0	1 (1.1)	
Yes, as long as syringe is refrigerated *	30 (31.6)	91 (95.8)	<0.001
No, syringes are for a single expressing use only	30 (31.6)	3 (3.2)	
Not sure	35 (36.8)	0	
How much colostrum would you expect to collect in the first session of hand expressing?			
A lot (>10 mL)	0	0	
A moderate amount (between 1–10 mLs)	0	2 (2.1)	
A little (about 1 mL)	25 (26.3)	23 (24.23)	<0.001
Generally nothing at all	8 (8.4)	0	
Everybody will be different *	42 (44.2)	70 (73.7)	
Not sure	20 (21.1)	0	
If you can't gather any colostrum during expressing, does this mean that you will have trouble breastfeeding?			
Yes	1 (1.1)	0	
Probably	3 (3.2)	0	<0.001
Probably not	13 (13.7)	9 (9.5)	
No *	53 (55.8)	85 (89.5)	
Not sure	25 (26.3)	1 (1.1)	
Should hand expressing be painful?			
Yes sometimes	7 (7.4)	1 (1.1)	
No *	52 (54.7)	92 (96.8)	<0.001
Not sure	36 (37.9)	2 (2.1)	
TOTAL KNOWLEDGE SCORE (mean ± SD correct/7)	3.05 ± 1.70	6.32 ± 0.76	<0.001

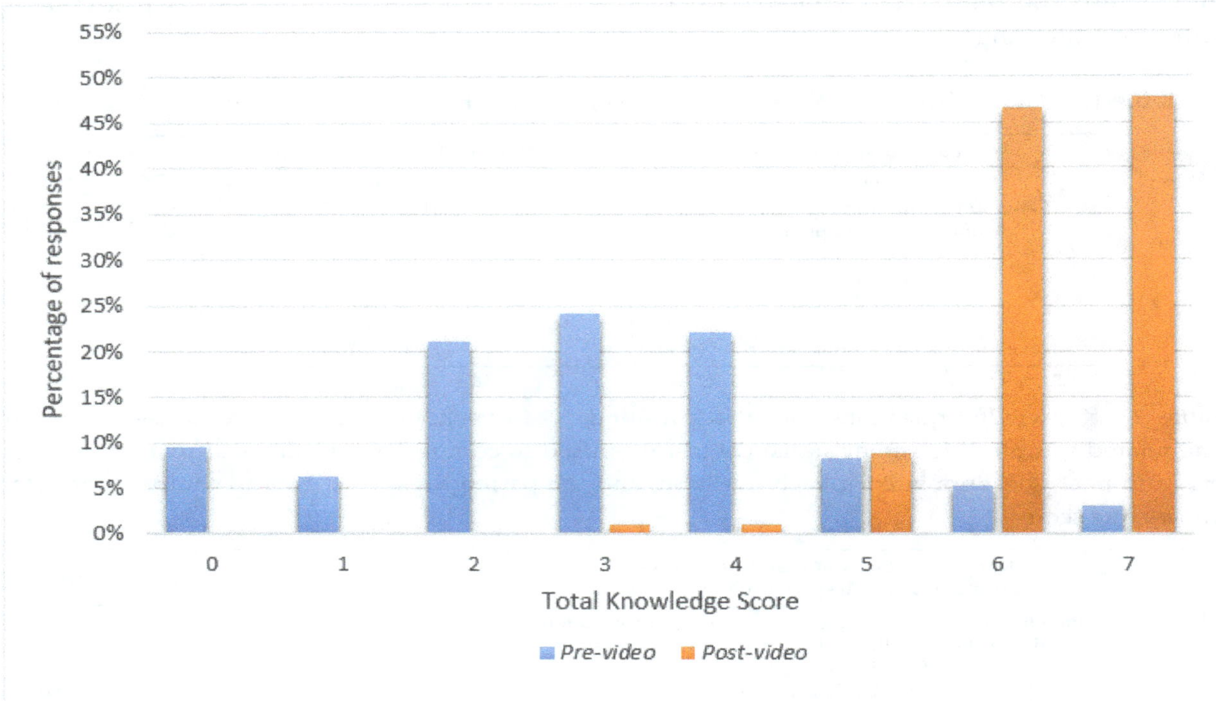

Figure 1. Chart of antenatal expressing of colostrum total knowledge scores scale pre- and post-video (minimum possible score = 0; maximum possible score = 7, n = 95).

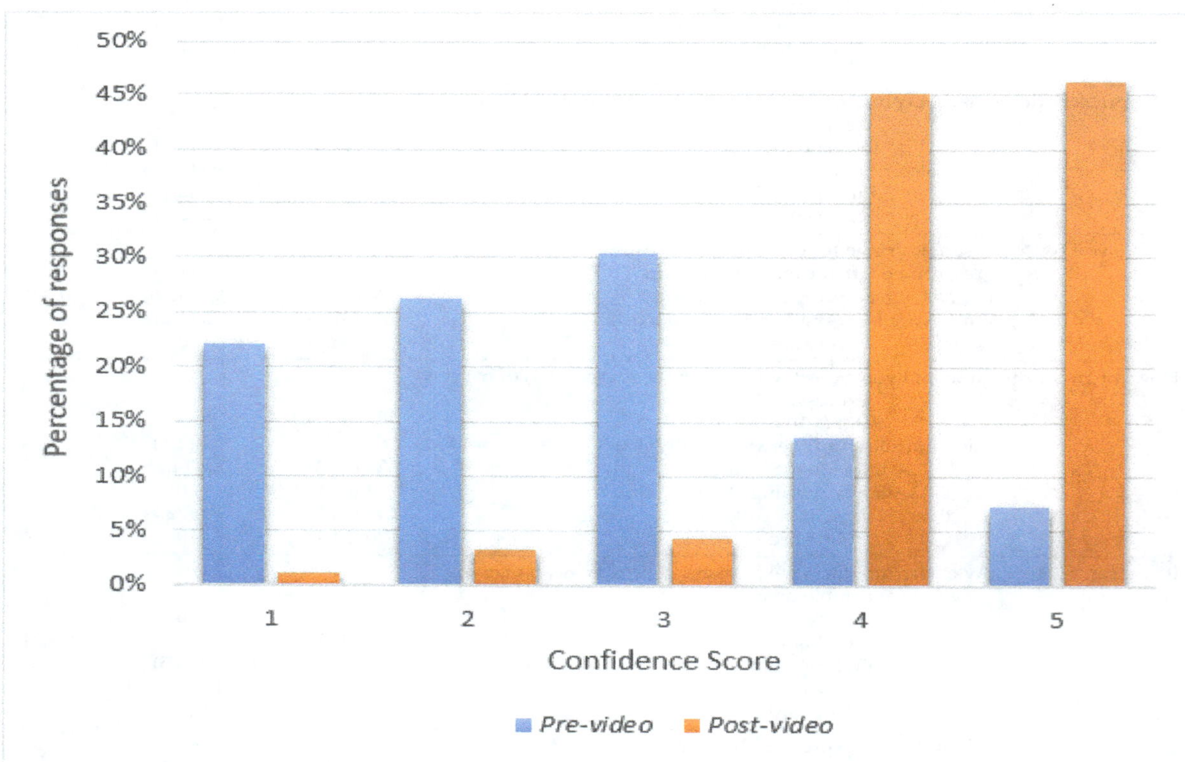

Figure 2. Chart of confidence scale pre- and post-video: How confident do you feel at the moment about hand expressing in pregnancy? (Minimum possible score = 1, representing very unconfident; maximum possible score = 5, representing very confident, n = 93).

When asked what they liked most about the video, 90 out of 95 respondents chose to write a full text response, which was subsequently grouped into one of five categories. The most common response was that the video was informative/interesting/detailed (32.6%). The inclusion of a practical demonstration (22.1%) in a real situation, and the use of real pregnant women (20.0%) were the next most frequently cited responses. Respondents also commented that the video was easy to understand and used clear explanations (15.8%). Others liked the video being "unrushed", "comfortable" or "relaxed" (3.2%). One respondent answered that they liked "everything" (1.1%). Specific quotes relating to the responses are shown in Table 3.

Table 3. Most common full text responses provided by pregnant women when giving their evaluation of the antenatal colostrum expressing video.

Response	Illustrative Quote
Aspects most liked about the video (n = 90/95 responded with full text response)	
The video was informative and interesting	*"Very informative, covering all aspects."* (#44, 26 yo, 2 previous children, has breastfed previously) *"I found it very interesting and helpful. I will definitely be asking my midwife if I can do it when I turn 37 weeks."* (#32, 36 yo, 1 previous child, has breastfed previously)
A practical demonstration using real women	*"Real women showing how to actually do it rather than cartoons or crochet breasts. Also that one woman had flat nipples like mine and was able to express which makes me hopeful."* (#23, 30 yo, 1 previous child, no previous breastfeeding). *"It was good to see the spectrum of colostrum colour and volume. Good to see techniques. Good to see a primip and multip."* (#52, 39 yo, no previous children). *"Close ups of colostrum and technique as well as how to collect on your own."* (#60, 35 yo, no previous children).
Easy to understand	*"Easy to understand. And the first video I've watched where they've shown how to collect one handed using the syringe too."* (#22, 32 yo, 1 previous child, has breastfed previously) *"Clear and explained well. Went over important bits twice"* (#21, 28 yo, 1 previous child, no previous breastfeeding)
Feelings about the use of real pregnant women in the video (n = 92/95 responded with full text response)	
More comforted about the process of antenatal expressing	*"I felt like I could relate to them more."* (#32, 36 yo, 1 previous child, has breastfed previously) *"It was much more reassuring seeing real pregnant mums"* (#13, 33 yo, 2 previous children, has breastfed before) *"Comforting to know it was real people learning the skill"* (#73, 34 yo, no previous children)
A realistic approach	*"Excellent and helpful because both were different i.e.) different sized breasts, one had breastfed before the other was a first time mum"* (#1, 29 yo, no previous children) *"It was good to see colostrum actually being expressed rather than someone imitating the process be it through use of an actor or prop."* (#76, 35 yo, no previous children).

refers to subject number. Yo = years old.

When asked what they didn't like about the video, the most common response was that it was too long (8.4%). This was followed by requests for more information (7.4%), including requests for information on why colostrum would be used, a visual example of when colostrum is not able to be collected using breast massage, when to stop collecting, and a reference diagram. Two women opposed the term "girls" used as a colloquial term in the video by the lactation consultant. Other comments included that it was hard to read the accompanying text and watch at the same time, that there was a need for more eye contact, and that it was hard to hear in places (1.1% for all).

When specifically asked about the length of the video, 78.9% of women found it appropriate, while 17.9% found it too long and 1.1% found it too short.

A total of 92 out of 95 women responded to the free text answer question about how they felt about the use of real women in the video, and all responded positively. Comments reflected women feeling more comforted about the process, even for those who had breastfed before, and finding a realistic approach helpful from a learning perspective (see Table 3).

A total of 93 out of 95 women responded to questions on video satisfaction which were determined on a continuous sliding scale of 1 (very unsatisfied), to 5 (very satisfied). All three aspects and overall satisfaction scored a median of 5.00, with a small interquartile range (IQR): depth of information covered (IQR 4.10–5.00, with 53.8% of respondents scoring 5), clarity of voices (IQR 4.10–5.00, 53.8% scoring 5), quality of images (IQR 4.25–5.00, 59.1% scoring 5), overall satisfaction (IQR 4.20–5.00, 53.8% scoring 5). Free text comments in this section indicated some minor dissatisfaction with the volume of voices, being told breastfeeding is best, a preference for non-scrolling text, a request for more information around how to administer the collected colostrum to a baby, the video being too long and a request for more specific information on hand placement.

When asked for additional suggestions for improvement of the video, three responses were received. These were the inclusion of a diagram of exactly where to place the hands with distance from the nipple and direction of pressure improvement, better music, and more focus on the syringe during the demonstration.

After viewing the video, approximately a fifth of women still had questions about ACE. Most questions related to safety, current health service recommendations for ACE and evidence around using ACE:

"Do all hospitals recommend doing this?"
"Can I start at 36 weeks?"
"Is it recommended for all uncomplicated pregnancies?"
"Have any studies been done on women who have previously experienced low supply to see if antenatal hand expressing helps?"
"Will this bring on early labour?"
"Will it help with establishing a good milk supply?"

This issue of safety and evidence can be better clarified as more research is done in the area.

Other questions focused on the use of stored colostrum, and have since been addressed in a revised version of the video:

"Should I give my baby the expressed colostrum even if he is feeding well?"
"How long can you store it frozen?"
"How do you defrost it?"

There were also questions specifically regarding expressing with gestational diabetes mellitus (GDM):

"What is the best time of day to express if you have gestational diabetes—does it matter if it's done before or after a meal?"
"What are the benefits for GDM?"

In addition, one mother asked what to do if ACE was hurting, and another asked what to do if they try ACE and do not produce any colostrum.

After viewing the video, women were also asked whether they would be likely to recommend the video to pregnant family or friends, if hand expression of colostrum was suggested by their healthcare provider. Responses were gauged using a five-point Likert scale ranging from "definitely yes" to "definitely not". Almost all women responded "definitely yes" (59.1%) or "probably yes" (37.6%), with 2.2% responding "might or might not" and 1.1% responding "probably not". No women selected "definitely not".

4. Discussion

The online video was effective in significantly increasing both knowledge and confidence around antenatal expressing of colostrum. The average knowledge score doubled in the post-video questionnaire, from 3.05 ± 1.70 to 6.32 ± 0.76, from a possible total score of 7. After viewing the video, the majority of women were able to correctly answer each knowledge question. The knowledge areas showing the largest improvements were when to start ACE (from 42.1% correct to 98.9% correct), and how often to express per day (from 26.3% correct to 94.7% correct). This observed increase in knowledge validates the most popular comments regarding what was liked about the video, which focused on the video being informative, detailed and interesting. If a learner finds the subject content interesting, this facilitates the learning process and makes them more likely to retain the information [10].

Reported confidence in using ACE also showed a substantial increase, from a mean score of 2.56 to 4.32 out of a possible 5. It is important to see an increase in confidence alongside an increase in knowledge, as knowledge alone is not necessarily enough to result in a change to practice. Self-confidence in applying skills, also known as a sense of competence, is recognised in the literature as being important when implementing health-related behaviour changes [11]. Importantly, self-confidence, along with expectations, can influence a mother's judgement on her ability to breastfeed [12]. The use of real pregnant women in the video, as opposed to the use of breast models or actors, likely helped women to feel more confident—it was noted by the respondents as being the second most common liked aspect of the video. As in real life, the women in the video had differently shaped breasts and nipples, and this resonated with some respondents. Observational learning improves maternal breastfeeding confidence postpartum [12], and our results suggest that observational learning via video is also valuable during the prenatal period for improving confidence with hand expressing. Self-confidence encompasses both self-efficacy and self-esteem. Self-efficacy refers to an individual's belief in his or her capacity to perform behaviours necessary to accomplish a specific task or achieve a certain outcome. Bandura's theoretical sources of self-efficacy includes vicarious experience (alongside enactive mastery experience, verbal/social persuasion, and physiological and affective states), which refers to the learning of behaviour from observing others, such as watching videos of the behaviour [13,14]. This theory supports the concept that women who watch the ACE video and see women similar to themselves successfully expressing are more likely to succeed, due to an increased belief that they too possess the capabilities to master the skill of expressing in pregnancy.

The most common criticisms were that the video was too long and that it lacked some minor information, although these were an exception, with less than 20% of women expressing dislikes when prompted. When specifically asked about the length of the video, 17% reported that it was too long. The length of the video allowed for a complete demonstration and a relaxed atmosphere, which was noted as positive by some women, however it was possible to shorten it by speeding up some sections, particularly around the demonstration. Other aspects of video satisfaction indicated that it was well-received in terms of clarity of voices, quality of images and depth of information covered.

We have since updated the video to cut out unnecessary and repetitive sections, reducing it to 15 min. We have also added additional information in the form of text notes at relevant times throughout the video.

Overall, 97% of women in this video evaluation stated that they would be likely to recommend it to pregnant family or friends, if hand expression of colostrum was suggested by their healthcare provider. Family and friend recommendations can have an important impact on public health strategies. Eighty-three percent of online respondents across 60 different countries said that they completely or somewhat trusted the recommendations of friends and family, according to Nielsen's Global Trust in Advertising Report in 2015 [15]. The high level of recommendation demonstrated in our findings suggests that women valued the information they received from the video enough to share it with others.

An online video provides unique advantages for instruction over a traditional face-to-face format. Being online allows pregnant women to view the video at a time and location convenient for them. This is particularly valuable for mothers who already have children, along with those located in remote areas. Another advantage of a video is the ability to pause and replay certain sections according to the viewer's needs and understanding. Videos have become increasingly popular in education, and many universities now offer online instruction, incorporating videos and recorded lectures. Disadvantages also exist with video instruction, notably technical issues with glitches in internet bandwidth and connectivity [16]. In 2018, about 88% of the Australian population were active internet users, with an average of 5 h and 34 min spent on the internet daily [17]. A high-quality video with professional sound and lighting is key to better engage learners, as is audio/visual elements to the video that support the content above and beyond the use of text [18]. Results of our evaluation suggested that our ACE video is likely to be viewed as a valuable tool by pregnant women.

Risk of self-selection bias was an important potential limitation of this study, with women who were interested in ACE being more likely to participate. In addition, the women who participated in our study had a relatively narrow age range. These factors limited our ability to generalise our results to a wider population.

Our findings have important implications for the use of ACE video instruction for future research, and potential public health initiatives leading on from this. Many mothers introduce formula due to a perception of poor milk supply [19], and cite a previously unsuccessful breastfeeding experience, poor breastmilk or difficulties breastfeeding as reasons for ceasing breastfeeding early [20]. A mother's attitude towards breastfeeding has been shown to be a strong predictor of breastfeeding duration. This is shaped by personal factors including personal experience, exposure to positive role models and societal value [21]. Performing ACE and the storage of frozen colostrum in the weeks prior to birth has been demonstrated to build confidence with breastfeeding [22]. Instruction on ACE during pregnancy, alongside general instruction on breastfeeding routinely provided in antenatal classes, may help to build a positive attitude toward breastfeeding. Our video has been specifically designed for this purpose, and results from this study suggest that it is an acceptable and economical way to allow the efficacy and safety of ACE to be tested in future research. Future research may also investigate a potential role of this video in the education of healthcare practitioners working in maternal and infant health, who also have a need to increase knowledge, skills, and attitudes to assist breastfeeding families.

Author Contributions: R.G., J.C. and T.A.O. were involved in the study design and video scripting, C.M. produced and edited the video, T.A.O. analysed the data, T.A.O. and R.G. interpreted the findings, T.A.O. drafted the manuscript. All authors critically reviewed the manuscript and approved the final version submitted for publication.

Acknowledgments: The authors would like to thank the pregnant mothers who participated in this evaluation. We would also like to acknowledge our valuable community reference group including Raenee Polmear, Pia Kaczor and Emma Connolly. We are particularly grateful to the two pregnant mothers who graciously agreed to feature in our video and made this project possible—thank-you!

Appendix A Video Stills

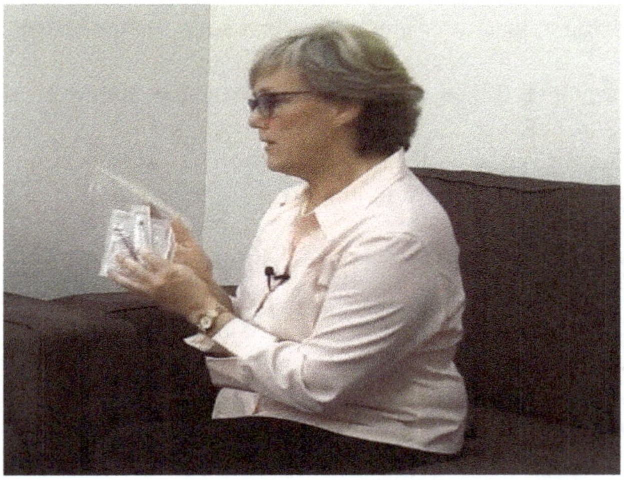

Figure A1. The lactation consultant discusses syringes and storage.

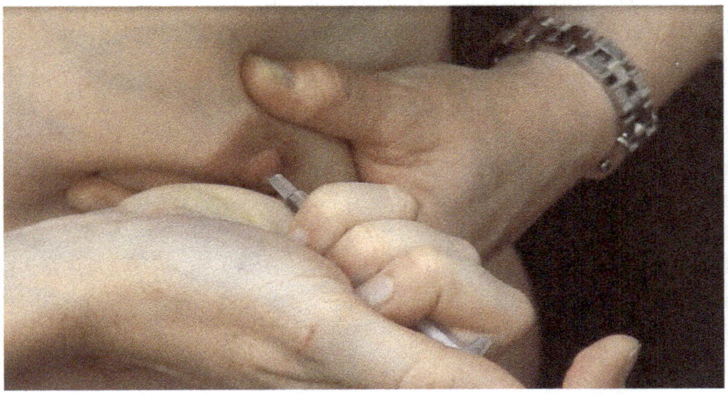

Figure A2. Close up of the colostrum collection during one of the demonstrations.

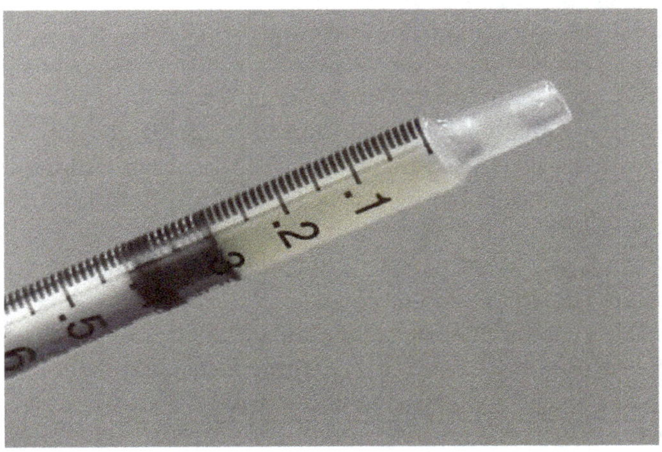

Figure A3. Close up of collected colostrum.

References

1. Chantry, C.J.; Dewey, K.G.; Peerson, J.M.; Wagner, E.A.; Nommsen-Rivers, L.A. In-hospital formula use increases early breastfeeding cessation among first-time mothers intending to exclusively breastfeed. *J. Pediatr.* **2014**, *164*, 1339–1345.e1335. [CrossRef] [PubMed]

2. Chapman, T.; Pincombe, J.; Harris, M. Antenatal breast expression: A critical review of the literature. *Midwifery* **2013**, *29*, 203–210. [CrossRef] [PubMed]
3. Cox, S. Expressing and storing colostrum antenatally for use in the newborn period. *Breastfeed. Rev.* **2006**, *14*, 11–16. [PubMed]
4. Kavanagh, J.; Kelly, A.; Thomas, J. Breast stimulation for cervical ripening and induction of labour. *Cochrane Database Syst. Rev.* **2005**, *20*, CD003392.
5. Singh, N.; Tripathi, R.; Mala, R.; Yedla, N. Breast stimulation in low-risk primigravidas at term: Does it aid in spontaneous onset of labour and vaginal delivery? A pilot study. *Biomed Res. Int.* **2014**, 695037. [CrossRef] [PubMed]
6. Demirel, G.; Guler, H. The effect of uterine and nipple stimulation on induction with oxytocin and the labor process. *Worldviews Evid.-Based Nurs.* **2015**, *12*, 273–280. [CrossRef] [PubMed]
7. Forster, D.A.; Moorhead, A.M.; Jacobs, S.E.; Davis, P.G.; Walker, S.P.; McEgan, K.M.; Opie, G.F.; Donath, S.M.; Gold, L.; McNamara, C.; et al. Advising women with diabetes in pregnancy to express breastmilk in late pregnancy (diabetes and antenatal milk expressing [DAME]): A multicentre, unblinded, randomised controlled trial. *Lancet* **2017**, *389*, 2204–2213. [CrossRef]
8. Binns, C.W.; Fraser, M.L.; Lee, A.H.; Scott, J. Defining exclusive breastfeeding in Australia. *J. Paediatr. Child Health* **2009**, *45*, 174–180. [CrossRef] [PubMed]
9. Connolly, E.L.; Reinkowsky, M.; Giglia, R.; Sexton, B.; Lyons-Wall, P.; Lo, J.; O'Sullivan, T.A. Education on antenatal colostrum expression and the baby friendly health initiative in an Australian hospital: An audit of birth and breastfeeding outcomes. *Breastfeed. Rev.* **2019**, 21–30.
10. Hidi, S. Interest and its contribution as a mental resource for learning. *Rev. Educ. Res.* **1990**, *60*, 549–571. [CrossRef]
11. Ryan, R.M.; Patrick, H.; Deci, E.L.; Williams, G.C. Facilitating health behaviour change and its maintenance: Interventions based on self-determination theory. *Eur. Health Psychol.* **2008**, *10*, 2–5.
12. Dennis, C.-L. Theoretical underpinnings of breastfeeding confidence: A self-efficacy framework. *J. Hum. Lact.* **1999**, *15*, 195–201. [CrossRef] [PubMed]
13. Bandura, A. Social learning through imitation. In *Nebraska Symposium of Motivation*; Jones, M.R., Ed.; University of Nebraska Press: Lincoln, OR, USA, 1962; pp. 211–269.
14. Bandura, A. *Social Foundations of Thought and Action: A Social Cognitive Theory*; Prentice Hall: Englewood Cliffs, NJ, USA, 1986.
15. The Nielsen Company. The Nielsen Global Survey of Trust in Advertising. Available online: http://www.nielsen.com/content/dam/nielsenglobal/apac/docs/reports/2015/nielsen-global-trust-in-advertising-report-september-2015.pdf (accessed on 21 May 2018).
16. Hartsell, T.; Yuen, S. Video streaming in online learning. *AACE J.* **2006**, *14*, 31–43.
17. Despinola, C. 2018 Digital Report—Australia. Available online: https://wearesocial.com/au/blog/2018/02/2018-digital-report-australia (accessed on 21 September 2018).
18. Hibbert, M. What Makes an Online Instructional Video Compelling? Available online: https://er.educause.edu/articles/2014/4/what-makes-an-online-instructional-video-compelling (accessed on 21 May 2018).
19. Inch, S.; Renfrew, M.J. Common breastfeeding problems. In *Effective Care in Pregnancy and Childbirth*, 2nd ed.; Enkin, M., Keirse, M., Renfrew, M.J., Eds.; Oxford University Press: Oxford, UK, 1995; Volume 2.
20. Australian Institute of Health and Welfare. *2010 Australian National Infant Feeding Survey: Indicator Results*; AIHW: Canberra, Australia, 2011.
21. Cox, K.; Giglia, R.; Binns, C.W. The influence of infant feeding attitudes on breastfeeding duration: Evidence from a cohort study in rural Western Australia. *Int. Breastfeed. J.* **2015**, *10*, 1–9. [CrossRef] [PubMed]
22. Brisbane, J.; Giglia, R. Experiences of expressing and storing colostrum antenatally: A qualitative study of mothers in regional Western Australia. *J. Child Health Care* **2015**, *19*, 206–215. [CrossRef] [PubMed]

7

Lactoferrin in Human Milk of Prolonged Lactation

Matylda Czosnykowska-Łukacka [1,*,†], Magdalena Orczyk-Pawiłowicz [2,*,†], Barbara Broers [1] and Barbara Królak-Olejnik [1]

1 Neonatology Department, Wroclaw Medical University, Borowska 213, 50-556 Wroclaw, Poland; barsamut@gmail.com (B.B.); barbara.krolak-olejnik@umed.wroc.pl (B.K.-O.)
2 Department of Chemistry and Immunochemistry, Wroclaw Medical University, M. Skłodowskiej-Curie 48/50, 50-369 Wrocław, Poland
* Correspondence: matylda.czosnykowska-lukacka@umed.wroc.pl (M.C.-Ł.); magdalena.orczyk-pawilowicz@umed.wroc.pl (M.O.-P.)
† These authors contributed equally to this work.

Abstract: Among the immunologically important bioactive factors present in human milk, lactoferrin (Lf) has emerged as a key player with wide-ranging features that directly and indirectly protect the neonate against infection caused by a variety of pathogens. The concentration of Lf in human milk is lactation-stage related; colostrum contains more than 5 g/L, which then significantly decreases to 2–3 g/L in mature milk. The milk of mothers who are breastfeeding for more than one year is of a standard value, containing macronutrients in a composition similar to that of human milk at later stages. The aim of this study was to evaluate lactoferrin concentration in prolonged lactation from the first to the 48th month postpartum. Lactating women (n = 120) up to 48 months postpartum were recruited to the study. The mean value of lactoferrin concentration was the lowest in the group of 1–12 months of lactation (3.39 ± 1.43 g/L), significantly increasing in the 13–18 months group (5.55 ± 4.00 g/L; $p < 0.006$), and remaining at a comparable level in the groups of 19–24 month and over 24 months (5.02 ± 2.97 and 4.90 ± 3.18 g/L, respectively). The concentration of lactoferrin in mother's milk also showed a positive correlation with protein concentration over lactation from the first to the 48th month ($r = 0.3374$; $p = 0.0002$). Our results demonstrate the high immunology potential of human milk during prolonged lactation and that Lf concentration is close to the Lf concentration in colostrum. Evidence of stable or rising immunoprotein levels during prolonged lactation provides an argument for foregoing weaning; however, breastfeeding must be combined with solid foods meet the new requirements of a rapidly growing six-month or older baby.

Keywords: breastfeeding; lactoferrin; prolonged lactation; child nutrition

---

1. Introduction

Human milk (HM) serves as the gold standard in newborn and infant nutrition. Apart from the main nutrients, HM contains many bioactive proteins, growth factors, cells, and other constituents, which are crucial in the modulation of the development of a competent immune system to protect the term and preterm newborn against pathogens [1]. Among the immunologically important bioactive factors present in human milk, lactoferrin has emerged as a key player with wide-ranging features that directly and indirectly protect the neonate against infection caused by bacteria and other microorganisms.

Lactoferrin (or lactotransferrin, Lf) is an approximately 78 kDa glycoprotein from the transferrin family of proteins. Lf was first identified by Sørensen and Sørensen in 1939 in bovine milk as a red protein in whey [2], and later isolated in 1960 from both human and bovine milk [3–5]. Lf is expressed and secreted by epithelial cells in the main physiological secretions [6–8]. Lf plays a key role in specialized systems to bind iron, affecting cellular proliferation and differentiation, dependent on the degree of iron saturation [9,10]. Clinical trials have demonstrated roles for Lf in the prevention of diarrhea [11,12], neonatal sepsis, and necrotizing enterocolitis in preterm infants [13–15]. Lf may significantly impact development as well as the well-being of infants and later outcomes, which are directly related to breastfeeding. Maternal factors may affect the concentration of Lf in human milk, but affect infant factors as well. Lf concentrations are consistently highest in colostrum, then decrease gradually. However, the specific factors that are related to the Lf concentration in breast milk are unknown. Factors such as geographical location, ethnic origin, genetic polymorphisms, socio-economic status, nutritional status, as well as infants infections, type of delivery, and prematurity have been considered [16–18].

In human milk, Lf is the most abundant protein in the whey fraction [7]. The concentration of Lf in human milk is lactation-stage related: colostrum contains more than 5 g/L, which then significantly decreases to 2–3 g/L in mature milk. Multiple studies have evaluated Lf concentrations in human colostrum and mature milk and in term and preterm milk [7,19,20].

Lf elicits antibacterial effects against bacteria; however, Lf has protective activity due to the high affinity to iron. The iron-free form of Lf (apo-Lf) is a cause of iron deficiency in microorganisms as iron is required for life and growth rate [21]. Research has shown that the direct interaction between Lf and bacteria results in a bactericidal effect [22]. Lf associates with the lipoprotein of bacterial cells and forms receptor complexes. The binding of Lf inhibits the iron intake of bacteria or removes the protective effect of the membrane. Lf causes the release of lipopolysaccharides from the cell's wall, increases permeability of the membrane, and finally kills the Gram-negative bacteria. Lf binds the anionic molecules (e.g., lipoteichoic acid) on the cell surface of Gram-positive bacteria with greater effectiveness than lysozymes and antibiotics [23]. The antiviral effect of Lf is observed in the early phase of infection by inhibition of the growth of viruses. Lf and Lf-derived peptides can effectively act on a broad spectrum of fungal species, such as *Candida albicans*, *Candida krusei*, and *Aspergillus fumigatus* [24] by increasing membrane permeability, which leads to their death and additionally produces iron deprivation effects. Lf has a positively charged surface, which produces an anti-inflammatory effect. Lf interacts with proteoglycans on the surface of immune cells. This association can trigger signaling pathways that lead to physiological anti-inflammatory responses [25,26].

With reference to the research on the evolution of mammals, the protective function was the first in the ancestral mammary gland, which subsequently evolved to nourish the offspring. The protective components of milk remain highly conserved [27,28].

Breast milk after one year of lactation has nutritional value for children [29]. According to our previous results, the milk of mothers who breastfeed their children over one year or even over two years is standard value milk, and its macronutrient quantity composition is comparable mother's milk up to the first year of lactation [29]. However, further detailed quantitative data on the concentration and variability of the most important bioactive and immunomodulatory human milk proteins are necessary. The aim of this study was to evaluate lactoferrin concentration, the main glycoprotein with anti-pathogen activity, in breast milk during prolonged lactation from 1–48 months of lactation and to identify if any correlation exists between lactoferrin and protein concentrations during a healthy mother's lactation period. This is particularly important because Lf is an element providing innate immunity that is transferred to the breastfed infants and is crucial in the shaping and development of its immature immunological system.

2. Material and Methods

Mothers during lactation were recruited to the study from February 2017 to June 2018 using local groups for breastfeeding women on Facebook. We enrolled 120 participants in the study. The mother's age, socioeconomic status, race, health status, concomitant medications, parity, the mode of delivery, and frequency of breastfeeding were recorded. Milk samples were collected at the Regional Human Milk Bank and University Hospital (Wroclaw, Poland) between 08:00 and 14:00. Providing an interval of a few hours provides greater uniformity of samples. Considering efficiency of milk expression, an electric breast pump was used (Medela Symphony, Baar, Switzerland). Each mother received a sterile set and cup for milk collection. Samples for analyses ware taken immediately after complete emptying of the breast (two aliquots of 2–3 mL each). One session of milk expression should not deprive the infant of their nutritionally required volume. Milk samples were divided into four groups according to months postpartum: the first group was up to 12 months ($n = 24$), second group from 13 to18 months ($n = 33$), third group from 19 to 24 months ($n = 37$) and last group beyond 24 months ($n = 26$). The milk samples after collection were immediately cooled and frozen in −20 °C. This study received ethical approval Nr KB–65/2018 from the University Ethics Committee. Informed and written consent was provided by all participants before sample collection.

2.1. *Analysis of the Samples*

Each sample was initially heated at 40 °C as recommended by the human milk analyzer producer and homogenized using a sonicator (Sonicator®, MIRIS, Uppsala, Sweden) at 1.5 s/mL, to separate the lipid phase and avoid protein aggregation. Each aliquot was homogenized differently immediately prior to measurement. Analyses were performed in triplicate. Breast milk macronutrient concentration was measured using a human milk analyzer (HMA) (MIRIS, Uppsala, Sweden) calibrated previously with human milk standards. The HMA is based on mid-infrared spectroscopy, enabling the assessment of fat, protein, lactose, energy, and total solids content. Protein is the protein content based on the total amount of nitrogen (N) in a sample. This means that non-protein nitrogen (NPN) compounds are also included in this value. "True protein" is corrected for this and represents only the content of actual protein, hence the denotation "true". The Miris HMA (Uppsala, Sweden) measures both crude protein and true protein to avoid misunderstandings. The obtained results are expressed in g/L. A detailed description of the measurement method was described in previous study [29].

2.2. *Skim Milk Sample Preparation*

All collected samples of mother's milk were immediately transferred to the dedicated plastic tubes WHAT for freezing and stored at −20 °C until analysis. To obtain the aqueous phase of milk (skim milk), all milk samples were centrifuged at 3500× g at 4 °C for 35 min. Next, the milk fat layer and cells were removed [30]. The skim milk samples were aliquoted and stored at −20 °C. All milk samples were handled by the same person. Before the determinations of lactoferrin concentration, the skim milk samples were thawed at room temperature for one hour.

2.3. *Analysis of Lactoferrin in Skim Milk*

The concentration of lactoferrin in skim milk samples was determined according to a modified procedure reported previously [31]. For testing, 100 µL of 5×10^3, 10×10^3, 25×10^3, and 50×10^3 fold diluted skim milk samples and parallel standard of lactoferrin derived from human milk in concentrations ranging from 0.8 to 50 ng per 100 µL (Sigma Aldrich, St. Louis, MO, USA) in Tris-HCl buffer with sodium chloride (pH = 7.5) were added to the individual microtiter plate wells (Nunc International, Naperville, IL, USA) and incubated for 2 h at 37 °C. The concentration of lactoferrin was analyzed using rabbit anti-human lactoferrin antibodies phosphatase-labeled (Jackson ImmunoResearch Europe Ltd., Ely, UK) in TRIS-HCl buffer (pH = 7.5) with 0.2% Tween 20 for 1 h at 37 °C and then detected by the reaction with phosphatase's substrate, 4-nitrophenyl phosphate, disodium salt (SERVA, Heidelberg, Germany). The absorbance was measured after stopping the enzymatic reaction in a Stat Fax 2100 for Microplate Reader (Awareness Technology Inc., Palm City, FL, USA) using a 405 nm filter and 630 nm as the reference filter. The background absorbance for the ELISA test was low (below 0.04 AU) when Tris-buffered saline was added to the microtiter plate well instead of milk or lactoferrin standard samples. As the negative control, a human albumin (Sigma, St. Louis, MO, USA) was used. All skim milk samples were assayed at four different skim milk sample dilutions in duplicate. The intra-assay and inter-assay coefficients of variation were 4.8% and 5.6%, respectively.

2.4. Statistical Analysis

The statistical analysis was performed using the TIBCO STATISTICA 13.3 software package (StatSoft, Inc., Tulsa, OK, USA). The chi-square test was used for comparison the study population data. Due to the higher interindividual differences reported for many factors of human milk as well as the unequal sample size in the analyzed groups, nonparametric tests were used for analysis. Comparisons between analyzed groups were performed using the Kruskal–Wallis test. The obtained data are presented as the mean ± SD and the median with 25th–75th percentiles. To determine whether any relationships existed among the concentration of lactoferrin and analyzed factors, the correlations were evaluated according to Spearman's coefficient. A p-value lower than 0.05 was considered significant. The charts were prepared using linear regression with a 95% confidence level.

3. Results

The key characteristics of the cohort are detailed in Table 1. All infants were exclusively breastfed up to six months.

Table 1. Characteristics of the study population.

Outcome and Exposure Variables Breastfeeding	Breastfeeding ≤12 Months n = 24% (n/N)	Breastfeeding >12 Months n = 96% (n/N)	χ^2	p-Value	
Maternal age % (n/N)					
25–29	50 (12/24)	33 (31/94)			
30–34	41.7 (10/24)	45 (41/94)	2.672	0.139	NS
35+	8.3 (2/24)	22 (22/94)			
Race/ethnicity					
Caucasian	100 (24/24)	100 (96/96)	-	-	-
Socioeconomic status and education					
Secondary education	12.5 (3/24)	20 (16/96)	0.25	0.617	NS
High education	87.5 (21/24)	83.3 (80/96)			
Parity					
1	79 (19/24)	67.7 (65/96)			
2	21 (5/24)	33.3 (32/96)	1.628	0.22	NS
3	0 (0/24)	2 (2/96)			
Birth weight					
Appropriate for Gestational Age (AGA)	100 (24/24)	100 (96/96)	-	-	-
gestational age					
34–37	4.2(1/24)	1. (1/96)	1.144	0.285	NS
>37	95.8(23/24)	99 (95/96)			
Medicines during lactation					
No medications	71(17/24)	66 (63/96)			
Thyroxine	21(5/24)	29 (28/96)	0.884	0.643	NS
Others	8(2/24)	5 (5/96)			
Maternal diet during lactation					
Vegan/vegetarian	0 (0/24)	8 (8/96)			
Dairy-free diet	21 (5/24)	7 (7/96)	-	-	-
Gluten-free diet	0 (0/24)	3 (3/96)			
Complementary foods introduction above 6 months of life	NA	94 (90/96)	-	-	-

χ^2 test at $p < 0.05$; NA—Not assessed, NS—Not significant. -: not calculated

3.1. Lactoferrin

To determine if the concentration of lactoferrin in mother's milk is connected with the month of prolonged lactation, the correlation was calculated; however, the obtained result showed no correlation ($r = 0.1675$; $p = 0.0674$) with prolonged lactation from the first to the 48th month, as shown in Figure 1A.

The mean value of lactoferrin concentration was the lowest value in the group of 12 months of lactation (3.39 ± 1.43 g/L), significantly increasing in the 13–18 months group (5.55 ± 4.00 g/L; $p < 0.006$)

and remaining stable thereafter in the groups of 19–24 months and over 24 months (5.02 ± 2.97 and 4.90 ± 3.18 g/L, respectively) (Table 2).

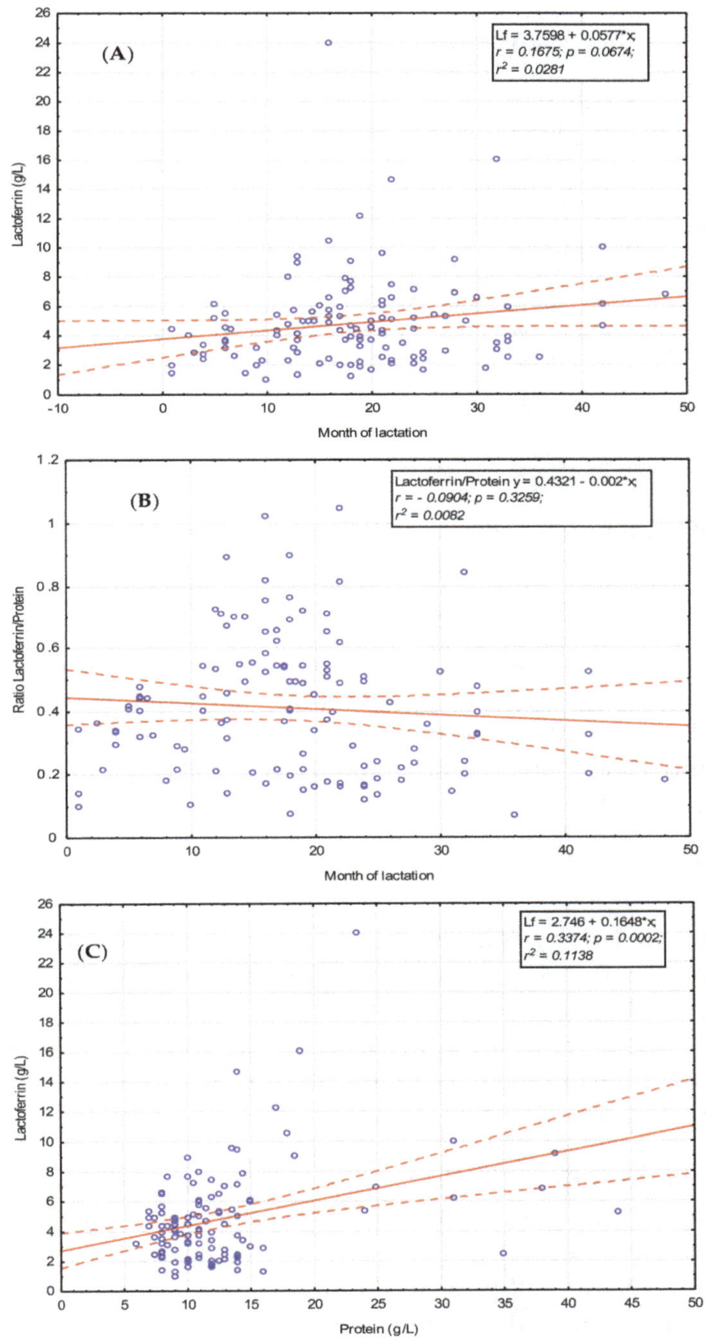

Figure 1. The correlation of (**A**) lactoferrin and (**B**) the ratio of lactoferrin to protein concentration with lactation progression from the 1st to the 48th month and (**C**) the correlation of lactoferrin and protein concentrations for all analyzed samples. A solid line indicates linear regression, and 95% confidence intervals are shown by dotted lines; blue hollow—individual samples; solid circle—2 or more individual samples with the same or very close values. *: multiplied

Table 2. Lactoferrin and protein concentrations in breast milk during prolonged lactation.

Breast Milk. Lactoferrin/Protein Content	Lactation			
	1–12 Months $n = 24$	13–18 Months $n = 33$	19–24 Months $n = 37$	>24 Months $n = 26$
Lactoferrin (g/L)	3.39 ± 1.43 3.24 2.30–4.47	5.55 ± 4.00 * 4.92 3.69–6.08 $p < 0.006$	5.02 ± 2.97 4.42 3.16–6.53	4.90 ± 3.18 4.29 2.49–6.18
Protein (g/L)	10.5 ± 2.3 10.0 8.5–12.8	10.4 ± 3.4 9.0 8.0–11.0	11.2 ± 2.7 ** 11.0 9.5–12.0 $p < 0.05$	19.1 ± 10.7 *** 14.3 12.0–25.0 $p < 0.0001$
Lactoferrin/Protein ratio	0.32 ± 0.12 0.33 0.25–0.41	0.49 ± 0.21 * 0.54 0.36–0.65 $p < 0.002$	0.43 ± 0.21 0.45 0.22–0.54	0.29 ± 0.17 *** 0.24 0.18–0.36 $p < 0.009$

Values are given as the mean ± SD, median and 25th–75th percentiles. The Mann–Whitney U-test was used for statistical calculations, and a p-value lower than 0.05 was considered significant. Significantly different from the milk group of: * 1–12 months of lactation, ** 13–18 months of lactation, *** 19–24 months of lactation.

3.2. Total Protein

The concentration of protein in mother's milk was positively correlated with prolonged lactation during the analyzed period up to 48 months; however, the correlation coefficient value was weak ($r = 0.25$; $p < 0.05$).

The mean values of protein concentrations were comparable in the groups of 1–12 and 13–18 months of lactation (10.5 ± 2.3 and 10.4 ± 3.4 g/L, respectively). In subsequent analyzed lactation periods, i.e., 19–24 and over 24 months of lactation, protein concentrations significantly increased and reached 11.2 ± 2.7 g/L ($p < 0.05$) and 19.1 ± 10.7 g/L ($p < 0.0001$), respectively (Table 2).

3.3. Lactoferrin/Protein Ratio

To identify the existence of any relationship between the concentration of lactoferrin and the concentration of total protein, the correlation coefficient was calculated. Mother's milk lactoferrin was positively correlated with protein concentration ($r = 0.3374$; $p = 0.0002$), as shown in Figure 1B, for the analyzed set of samples derived for 1–48 months of lactation. However, for both lactoferrin and protein concentrations, high interindividual differences among mothers were observed and this result may be characteristic for our particular data set only.

In contrast, the calculated coefficient of lactoferrin to the protein concentration (Lf/Protein) showed no correlation with lactation progression for 1–48 months ($r = -0.0904$; $p = 0.3259$) as shown in Figure 1C. The calculated coefficient of Lf/Protein in the group of 1-12 months of lactation reached 0.32 ± 0.12, significantly increasing in the 13–18-month group (0.49 ± 0.21, $p < 0.002$) and remaining at a comparable level in the 19–24-month group (0.43 ± 0.21), decreasing in the >24 months group to 0.29 ± 0.17 ($p < 0.009$; Table 2, Figure 2).

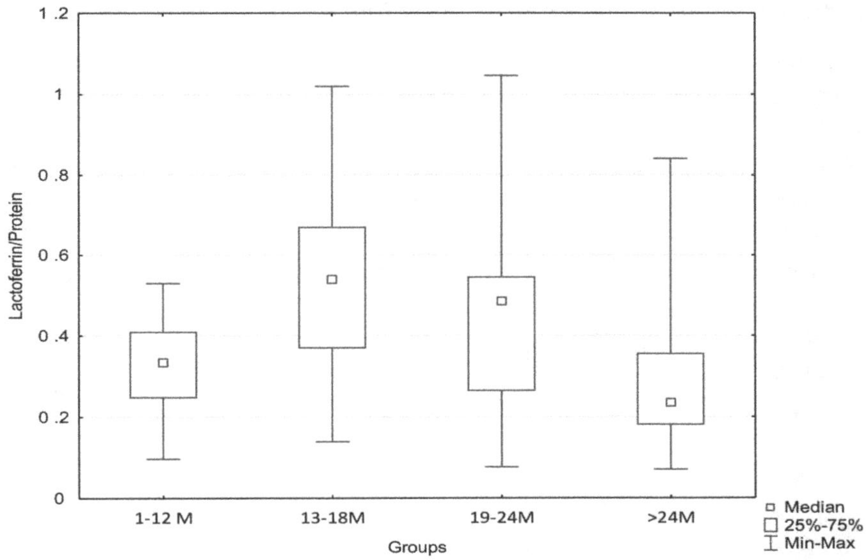

Figure 2. The coefficient of lactoferrin to the protein concentration in the four groups analyzed: Group1 up to 12 months (n = 24), group 2 from 13 to 18 months (n = 33), group 3 from 19 to 24 months (n = 37), and group 2 above 24 months (n = 26).

3.4. Lactoferrin Concentration in Relation to Macronutrients

The dependencies between lactoferrin concentration and macronutrients in mother's milk were analyzed throughout the whole lactation period, 1–12, 13–18, 19–24, and >24 months of lactation. The values of the calculated coefficient, which are statistically significant ($p < 0.05$), are given in Table 3. In contrast with the lack of correlation between lactoferrin concentration and month of lactation for 1–48 months of lactation, a positive correlation was found for prolonged lactation, specifically above 24 months. The concentration of lactoferrin over 24 months is negatively correlated negatively with the concentration of carbohydrates ($r = -0.50$) and positively with the concentration of fat ($r = 0.58$), protein ($r = 0.56$), true protein ($r = 0.58$), dry mass ($r = 0.65$), and energy ($r = 0.65$). A statistically significant negative correlation was found between lactoferrin concentration and carbohydrates ($r = -0.32$) and positive correlations between lactoferrin and fat ($r = 0.19$), protein ($r = 0.25$), true protein ($r = 0.24$), dry mass ($r = 0.18$), and energy ($r = 0.19$) in the lactation from month 1 to 48. However, the correlations observed were much stronger in prolonged lactation above the month 24. In contrast, no correlations were found in the other analyzed periods of lactation, namely up to month 12, months 13–18, and 19–24.

Table 3. Correlations between lactoferrin and macronutrients over prolonged lactation from month 1 to 48 and for particular periods.

	Correlation Coefficient (r Value *)				
	Lactoferrin				
	1–48 months	1–12 months	13–18 months	19–24 months	Over 24 months
Duration of lactation	NS	NS	NS	NS	0.39
Carbohydrate	–0.32	NS	NS	NS	–0.50
Fat	0.19	NS	NS	NS	0.58
Protein	0.25	NS	NS	NS	0.56
True protein	0.24	NS	NS	NS	0.58
Dry mass	0.18	NS	NS	NS	0.65
Energy	0.19	NS	NS	NS	0.65

The values of r were calculated according to Spearman's method corresponding to the correlation between the concentrations of lactoferrin and macronutrients over prolonged lactation from month 1 to 48. * all r values are statistically significant with $p < 0.05$. NS—Not significant.

3.5. Lactoferrin Concentration in Breast Milk in Relation to the Number of Feedings

The relationship between lactoferrin concentration of mother's milk and the number of feedings during the analyzed period from month 13 to 48 and the three stages of prolonged lactation, namely months 13–18, 19–24, and >24 of lactation were analyzed. We found no significant correlations for months 13–48 (Figure 3A) as well as for months 13–18 and 19–24; however, for lactation over 24 months, we observed a weak negative tendency between the number of feedings and lactoferrin concentration ($r = -0.26$; $p = 0.2868$; Figure 3B). Additionally, we found no correlation between lactoferrin concentration and maternal age, parity, or time of delivery-gestational age.

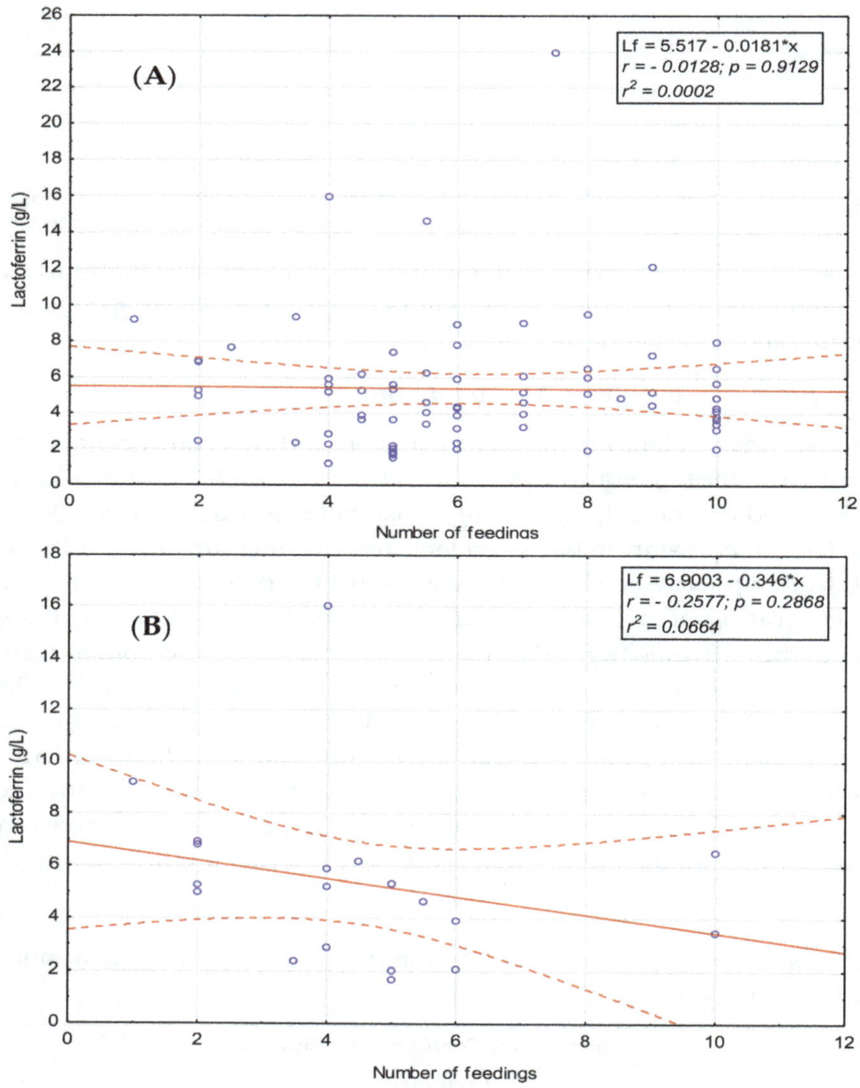

Figure 3. Relationship between the concentration of lactoferrin and the number of feedings mother's milk (**A**) during 13–48 months of lactation, (**B**) over 24 months of lactation. A solid line indicates linear regression, and 95% confidence intervals are shown by dotted lines; blue hollow—individual samples. *: multiplied.

4. Discussion

HM is a dynamic fluid that changes significantly in its composition from the onset of lactation to prolonged lactation above one year postpartum [29,32]. Total milk protein concentration decreases during the lactation period, but this trend is not general for all proteins. In our previous work, we demonstrated that macronutrients concentrations change in prolonged lactation. As a continuation of the previous study, lactoferrin changes in prolonged lactation were assessed in this study. During the first month of lactation, Lf decreases and then remains relatively stable [33]. The highest content of Lf is in colostrum at 5.5 g/L, whereas mature milk contains only 1.5–3.0 g/L, dependent on the stage of lactation in the first year postpartum [32,34,35]. Affolter et al. [36] reported that the concentration of lactoferrin decreases over the lactation period from the fifth day to eight months from 3.30 to 1.17 g/L. However, this decrease was constant during lactation until one to two months (1.24 g/L), and then stabilized until the eighth month. Changes in Lf content may reflect various biological functions of milk during different stages of newborn and infant development [33].

Our results show that the Lf concentration during prolonged lactation ranges from 4.9 to 5.02 g/L. Previous studies have shown that Lf concentration is negatively correlated with the volume of milk expression as well as the stage of lactation and parity [33,37]. The results showed the highest Lf content was recorded between 12 and 24 months of lactation. Above 24 months, concentration decreases, although not significantly, to 4.9 g/L. To the best of our knowledge, this is the first study assessing Lf concentration in human milk during prolonged lactation. These data have shown that Lf content above 12 months of lactation is higher and close to the Lf concentration in colostrum.

The concentration of lactoferrin in mother's milk showed a positive correlation with protein concentration over lactation from the early stage until four years postpartum. The coefficient of Lf concentration to protein did not show a correlation with lactation progression. Lf concentration and milk compositions are influenced by various factors such as health conditions and/or biochemical indicators of blood [33–36].

A notable inter-individual variability of lactoferrin content has also been observed, suggesting a lack of tight regulation in the synthesis and/or blood-to-mammary gland transfer of this protein [34]. Thereby, milk enhances the survival of offspring by promoting immunological competence. The rising concentrations of bioactive proteins, which occur as lactation progresses, are likely a physiological response to the diverse environmental demands of the human baby, which progressively acquires nutritional independence [38].

Raw mother's milk contains a relatively high concentration of Lf, which leads to more effective inhibition of growth of pathogenic bacteria in comparison to pasteurized mother's milk. As shown by Woodman et al. [38], human Lf is much more effective than bovine Lf in the inhibition of bacterial growth, although higher doses of bovine Lf also showed activity against *Bifidobacterium breve* and *Staphylococcus epidermidis*. Given the above, we suggest that human milk from prolonged lactation, which contains a comparable level of Lf, might be considered an alternative source of milk/lactoferrin provided in the feeding of preterm infants, although further detailed analysis is needed. Different methods used to preserve human milk bioactivity significantly impact Lf concentration [31]. Only further studies involving detailed tests of lactoferrin concentration in milk samples from prolonged lactation before and after pasteurization will help answer this question.

The strength of our study is that it is a unique and well-characterized collection of milk samples of mothers with prolonged lactation of up to 48 months, which impacts the credibility of the results obtained. To determine Lf concentration, a specific immunological method, ELISA, was used to prevent obtaining of false positive results. A limitation of our study is the homogeneous test group, which may not enable drawing a causal relationship between the factors that can influence milk Lf concentration, since, as reported by Yang et al. [33], milk Lf concentrations varies amongst different geographical regions in the Chinese population.

Evidence of stable or increasing immunoprotein levels during prolonged lactation provides the additional argument for allowing non-weaning; however, breastfeeding must be combined with solid foods to meet all the new requirements of a rapidly growing six-month or older baby. A number of clinical trials have been conducted to determine the influence of Lf on the protection against neonatal infections [39,40]. Based on published studies of Lf supplementation in preventing infection, determining the Lf concentration during lactation is important not only in the first six months. If the concentration changes during the lactation phase, colostrum has the highest Lf concentration, and decreases significantly during days after delivery. We now know that the milk of long-nursing mothers has a similar concentration to that in colostrum. Physicians should consider this to encourage exclusive breastfeeding, especially in risk groups such as premature babies [41].

To the best of our knowledge, based on the Internet databases such as Web of Science and pubmed, this is the first large-scale study performed on lactoferrin concentration in breast milk during prolonged lactation and the influence of various factors on its concentration. Coincident with the lack of public acceptance of breastfeeding beyond the first or even the second year, these findings have been ignored for decades.

5. Conclusions

Results show that the Lf concentration during prolonged lactation ranges from 4.9 to 5.02 g/L. The highest Lf content was recorded between 12 and 24 months of lactation. Above 24 months, concentration decreases, although not significantly. These data have shown that Lf content above 12 months of lactation is close to the Lf concentration in colostrum.

Author Contributions: M.C.-Ł. and M.O.-P.: These authors contributed equally to this work. Conceptualization, M.C.-Ł., M.O.P. and B.K.-O.; Methodology, M.O.-P. and M.C.-Ł.; Formal Analysis, M.O.-P. and M.C.-Ł.; Writing-Original Draft Preparation, M.C.-Ł. B.K.-O., M.O.-P. and. B.B.; Writing—Review & Editing, B.K.-O., M.O.-P.; Visualization, M.O.-P.; Supervision, B.K.-O.

Acknowledgments: We would like to thank Zuzanna Sycz and the mothers who came to the Regional Human Milk Bank in University Hospital in Wrocław and expressed breast milk to the study. We would like to also thank Robin and Barbara Royle for their help in the language correction of the text.

References

1. Ballard, O.; Morrow, A.L. Human milk composition: Nutrients and bioactive factors. *Pediatr. Clin. N. Am.* **2013**, *60*, 49–74. [CrossRef] [PubMed]
2. Sorensen, M.; Sorensen, S.P.L. The proteins in whey. *Compte Rendu Trav. Lab. Carlsberg* **1939**, *23*, 55–99.
3. Groves, M.L. The isolation of a red protein from milk. *J. Am. Chem. Soc.* **1960**, *83*, 3345–3350. [CrossRef]
4. Johansson, B. Isolation of an iron-containing red protein from human milk. *Acta Chem. Scand.* **1960**, *14*, 510–512. [CrossRef]
5. Montreuil, J.; Tonnelat, J.; Mullet, S. Preparation and properties of lactosiderophilin (lactotransferrin) of human milk. *Biochim. Biophys. Acta* **1960**, *45*, 413–421. [CrossRef]
6. Rosa, L.; Cutone, A.; Lepanto, M.S.; Paesano, R.; Valenti, P. Lactoferrin: A Natural Glycoprotein Involved in Iron and Inflammatory Homeostasis. *Int. J. Mol. Sci.* **2017**, *18*, 1985. [CrossRef] [PubMed]
7. Liao, Y.; Alvarado, R.; Phinney, B.; Lönnerdal, B. Proteomic characterization of human milk whey proteins during a twelve-month lactation period. *J. Proteome Res.* **2011**, *10*, 1746–1754. [CrossRef]
8. Lönnerdal, B.; Iyer, S. Lactoferrin: Molecular structure and biological function. *Annu. Rev. Nutr.* **1995**, *15*, 93–110. [CrossRef]
9. Vogel, H.J. Lactoferrin, a bird's eye view. *Biochem. Cell Biol.* **2012**, *90*, 233–244. [CrossRef]
10. Lönnerdal, B. Nutritional roles of lactoferrin. *Curr. Opin. Clin. Nutr. Metab. Care* **2009**, *12*, 293–297. [CrossRef]
11. Zavaleta, N.; Figueroa, D.; Rivera, J.; Julia, S.; Segundo, A.; Bo, L. Efficacy of rice-based oral rehydration solution containing recombinant human lactoferrin and lysozyme in Peruvian children with acute diarrhea. *J. Pediatr. Gastroenterol. Nutr.* **2007**, *44*, 258–264. [CrossRef] [PubMed]
12. Ochoa, T.J.; Chea-Woo, E.; Baiocchi, N.; Pecho, I.; Campos, M.; Prada, A.; Valdiviezo, G.; Lluque, A.; Lai, D.; Cleary, T.G. Randomized double-blind controlled trial of bovine lactoferrin for prevention of diarrhea in children. *J. Pediatr.* **2013**, *162*, 349–356. [CrossRef] [PubMed]
13. Manzoni, P.; Rinaldi, M.; Cattani, S.; Pugni, L.; Romeo, M.G.; Messner, H.; Stolfi, I.; Decembrino, L.; Laforgia, N.; Vagnarelli, F.; et al. Bovine lactoferrin supplementation for prevention of late-onset sepsis in very low-birth-weight neonates: A randomized trial. *JAMA* **2009**, *302*, 1421–1428. [CrossRef] [PubMed]

14. Manzoni, P.; Garcia Sanchez, R.; Meyer, M.; Stolfi, I.; Pugni, L.; Messner, H.; Cattani, S.; Betta, P.M.; Memo, L.; Decembrino, L. Exposure to gastric acid inhibitors increases the risk of infection in preterm very low birth weight infants but concomitant administration of lactoferrin counteracts this effect. *J. Pediatr.* **2018**, *193*, 62–67. [CrossRef] [PubMed]
15. Pammi, M.; Suresh, G. Enteral lactoferrin supplementation for prevention of sepsis and necrotizing enterocolitis in preterm infants. *Cochrane Database Syst. Rev.* **2017**, *6*, CD007137. [CrossRef] [PubMed]
16. Mastromarino, P.; Capobianco, D.; Campagna, G.; Laforgia, N.; Drimaco, P.; Dileone, A.; Baldassarre, M.E. Correlation between lactoferrin and beneficial microbiota in breast milk and infant's feces. *Biometals* **2014**, *27*, 1077–1086. [CrossRef] [PubMed]
17. Broadhurst, M.; Beddis, K.; Black, J.; Henderson, H.; Nair, A.; Wheeler, T. Effect of gestation length on the levels of five innate defence proteins in human milk. *Early Hum. Dev.* **2015**, *91*, 7–11. [CrossRef]
18. Villavicencio, A.; Rueda, M.S.; Turin, C.G.; Ochoa, T.J. Factors affecting lactoferrin concentration in human milk: How much do we know? *Biochem. Cell Biol.* **2016**, *95*, 12–21. [CrossRef]
19. Ronayne de Ferrer, P.A.; Baroni, A.; Sambucetti, M.E.; López, N.E.; Cernadas, J.M.C. Lactoferrin levels in term and preterm milk. *J. Am. Coll. Nutr.* **2000**, *19*, 370–373. [CrossRef]
20. Lönnerdal, B. Law infant nutrition: Bioactive proteins of human milk and implications for composition of infant formulas. *Am. J. Clin. Nutr.* **2014**, *99*, 712S–717S. [CrossRef]
21. Law, B.A.; Reiter, B. The isolation and bacteriostatic properties of lactoferrin from bovine milk whey. *J. Dairy Res.* **1977**, *44*, 595–599. [CrossRef] [PubMed]
22. Ostan, N.K.; Yu, R.H.; Ng, D.; Lai, C.C.-L.; Pogoutse, A.K.; Sarpe, V.; Hepburn, M.; Sheff, J.; Raval, S.; Schriemer, D.C.; et al. Lactoferrin binding protein B–a bi-functional bacterial receptor protein. *PLoS Pathog.* **2017**, *13*, e1006244. [CrossRef] [PubMed]
23. Barbiroli, A.; Bonomi, F.; Capretti, G.I.; Iametti, S.; Manzoni, M.; Piergiovanni, L.; Rollini, M. Antimicrobial activity of lysozyme and lactoferrin incorporated in cellulose-based food packaging. *Food Control* **2012**, *26*, 387–392. [CrossRef]
24. Zarember, K.A.; Sugui, J.A.; Chang, Y.C.; Kwon-Chung, K.J.; Gallin, J.I. Human polymorphonuclear leukocytes inhibit Aspergillus fumigatus conidial growth by lactoferrin-mediated iron depletion. *J. Immunol.* **2007**, *178*, 6367–6373. [CrossRef]
25. Legrand, D. Overview of Lactoferrin as a Natural Immune Modulator. *J. Pediatr.* **2016**, *173*, S10–S15. [CrossRef] [PubMed]
26. Wang, B.; Timilsena, Y.P.; Blanch, E.; Adhikari, B. Lactoferrin: Structure, Function, Denaturation and Digestion. *Crit. Rev. Food Sci. Nutr.* **2019**, *59*, 580–596. [CrossRef]
27. Hassiotou, F.; Geddes, D.T. Immune Cell–Mediated Protection of the Mammary Gland and the Infant during Breastfeeding. *Adv Nutr.* **2015**, *6*, 267–275. [CrossRef] [PubMed]
28. Vorbach, C.; Capecchi, M.R.; Penninger, J.M. Evolution of the mammary gland from the innate immune system? *Bioessays* **2006**, *28*, 606–616. [CrossRef]
29. Czosnykowska-Łukacka, M.; Królak-Olejnik, B.; Orczyk-Pawiłowicz, M. Breast Milk Macronutrient Components in Prolonged Lactation. *Nutrients* **2018**, *10*, 1893. [CrossRef]
30. Orczyk-Pawiłowicz, M.; Hirnle, L.; Berghausen-Mazur, M.; Kątnik-Prastowska, I.M. Lactation stage-related expression of sialylated and fucosylated glycotopes of human milk α-1-acid glycoprotein. *Breastfeed Med.* **2014**, *9*, 313–319. [CrossRef]
31. Wesolowska, A.; Sinkiewicz-Darol, E.; Barbarska, O.; Strom, K.; Rutkowska, M.; Karzel, K.; Rosiak, E.; Oledzka, G.; Orczyk-Pawiłowicz, M.; Rzoska, S.; et al. New Achievements in High-Pressure Processing to Preserve Human Milk Bioactivity. *Front. Pediatr.* **2018**, *16*, 323. [CrossRef] [PubMed]
32. Rai, D.; Adelman, A.S.; Zhuang, W.; Rai, G.P.; Boettcher, J.; Lönnerdal, B. Longitudinal changes in lactoferrin concentrations in human milk: A global systematic review. *Crit. Rev. Food Sci. Nutr.* **2014**, *54*, 1539–1547. [CrossRef] [PubMed]
33. Yang, Z.; Jiang, R.; Chen, Q.; Wang, J.; Duan, Y.; Pang, X.; Jiang, S.; Bi, Y.; Zhang, H.; Lönnerdal, B.; et al. Concentration of Lactoferrin in Human Milk and Its Variation during Lactation in Different Chinese Populations. *Nutrients* **2018**, *10*, 1235. [CrossRef] [PubMed]
34. Haschke, F.; Haiden, N.; Thakkar, S.K. Nutritive and bioactive proteins in breastmilk. *Ann. Nutr. Metab.* **2016**, *69*, 16–26. [CrossRef] [PubMed]

35. Garcia-Rodenas, C.L.; De Castro, C.A.; Jenni, R.; Thakkar, S.K.; Beauport, L.; Tolsa, J.-F.; Fischer-Fumeaux, C.J.; Affolter, M. Temporal changes of major protein concentrations in preterm and term human milk. A prospective cohort study. *Clin. Nutr.* **2019**, *38*, 1844–1852. [CrossRef] [PubMed]
36. Affolter, M.; Garcia-Rodenas, C.; Vinyes-Pares, G.; Jenni, R.; Roggero, I.; Avanti-Nigro, O.; de Castro, C.A.; Zhao, A.; Zhang, Y.; Wang, P.; et al. Temporal changes of protein composition in breast milk of Chinese Urban mothers and impact of caesarean section delivery. *Nutrients* **2016**, *8*, 504. [CrossRef] [PubMed]
37. Trend, S.; Strunk, T.; Lloyd, M.; Kok, C.H.; Metcalfe, J.; Geddes, D.T.; Lai, C.T.; Richmond, P.; Doherty, D.A.; Simmer, K.; et al. Levels of innate immune factors in preterm and term mothers' breast milk during the 1st month postpartum. *Br. J. Nutr.* **2016**, *115*, 1178–1193. [CrossRef]
38. Woodman, T.; Strunk, T.; Patole, S.; Hartmann, B.; Simmer, K.; Currie, A. Effects of lactoferrin on neonatal pathogens and Bifidobacterium breve in human breast milk. *PLoS ONE* **2018**, *13*, e0201819. [CrossRef]
39. Ochoa, T.J.; Pezo, A.; Cruz, K.; Chea-Woo, E.; Cleary, T.G. Clinical studies of lactoferrin in children. *Biochem. Cell Biol.* **2012**, *90*, 457–467. [CrossRef] [PubMed]
40. Siqueiros-Cendón, T.; Arévalo-Gallegos, S.; Iglesias-Figueroa, B.F.; García-Montoya, I.A.; Salazar-Martínez, J.; Rascón-Cruz, Q. Immunomodulatory effects of lactoferrin. *Acta Pharmacol. Sin.* **2014**, *35*, 557–566. [CrossRef]
41. Newburg, S.; Walker, W.A. Protection of the neonate by the innate immune system of developing gut and of human milk. *Pediatr. Res.* **2007**, *61*, 2. [CrossRef] [PubMed]

8

Concentrations of Water-Soluble Forms of Choline in Human Milk from Lactating Women in Canada and Cambodia

Alejandra M. Wiedeman [1,2], Kyly C. Whitfield [1,2,3], Kaitlin M. March [1,2], Nancy N. Chen [1,2], Hou Kroeun [4], Ly Sokhoing [4], Prak Sophonneary [5], Roger A. Dyer [2], Zhaoming Xu [1], David D. Kitts [1], Timothy J. Green [1,2,6], Sheila M. Innis [2,†] and Susan I. Barr [1,*]

1 Food, Nutrition, and Health Program, The University of British Columbia, Vancouver, BC V6T 1Z4, Canada; awiedeman@bcchr.ca (A.M.W.); kyly.whitfield@msvu.ca (K.C.W.); kaitlin.march@cw.bc.ca (K.M.M.); nnchen30@gmail.com (N.N.C.); zhaoming.xu@ubc.ca (Z.X.); david.kitts@ubc.ca (D.D.K.); tim.green@sahmri.com (T.J.G.)
2 BC Children's Hospital Research Institute, Vancouver, BC V5Z 4H4, Canada; radyer@mail.ubc.ca (R.A.D.); sinnis@mail.ubc.ca (S.M.I.)
3 Department of Applied Human Nutrition, Mount Saint Vincent University, Halifax, NS B3M 2J6, Canada
4 Helen Keller International—Cambodia Country Office, Phnom Penh 12301, Cambodia; hkroeun@hki.org (H.K.); lsokhoing@hki.org (L.S.)
5 National Nutrition Programme, Maternal and Child Health Centre, Ministry of Health, Phnom Penh 12202, Cambodia; sophonprak@gmail.com
6 South Australia Health and Medical Research Institute, Adelaide, SA 5000, Australia
* Correspondence: susan.barr@ubc.ca
† Deceased.

Abstract: Choline has critical roles during periods of rapid growth and development, such as infancy. In human milk, choline is mostly present in water-soluble forms (free choline, phosphocholine, and glycerophosphocholine). It is thought that milk choline concentration is influenced by maternal choline intake, and the richest food sources for choline are of animal origin. Scarce information exists on milk choline from countries differing in animal-source food availability. In this secondary analysis of samples from previous trials, the concentrations of the water-soluble forms of choline were quantified by liquid chromatography-tandem mass spectrometry in mature milk samples collected from lactating women in Canada (n = 301) and in Cambodia (n = 67). None of the water-soluble forms of choline concentrations in milk differed between Canada and Cambodia. For all milk samples (n = 368), free choline, phosphocholine, glycerophosphocholine, and the sum of water-soluble forms of choline concentrations in milk were (mean (95%CI)) 151 (141, 160, 540 (519, 562), 411 (396, 427), and 1102 (1072, 1133) μmol/L, respectively. Theoretically, only 19% of infants would meet the current Adequate Intake (AI) for choline. Our findings suggest that the concentrations in milk of water-soluble forms of choline are similar in Canada and Cambodia, and that the concentration used to set the infant AI might be inaccurate.

Keywords: choline; phosphocholine; glycerophosphocholine; lactation; human milk; infants; adequate intake; dietary recommendations; Canada; Cambodia

1. Introduction

Choline is an essential nutrient with important roles during periods of rapid growth and development, such as early infancy [1–3]. Choline has a wide range of functions, including serving as a precursor for the synthesis of acetylcholine, phospholipids critical for cell membranes, surfactants important in lung maturity, bile formation, and betaine, which is an osmolyte and a methyl group donor [4,5]. In humans, large amounts of choline are present in milk, mainly as the water-soluble forms free choline, phosphocholine, and glycerophosphocholine, contributing an average of 84% of the total choline, whereas the lipid-soluble (phosphatidylcholine and sphingomyelin) forms account for the remaining 16% [6–10]. It has been reported that milk choline concentrations are positively associated with circulating choline concentrations in infants [7], and elevated circulating choline, as free choline, might enhance free choline uptake across the blood-brain barrier [11,12]. The authors of a recent observational study suggest that higher milk free choline concentration (mean 158 μmol/L) is associated with better infant recognition memory (latency at central leads, $\beta = 1.90$, $R^2 = 0.30$, $p < 0.01$) adjusted by other milk nutrients at an age of six months [13].

The World Health Organization recommends exclusive breastfeeding for the first six months to promote optimal growth of the infant [14]. Generally, the average concentration of nutrients in mature milk from healthy, well-nourished mothers, in conjunction with the average volume consumed by fully breast-fed infants, is used to set dietary recommendations for infancy and to determine the additional amount of the nutrient over the recommendation for non-lactating women for lactation [1]. For early infancy (0–6 months), the Adequate Intake (AI) for choline was set at 125 mg/day (equivalent to 1500 μmol/L and an assumed volume of 780 mL) [1]. Milk choline concentrations are thought to reflect habitual maternal dietary choline intake [15,16], with foods of animal origin being the richest source of choline [17].

Limited data are available on choline concentration in mature human milk, including reports from the United States [6,8,10,18], Turkey [7,9], Canada [19], Japan [20], Korea [21], Sweden [22], and Ecuador [15]. Nevertheless, sample sizes in these studies are small (n = 1–75), and include milk samples collected after a full-term, pre-term, or mixed birth term pregnancy. Moreover, the available data on milk choline are generally from high-income countries where maternal animal-source food availability [23] and consumption is greater than in middle- and low-income countries [24,25].

In this study, we used secondary data from recent randomized controlled trials (none of which provided choline), in which mature milk samples were collected from lactating women in Canada and Cambodia, two countries differing in dietary food source availability [23]. Our primary aim was to assess the concentration of the water-soluble forms of choline. In addition, we also explored the associations between maternal dietary choline intake and milk concentrations of water-soluble forms of choline in a subset of the Canadian participants. We found that the concentrations of milk water-soluble forms of choline did not significantly differ between Canada and Cambodia, despite lower likely choline intakes in Cambodia, and that maternal total dietary choline intake was not significantly associated with the concentration of water-soluble forms of choline in milk in a subset of the Canadian participants.

2. Materials and Methods

2.1. *Study Participants and Sample Collection*

The present study was a secondary cross-sectional analysis of previous randomized controlled trials conducted in Canada and Cambodia [26–28]. In all the trials, convenience samples of mature milk were collected from apparently healthy lactating women (18–45 year) who had low-risk pregnancies, uncomplicated deliveries, and gave birth to healthy, full-term infants. All subjects gave their informed consent for inclusion before they participated in the studies. The studies were conducted in accordance with the Declaration of Helsinki. Demographic characteristics including age, ethnicity, education, and household income were collected from the participants.

2.1.1. Canadian Samples

In Canada, participants were enrolled in two supplementation trials (neither of which contained choline) and have been previously described [26,27]. In the first trial, women had consumed a daily supplement containing docosahexaenoic acid or placebo from 16 weeks gestation through to the end of pregnancy [26]. In the second trial, women had consumed a daily prenatal multivitamin and mineral supplement and were randomly assigned to one of three vitamin D supplement groups between 13–24 weeks gestation through to eight weeks postpartum [27]. The University of British Columbia Children's and Women's Research Ethics Board approved these trials (H08-70242 and H09-01261).

Canadian participants provided a single mature milk sample at eight weeks postpartum. In the first trial, hindmilk samples were collected at the participant's house into pre-labeled tubes and stored in a home freezer for up to three days before being stored at −80 °C [26]. For the present study, a total of 147 milk samples from the first trial were available for analysis. In the second Canadian trial, a full breast expression from the breast that had not been most recently emptied was collected during a clinical visit and stored at −80 °C [27]. For the present study, a total of 154 milk samples from the second trial were available for analysis.

2.1.2. Cambodian Samples

In Cambodia, women had been consuming either a thiamine-fortified or placebo fish sauce, containing insignificant choline content [17], ad libitum for six months before milk collection [28]. The Cambodian National Ethics Committee for Health Research (245 NECHR) approved this trial.

Participants provided a single mature milk sample between three to 28 weeks postpartum as a full breast expression from the breast that had not been most recently emptied in their villages in Prey Veng. The milk samples were transported on ice to the National Institute of Public Health in Phnom Penh (<5 h) for storage at −80 °C until being shipped on dry ice to the University of British Columbia for analysis. For the present study, a total of 67 milk samples from Cambodia were available for analysis.

2.2. *Biochemical Analysis*

For all milk samples (n = 368), the concentrations of the water-soluble forms of choline (free choline, phosphocholine, and glycerophosphocholine) were quantified in 20 µL aliquots by stable isotope dilution liquid chromatography-tandem mass spectrometry (LC-MS/MS), according to the method described in detail elsewhere [19]. The inter-assay and intra-assay coefficients of variation were: 4.8% and 1.4% for free choline, 5.4% and 0.2% for phosphocholine, and 3.6% and 2.1% for glycerophosphocholine, respectively.

2.3. *Dietary Choline Intake Assessment*

For all infants (n = 368), dietary choline intake was estimated using milk total choline concentration and daily reference intake volume, based on the methods used to set the AI for early infancy [1]. First, total choline in milk was calculated by multiplying the concentration of the sum of the water-soluble forms of choline of each participant by a conversion factor (1.19), based on the assumption that on average the water-soluble forms of choline make up 84% of total choline in human milk [6–9,13]. Then, dietary choline intake from milk was estimated using 780 mL/day as the reference volume of milk consumption of breastfed infants during their first six months [1].

In Canada, dietary intake during lactation was available for 143 of the participants enrolled in the first trial. Intake was estimated using a semi-quantitative food frequency questionnaire (FFQ), covering the intake of the previous month, administered at 16 and 36 weeks of gestation. Dietary intakes of choline were estimated using a nutrient analysis software (ESHA Food Processor SQL, version 10.14.41; Salem, OR) and the United States Department of Agriculture (USDA) database on the Choline Content of Common Foods (Version 2) [17]. A validation analysis indicated that compared to the mean of three 24 h recalls, the FFQ was a valid instrument to assess dietary choline intake: the energy-adjusted de-attenuated correlation coefficient was 0.70, only 7.5% were grossly misclassified (e.g., opposite tertiles), and weighted Cohen's kappa was 0.32 [29].

2.4. Statistical Analysis

All statistical analyses were performed using SPSS 22.0 (SPSS Inc., Chicago, IL, USA) and statistical significance was set at $p < 0.05$ for two-sided testing. Data normality was determined using the Kolmogorov-Smirnov test, and skewed distributed data was log-transformed before further analyses. The concentrations of water-soluble forms of choline in milk were compared within each trial, by randomization groups, using independent samples one-way analysis of variance (ANOVA) or Student's t-test, as appropriate. In Canada, the concentrations of water-soluble forms of choline in milk were compared between the two trials, by milk fraction collected (i.e., hindmilk versus a full breast expression), using independent samples Student's t-test. In Cambodia, the relationship between the concentration of water-soluble forms of choline in milk and weeks postpartum was assessed by Pearson's correlation coefficient.

Demographic characteristics including age, ethnicity, education, and household income were compared between the two groups, Canada and Cambodia, using independent samples Student's t-test for continuous variable and Fisher's exact test for categorical variables. Water-soluble forms of choline concentrations in milk were compared between Canadian and Cambodian participants using independent samples Student's t-test. The estimated total choline intake was compared with the corresponding AI by one sample Student's t-test. The relationships between maternal dietary choline intake during pregnancy and the concentrations of water-soluble forms of choline in milk samples at eight weeks postpartum were explored using Pearson's correlation coefficient, and Bonferroni's correction was used to adjust for multiple comparisons.

3. Results

A total of 301 milk samples from Canadian and 67 milk samples from Cambodian lactating women were included in this analysis. In Canada, the concentrations of individual and total water-soluble forms of choline in milk compared within each trial (randomization groups) and between the two trials (milk fraction collected) did not differ ($p > 0.05$ for all, Table S1), and therefore the participants from both Canadian trials are presented as one group. Among the Cambodian sample, the concentrations of individual and total water-soluble forms of choline in milk compared by randomization groups did not differ, and there was no need to control for weeks postpartum, as no statistically significant correlations were found with the concentrations of individual and total water-soluble forms of choline in milk ($p > 0.05$ for all, Table S2). Participant characteristics are shown in Table 1. Compared to Cambodian women, Canadian women differed in age, education, ethnicity, and household income ($p < 0.001$).

The concentrations of the individual and the sum of the water-soluble forms of choline in milk are presented in Table 2, and did not differ significantly when comparing milk samples between Canada and Cambodia ($p > 0.05$, for all). Although Canadian women were older than Cambodian women, maternal age was not correlated with milk choline concentrations (r = 0.014 to 0.065, $p > 0.05$, for all). Among all samples ($n = 368$), phosphocholine and glycerophosphocholine were the predominant compounds, contributing 49% and 37% to the sum of the water-soluble forms of choline in milk, respectively.

For infants, the estimated total choline intakes in Canada, Cambodia, and in both countries combined are presented in Table 3, and were significantly below the AI for choline for early infancy (125 mg/day; $p < 0.001$, for all). Based on these data, only 19% of infants in Canada and Cambodia would have met the current choline AI recommendation, compared to an expected value of ~50% [1]. For maternal intake, since the estimated choline intakes between gestational time points (16 and 36 weeks of gestation) did not differ ($p = 0.927$, Table S3) and were significantly correlated (r = 0.590, $p < 0.001$), only the second time point was used, as it was the closest to the milk collection. The estimated maternal total choline intake was significantly below the AI for choline for both pregnancy (450 mg/day) and lactation (550 mg/day) ($p < 0.001$ for both).

The correlation coefficients between the estimated choline intake and the concentrations of the water-soluble forms of choline in milk are presented in Table 4. The sum of the water-soluble forms of choline in milk was positively, but weakly, correlated with dietary total choline intake (r = 0.166,

$p = 0.048$), dietary free choline intakes ($r = 0.223$, $p = 0.007$), and dietary water-soluble forms of choline intake ($r = 0.182$, $p = 0.029$). After adjusting for multiple comparisons, the correlations were no longer significant (Bonferroni's correction $p > 0.006$, for all).

Table 1. Demographic characteristics of lactating women in Canada and Cambodia.

Demographic Characteristics	Canada ($n = 301$)	Cambodia ($n = 67$)	p Value [2]
Age (year) [1]	33.3 ± 4.1	26.1 ± 4.7	<0.001
Parity (n; %)			
1	161; 53%	34; 51%	0.720
2	112; 37%	24; 36%	
3 or more	28; 9%	9; 12%	
Education (n; %)			
None	0; 0%	6; 9%	<0.001
Some primary	0; 0%	31; 46%	
Some secondary	11; 4%	30; 44%	
Some postsecondary	290; 96%	0; 0%	
Ethnicity (n; %)			
European	234; 78%	-	<0.001
Asian	40; 13%	-	
Khmer	-	67; 100%	
Other	27; 9%	-	
Household income (n; %)			<0.001
<$20 000 CAD	10; 3%	67; 100%	
$20 000–50 000 CAD	47; 16%	-	
>$50 000 CAD	244; 81%	-	

[1] Data are presented as mean ± SD; [2] Continuous data were analyzed by independent samples Student's t-test, and categorical data analyzed by Fisher's exact test.

Table 2. Concentration of water-soluble forms of choline in milk samples of lactating women in Canada and Cambodia [1].

Forms of Choline Concentration (μmol/L)	All Women ($n = 368$)	Canada ($n = 301$)	Cambodia ($n = 67$)	p Value [2]
Free choline	151 (141, 160)	155 (144, 165)	143 (132, 154)	0.071
Phosphocholine	540 (519, 562)	535 (512, 559)	562 (513, 612)	0.336
Glycerophosphocholine	411 (396, 427)	416 (399, 434)	390 (356, 423)	0.178
Water-soluble choline [3]	1102 (1072, 1133)	1106 (1071, 1140)	1095 (1018, 1150)	0.686

[1] Data are presented as mean (95% CI), and concentrations were quantified using liquid chromatography-tandem mass spectrometry; [2] Group differences were analyzed by independent samples Student t-test after log-transformation; [3] Water-soluble choline corresponds to the sum of free choline, phosphocholine, and glycerophosphocholine.

Table 3. Estimated dietary total choline intake in Canada and Cambodia [1].

Dietary Intake	Infants [2]			Maternal Canada ($n = 143$) [3]
	All ($n = 368$)	Canada ($n = 301$)	Cambodia ($n = 67$)	
Total choline (mg/day)	106 (103, 109)	107 (103, 110)	105 (98, 111)	408 (390, 427)
AI (mg/day)	125	125	125	450
Above AI [4] (n; %)	71; 19	58; 19	13; 19	46; 32

[1] Dietary intake data are presented as mean (95% CI); [2] Total choline intakes were estimated assuming that water-soluble forms of choline contribute 84% to total choline and a reference milk intake of 780 mL/day; [3] Total choline intakes were estimated at 36 weeks of gestation using a food frequency questionnaire and the USDA database on choline content in common foods (version 2); [4] Since the AI reflects the average choline concentration of breastmilk from healthy lactating women, it is expected that ~50% of infants would have intakes above the AI. When mean intake equals the AI, it is assumed that the prevalence of inadequacy in the group is low; when mean intake is below the AI, no conclusions regarding adequacy can be drawn.

Table 4. Correlation between dietary choline intake during pregnancy and water-soluble forms of choline in milk from a subset of Canadian participants [1].

Dietary Intakes (n = 143)	Milk Choline Metabolites			
	Free Choline	Phospho-Choline	Glycerophospho-Choline	Water-Soluble Choline
Free choline	0.054	0.125	0.129	0.223 **
Phosphocholine	0.134	0.063	−0.007	0.128
Glycerophosphocholine	0.105	0.034	0.101	0.130
Water-soluble choline [2]	0.102	0.094	0.093	0.182 *
Phosphatidylcholine	−0.016	0.145	−0.056	0.091
Sphingomyelin	−0.031	0.147	−0.109	0.036
Lipid-soluble choline [3]	−0.016	0.150	−0.058	0.093
Total choline [4]	0.043	0.150	0.017	0.166 *

[1] Data are presented as Pearson's correlation coefficients after log-transformation, none of the observed associations were significant after Bonferroni's correction (0.05/8 = 0.006; $p > 0.006$, for all comparisons); [2] Water-soluble choline corresponds to the sum of free choline, phosphocholine, and glycerophosphocholine; [3] Lipid-soluble choline corresponds to the sum of phosphatidylcholine and sphingomyelin; [4] Total choline corresponds to the sum of all individual forms of choline; * $p < 0.05$, ** $p < 0.01$.

4. Discussion

An interesting finding from our study was that concentrations of the water-soluble forms of choline in mature milk did not differ between lactating women in Canada and Cambodia (1106 and 1095 μmol/L, respectively), regardless of differences in animal food availability [23] and different likely dietary choline intakes, as described for other low- and middle-income countries [24,25]. An earlier study, in 1982, reported that free choline concentration in milk was lower in lactating women in Ecuador (40% < 100 μmol/L) compared to the United States (55% > 300 μmol/L) [15]. However, free choline contributes an average of only 10% of the total choline in human milk [6–10], and it is unknown whether this difference would be physiologically relevant. Although dietary information was not collected, the authors hypothesized that the difference was a result of the low dietary choline intake in Ecuador [15].

Two recent choline supplementation studies reported that lactating women consuming choline supplemented diets (means of 930 or 1088 mg/day) with close to two-times the corresponding AI (550 mg/day) had significantly higher milk total choline concentrations (20%) compared to control groups (mean intakes of 364 or 480 mg/day) [8,10]. In our study, the mean dietary choline intake in Canada (408 mg/day) was closer to the amount of choline consumed in the control than the supplemented groups of previous studies [8,10]. Thus, the difference in the dietary choline intake between Canada and Cambodia may not have reached the range in which a difference in milk choline concentration would be observed. An alternative explanation for similar milk choline concentrations between Canadian and Cambodian women in our study may be that the mammary gland can obtain choline from both maternal circulation [30] and the endogenous synthesis of phosphatidylcholine through the phosphatidylethanolamine *N*-methyl transferase (PEMT) pathway [31]. Although it has been described that PEMT is mostly active in liver and kidney [32,33], its activity has also been identified in the epithelial cells of the mammary gland [34]. Consequently, this may contribute to ensuring that sufficient choline is excreted in milk to meet the choline demand for the rapidly growing and developing infant.

The estimated mean concentration of water-soluble forms of choline reported in our study was 1102 μmol/L (n = 368), which is in agreement with previously reported values in mature milk samples. In 1996, the first study including all individual forms of choline in mature milk from the United States reported a concentration of water-soluble forms of choline of 1048 μmol/L (n = 16) [6]. Two later studies from the same country have reported mean concentrations of water-soluble forms of choline of 987 and 1024 μmol/L (n = 28 and n = 48) [8,10], where choline quantification was conducted by LC-MS/MS as in our analysis. In Canada, our group recently reported on the concentration of water-soluble forms of choline in donor's milk with a slightly higher mean concentration of water-soluble forms of choline of 1275 μmol/L (n = 30) [19]. However, it is unknown whether the pasteurization process, which is routinely used in milk banks, has an impact on the total or individual forms of choline concentration in milk. In Turkey, slightly higher concentrations of water-soluble forms of choline in mature milk

(1189 and 1402 μmol/L) were reported in two studies ($n = 12$, $n = 54$), where choline was analyzed by less sensitive enzymatic methods [7,9].

Based on our results, the estimated total choline intake of the infants was 106 mg/day ($n = 368$), which is significantly below the corresponding AI for choline (125 mg/day) [1]. However, it is important to note that the AI for choline for infants of 0–6 months reflected a milk total choline concentration of 1500 μmol/L, which in fact was 20% higher than the mean concentration of total choline in human milk published at that time (1254 μmol/L) [6], and no rationale was provided as to why a higher concentration was used to set the AI during infancy instead of the observed average as per definition [35]. Accordingly, results categorized using the current AI for choline for infants of 0–6 months as a cut-off must be interpreted with caution, as the current recommendation may not accurately reflect the mean total choline concentration in human milk.

The milk choline concentrations reported in the present study are also relevant from a clinical perspective, as the nutrient content in human milk may be used as a guideline to develop human milk substitutes and enteral formulas for infants. Current guidelines for choline content in infant formula are 7–50 mg/100 kcal [36,37], which is equivalent to a wide range of choline intake ranging between 37–265 mg/day, based on milk consumption of 780 mL/day and energy content of 68 kcal/100 mL [36]. Most of the commercially available infant formulas add choline as free choline, which contributes 57% of total choline [17], compared to only 10% in human milk [6–10]. Accordingly, current infant formula composition does not mimic the profile of choline forms present in human milk; whether this is physiologically relevant is not known.

In this study, we found that the concentration of water-soluble forms of choline in milk was not significantly associated with maternal choline intake when estimated during pregnancy from a subset of the Canadian participants. In line with this finding, another study reported that choline intake was not associated with choline concentration in milk, except for a weak association with milk phosphatidylcholine ($R^2 = 0.11$, $p = 0.007$) [8]. It also could be possible that maternal intake during pregnancy was not the same as when the milk samples were collected at eight weeks postpartum. However, previous studies have observed a minor and non-significant variation in the maternal diet when comparing intakes during pregnancy and lactation periods (2–4% change) [38,39]. This is in agreement with the finding that total choline intakes at 16 and 36 weeks of gestation did not differ ($p = 0.927$) and were positively associated ($r = 0.590$, $p < 0.001$) in our study.

A potential limitation of the present study was that milk samples were collected at different time points during lactation among the Cambodian participants (3–28 weeks postpartum). However, it has been described that total choline concentration in milk increases from colostrum at birth to two weeks postpartum, and then stays stable beyond six months [7,20,21,40], and we found no association between total water-soluble choline concentration and week postpartum of the milk collection ($p = 0.915$). Additionally, we compared different milk fractions, hindmilk versus a full breast expression, which, at least for the water-soluble forms of choline, did not differ in the Canadian trials (Table S1, $p > 0.05$) and is in agreement with an earlier study that compared different milk fractions [18]. Another limitation was that only the water-soluble forms of choline were quantified, without including the lipid-soluble forms. However, the water-soluble forms of choline contribute an average of 84% of the total choline concentration in human milk, which is relatively stable based on the published data even among the supplemented groups [6–10]. In addition, the actual infant daily volume intake of human milk is unknown, and the reference intake volume (780 mL/day) used to set the AI for different nutrients, including choline, for early infancy was selected [1], which was obtained from earlier studies assessing infant's body weight before and after breastfeeding during the first six months of life [41–44]. Recently, a comparable value of the daily volume of human milk intake between two and five months has been published [45]. Moreover, no dietary information was collected in Cambodia and further studies need to be conducted to confirm the differences assumed in total choline intake.

5. Conclusions

The present study is the first to report water-soluble forms of choline concentrations in mature milk samples collected from lactating women in Cambodia and could be considered the largest study to date for choline assessment in human milk. In summary, we found that the concentrations of the water-soluble forms of choline in mature human milk samples did not differ between Canadian and Cambodian lactating women, despite lower likely choline intakes in Cambodia. The finding that the estimated dietary choline intake during early infancy was below the corresponding AI suggest that the current AI may not reflect the average choline concentration in human milk of healthy lactating women. Among a subset of the Canadian participants, maternal dietary choline was not significantly correlated to the milk water-soluble forms of choline.

Acknowledgments: Funding: Supported by the Canadian Institutes of Health Research and Grand Challenges Canada Stars in Global Health Round VI Phase I grant. A.M.W. received funding support through Doctoral Scholarship to study abroad, the Government of Chile, provided through Becas-Chile, and the Nutritional Research Fellowship, University of British Columbia. K.C.W. gratefully acknowledges funding support through the International Development Research Centre Doctoral Research Award, and K.C.W. and K.M.M. were supported by Canadian Institutes of Health Research Frederick Banting and Charles Best Canada Graduate Scholarships.

Author Contributions: The authors' contributions were as follows: S.M.I. and T.J.G. designed the research; K.C.W., K.M.M., N.N.C., H.K, L.S, and P.S. coordinated and conducted the studies from which the milk samples were obtained; R.A.D. contributed to laboratory analysis; and A.M.W. conducted laboratory and dietary analyses, analyzed data, and prepared the initial draft of the manuscript; Z.X., D.D.K., T.J.G., and S.I.B. provided critical input into the manuscript. All authors have read and approved the final version of the manuscript.

References

1. Institute of Medicine. *Dietary Reference Intakes for Thiamin, Riboflavin, Niacin, Vitamin B6, Folate, Vitamin B12, Pantothenic Acid, Biotin, and Choline*; The National Academy Press: Washington, DC, USA, 1998.
2. Zeisel, S.H.; Niculescu, M.D. Perinatal choline influences brain structure and function. *Nutr. Rev.* **2006**, *64*, 197–203. [CrossRef] [PubMed]
3. Zeisel, S.H.; da Costa, K.A. Choline: An essential nutrient for public health. *Nutr. Rev.* **2009**, *67*, 615–623. [CrossRef] [PubMed]
4. Zeisel, S.H.; Blusztajn, J.K. Choline and human nutrition. *Annu. Rev. Nutr.* **1994**, *14*, 269–296. [CrossRef] [PubMed]
5. Ueland, P.M. Choline and betaine in health and disease. *J. Inherit. Metab. Dis.* **2011**, *34*, 3–15. [CrossRef] [PubMed]
6. Holmes-McNary, M.Q.; Cheng, W.L.; Mar, M.H.; Fussell, S.; Zeisel, S.H. Choline and choline esters in human and rat milk and in infant formulas. *Am. J. Clin. Nutr.* **1996**, *64*, 572–576. [CrossRef] [PubMed]
7. Ilcol, Y.O.; Ozbek, R.; Hamurtekin, E.; Ulus, I.H. Choline status in newborns, infants, children, breast-feeding women, breast-fed infants and human breast milk. *J. Nutr. Biochem.* **2005**, *16*, 489–499. [CrossRef] [PubMed]
8. Fischer, L.M.; da Costa, K.A.; Galanko, J.; Sha, W.; Stephenson, B.; Vick, J.; Zeisel, S.H. Choline intake and genetic polymorphisms influence choline metabolite concentrations in human breast milk and plasma. *Am. J. Clin. Nutr.* **2010**, *92*, 336–346. [CrossRef] [PubMed]
9. Ozarda, Y.; Cansev, M.; Ulus, I.H. Breast milk choline contents are associated with inflammatory status of breastfeeding women. *J. Hum. Lact.* **2014**, *30*, 161–166. [CrossRef] [PubMed]
10. Davenport, C.; Yan, J.; Taesuwan, S.; Shields, K.; West, A.A.; Jiang, X.; Perry, C.A.; Malysheva, O.V.; Stabler, S.P.; Allen, R.H.; et al. Choline intakes exceeding recommendations during human lactation improve breast milk choline content by increasing PEMT pathway metabolites. *J. Nutr. Biochem.* **2015**, *26*, 903–911. [CrossRef] [PubMed]

11. Klein, J.; Koppen, A.; Loffelholz, K. Regulation of free choline in rat brain: Dietary and pharmacological manipulations. *Neurochem. Int.* **1998**, *32*, 479–485. [CrossRef]
12. Babb, S.M.; Ke, Y.; Lange, N.; Kaufman, M.J.; Renshaw, P.F.; Cohen, B.M. Oral choline increases choline metabolites in human brain. *Psychiatry Res.* **2004**, *130*, 1–9. [CrossRef]
13. Cheatham, C.L.; Sheppard, K.W. Synergistic effects of human milk nutrients in the support of infant recognition memory: An observational study. *Nutrients* **2015**, *7*, 9079–9095. [CrossRef] [PubMed]
14. World Health Organization. *The World Health Organization's Infant Feeding Recommendation*; WHO: Geneva, Switzerland, 2001.
15. Zeisel, S.H.; Stanbury, J.B.; Wurtman, R.J.; Brigida, M.; Fierro-Benitez, R. Choline content of mothers' milk in Ecuador and Boston. *N. Engl. J. Med.* **1982**, *306*, 175–176. [PubMed]
16. Allen, L.H. B vitamins in breast milk: Relative importance of maternal status and intake, and effects on infant status and function. *Adv. Nutr.* **2012**, *3*, 362–369. [CrossRef] [PubMed]
17. United States Department of Agriculture. *Database for the Choline Content of Common Foods, Release 2*; Agricultural Research Service: Washington, DC, USA, 2008.
18. Zeisel, S.H.; Char, D.; Sheard, N.F. Choline, phosphatidylcholine and sphingomyelin in human and bovine milk and infant formulas. *J. Nutr.* **1986**, *116*, 50–58. [CrossRef] [PubMed]
19. Moukarzel, S.; Soberanes, L.; Dyer, R.A.; Albersheim, S.; Elango, R.; Innis, S.M. Relationships among different water-soluble choline compounds differ between human preterm and donor milk. *Nutrients* **2017**, *9*, 696. [CrossRef] [PubMed]
20. Sakurai, T.; Furukawa, M.; Asoh, M.; Kanno, T.; Kojima, T.; Yonekubo, A. Fat-soluble and water-soluble vitamin contents of breast milk from Japanese women. *J. Nutr. Sci. Vitaminol.* **2005**, *51*, 239–247. [CrossRef] [PubMed]
21. Hanok Jeong, Y.S.; Chung, Y.-J. Choline and betaine concentrations in breast milk of Korean lactating women and the choline and betaine intakes of their infants. *Korean J. Nutr.* **2010**, *43*, 588–596. [CrossRef]
22. Wu, J.; Domellof, M.; Zivkovic, A.M.; Larsson, G.; Ohman, A.; Nording, M.L. NMR-based metabolite profiling of human milk: A pilot study of methods for investigating compositional changes during lactation. *Biochem. Biophys. Res. Commun.* **2016**, *469*, 626–632. [CrossRef] [PubMed]
23. Food and Agriculture Organization of the United Nations, Statistical Division. FAOSTAT Statistics Database. 2013. Available online: www.fao.org/faostat/en/#compare (accessed on 20 August 2017).
24. Gossell-Williams, M.; Fletcher, H.; McFarlane-Anderson, N.; Jacob, A.; Patel, J.; Zeisel, S. Dietary intake of choline and plasma choline concentrations in pregnant women in Jamaica. *West Indian Med. J.* **2005**, *54*, 355–359. [CrossRef] [PubMed]
25. Goon, S.; Dey, S.R. A 24-hour dietary recall for assessing the intake pattern of choline among Bangladeshi pregnant women at their third trimester of pregnancy. *Cent. Asian J. Glob. Health* **2014**, 3. [CrossRef]
26. Mulder, K.A.; King, D.J.; Innis, S.M. Omega-3 fatty acid deficiency in infants before birth identified using a randomized trial of maternal dha supplementation in pregnancy. *PLoS ONE* **2014**, *9*, e83764. [CrossRef] [PubMed]
27. March, K.M.; Chen, N.N.; Karakochuk, C.D.; Shand, A.W.; Innis, S.M.; von Dadelszen, P.; Barr, S.I.; Lyon, M.R.; Whiting, S.J.; Weiler, H.A.; et al. Maternal vitamin D(3) supplementation at 50 μg/d protects against low serum 25-hydroxyvitamin D in infants at 8 wk of age: A randomized controlled trial of 3 doses of vitamin D beginning in gestation and continued in lactation. *Am. J. Clin. Nutr.* **2015**, *102*, 402–410. [CrossRef] [PubMed]
28. Whitfield, K.C.; Karakochuk, C.D.; Kroeun, H.; Hampel, D.; Sokhoing, L.; Chan, B.B.; Borath, M.; Sophonneary, P.; McLean, J.; Talukder, A.; et al. Perinatal consumption of thiamine-fortified fish sauce in rural Cambodia: A randomized clinical trial. *JAMA Pediatr.* **2016**, *170*, e162065. [CrossRef] [PubMed]
29. Wiedeman Manriquez, A.M. Dietary Choline Intake and Biomarkers of Choline Status across the Life Cycle. Ph.D. Thesis, University of British Columbia, Vancouver, BC, Canada, 2017.
30. Chao, C.K.; Pomfret, E.A.; Zeisel, S.H. Uptake of choline by rat mammary-gland epithelial cells. *Biochem. J.* **1988**, *254*, 33–38. [CrossRef] [PubMed]
31. Vance, J.E.; Vance, D.E. Phospholipid biosynthesis in mammalian cells. *Biochem. Cell Biol.* **2004**, *82*, 113–128. [CrossRef] [PubMed]
32. Bremer, J.; Greenberg, D.M. Biosynthesis of choline in vitro. *Biochim. Biophys. Acta* **1960**, *37*, 173–175. [CrossRef]
33. Vance, D.E.; Walkey, C.J.; Cui, Z. Phosphatidylethanolamine *N*-methyltransferase from liver. *Biochim. Biophys. Acta* **1997**, *1348*, 142–150. [CrossRef]

34. Yang, E.K.; Blusztajn, J.K.; Pomfret, E.A.; Zeisel, S.H. Rat and human mammary tissue can synthesize choline moiety via the methylation of phosphatidylethanolamine. *Biochem. J.* **1988**, *256*, 821–828. [CrossRef] [PubMed]
35. Institute of Medicine. *Dietary Reference Intakes: Applications in Dietary Assessment*; The National Academies Press: Washington, DC, USA, 2000.
36. Koletzko, B.; Baker, S.; Cleghorn, G.; Neto, U.F.; Gopalan, S.; Hernell, O.; Hock, Q.S.; Jirapinyo, P.; Lonnerdal, B.; Pencharz, P.; et al. Global standard for the composition of infant formula: Recommendations of an ESPGHAN coordinated international expert group. *J. Pediatr. Gastroenterol. Nutr.* **2005**, *41*, 584–599. [CrossRef] [PubMed]
37. Codex Alimentarious Commision. *CODEX STAN 72-1981 for Infant Formula and Formulas for Special Medical Purposes Intended for Infants*; Codex Alimentarius: Geneva, Switzerland, 2007.
38. Lewis, E.D.; Subhan, F.B.; Bell, R.C.; McCargar, L.J.; Curtis, J.M.; Jacobs, R.L.; Field, C.J.; APoON Team. Estimation of choline intake from 24 h dietary intake recalls and contribution of egg and milk consumption to intake among pregnant and lactating women in Alberta. *Br. J. Nutr.* **2014**, *112*, 112–121. [CrossRef] [PubMed]
39. Pauwels, S.; Ghosh, M.; Duca, R.C.; Bekaert, B.; Freson, K.; Huybrechts, I.; Langie, S.A.S.; Koppen, G.; Devlieger, R.; Godderis, L. Maternal intake of methyl-group donors affects DNA methylation of metabolic genes in infants. *Clin. Epigenetics* **2017**, *9*, 16. [CrossRef] [PubMed]
40. Holmes, H.C.; Snodgrass, G.J.; Iles, R.A. Changes in the choline content of human breast milk in the first 3 weeks after birth. *Eur. J. Pediatr.* **2000**, *159*, 198–204. [CrossRef] [PubMed]
41. Hofvander, Y.; Hagman, U.; Hillervik, C.; Sjolin, S. The amount of milk consumed by 1–3 months old breast- or bottle-fed infants. *Acta Paediatr. Scand.* **1982**, *71*, 953–958. [CrossRef] [PubMed]
42. Butte, N.F.; Garza, C.; Smith, E.O.; Nichols, B.L. Human milk intake and growth in exclusively breast-fed infants. *J. Pediatr.* **1984**, *104*, 187–195. [CrossRef]
43. Neville, M.C.; Keller, R.; Seacat, J.; Lutes, V.; Neifert, M.; Casey, C.; Allen, J.; Archer, P. Studies in human lactation: Milk volumes in lactating women during the onset of lactation and full lactation. *Am. J. Clin. Nutr.* **1988**, *48*, 1375–1386. [CrossRef] [PubMed]
44. Allen, J.C.; Keller, R.P.; Archer, P.; Neville, M.C. Studies in human lactation: Milk composition and daily secretion rates of macronutrients in the first year of lactation. *Am. J. Clin. Nutr.* **1991**, *54*, 69–80. [CrossRef] [PubMed]
45. Gridneva, Z.; Rea, A.; Hepworth, A.R.; Ward, L.C.; Lai, C.T.; Hartmann, P.E.; Geddes, D.T. Relationships between breastfeeding patterns and maternal and infant body composition over the first 12 months of lactation. *Nutrients* **2018**, *10*, 45. [CrossRef] [PubMed]

9

Quantification of Nervonic Acid in Human Milk in the First 30 Days of Lactation: Influence of Lactation Stages and Comparison with Infant Formulae

Jiahui Yu [1,2], Tinglan Yuan [1,2], Xinghe Zhang [1,2], Qingzhe Jin [1,2], Wei Wei [1,2,*] and Xingguo Wang [1,2,*]

1. State Key Lab of Food Science and Technology, Jiangnan University, Wuxi 214122, China
2. International Joint Research Laboratory for Lipid Nutrition and Safety, Collaborative Innovation Center of Food Safety and Quality Control in Jiangsu Province, School of Food Science and Technology, Jiangnan University, Wuxi 214122, China

* Correspondence: weiw@jiangnan.edu.cn (W.W.); xingguow@jiangnan.edu.cn (X.W.)

Abstract: Nervonic acid (24:1 n-9, NA) plays a crucial role in the development of white matter, and it occurs naturally in human milk. This study aims to quantify NA in human milk at different lactation stages and compare it with the NA measured in infant formulae. With this information, optimal nutritional interventions for infants, especially newborns, can be determined. In this study, an absolute detection method that uses experimentally derived standard curves and methyl tricosanoate as the internal standard was developed to quantitively analyze NA concentration. The method was applied to the analysis of 224 human milk samples, which were collected over a period of 3–30 days postpartum from eight healthy Chinese mothers. The results show that the NA concentration was highest in colostrum (0.76 ± 0.23 mg/g fat) and significantly decreased ($p < 0.001$) in mature milk (0.20 ± 0.03 mg/g fat). During the first 10 days of lactation, the change in NA concentration was the most pronounced, decreasing by about 65%. Next, the NA contents in 181 commercial infant formulae from the Chinese market were compared. The NA content in most formulae was <16% of that found in colostrum and less than that found in mature human milk ($p < 0.05$). No significant difference ($p > 0.05$) was observed among NA content in formulae with different fat sources. Special attention was given to the variety of n-9 fatty acids in human milk during lactation, and the results indicated that interindividual variation in NA content may be primarily due to endogenous factors, with less influence from the maternal diet.

Keywords: n-9 fatty acid; nervonic acid; human milk fat; infant formula; lactational stage

---

1. Introduction

Human milk is generally regarded as the best source of nutrition for infants during their first six months of life [1]. Human milk contains 3%–5% fats, of which 98%–99% are triacylglycerols (TAGs), 0.26%–0.80% are phospholipids (PLs), and 0.25%–0.34% are sterols, as well as trace amounts of minor components, including monoacylglycerols (MAGs), diacylglycerols (DAGs), non-esterified fatty acids, and other substances [2]. Human milk fat is one of the most complex natural lipids with a unique fatty acids (FAs) composition. Nervonic acid (24:1 n-9, NA) is a very-long-chain monounsaturated fatty acid (>C_{20}) that naturally occurs in human milk (less than 2%) [3], but it has been rarely studied in the field of human nutrition.

NA is an essential constituent of the neuronal membrane [4] and plays a crucial role in problems such as early myelination [5], peroxisomal disorders [6,7], and undernourishment [8]. NA rapidly accumulates in the fetal brain at 32–37 weeks' gestation [9]. After birth, infants continue to obtain NA from human milk. Several publications have indicated that the NA concentration in human milk markedly decreases as lactation stages progress [10–12]. NA concentrations in colostrum (≤1 week postpartum) have been found to range from two- to six-fold higher than those in mature milk (>2 weeks and ≤16 weeks) [13,14]. The results suggested that the human brain heavily accumulates NA in the early days of life. Previous research identified that NA is an important fatty acid in the white matter and its deficiency in early development may damage the white matter [15]. The cause of the majority of preterm infants with cerebral palsy is mainly attributed to white matter diseases, such as periventricular leukomalacia [16,17].

The NA concentration in human milk is not routinely reported because NA quantitation is obscured by more abundant very-long-chain fatty acids when expressed percentage by weight of total fatty acids in gas chromatography (GC) analyses [18]. However, previous studies report that NA is detectable in human milk from different countries of the world, and a significantly higher NA content is present in colostrum compared to mature milk [11–13,19–21]. Very few data are available on the quantification of nervonic acid in human milk especially the amount in each lactation day.

The NA content in common vegetable oils is low, therefore infant formulae have much lower NA content compared with human milk [3], especially colostrum. However, relatively little attention has been paid to NA in infant formulae [22]. NA, together with docosahexaenoic acid (22:6 n-3, DHA) and arachidonic acid (20:4 n-6, AA), has a positive effect on the neural development of the neonate [23]. Nonetheless, the importance of DHA and AA in infant formulae have attracted researchers' attention [9,24,25], whereas few studies focus on the effect of NA in human milk and the comparison with infant formula which is potentially important.

This study aimed to develop an effective method for the quantification of NA concentration in human milk and systematically compare the NA concentration in human milk on different lactation days. The NA contents in infant formulae from three fat sources (cows' milk fat, goats' milk fat, and plant oil) were also studied. Special attention was given to the variation of three other n-9 FAs, including oleic acid (18:1 n-9, OA), eicosenoic acid (20:1 n-9, EiA) and erucic acid (22:1 n-9, EA), in human milk throughout lactation.

2. Materials and Methods

2.1. Standards and Chemicals

A standard mixture of 37 kinds of fatty acid methyl esters (FAMEs, from C_4 to C_{24}) was bought from Sigma-Aldrich (St. Louis, MO, USA). The standards methyl *cis*-15-tetracosenoate (24:1 n-9 FAME) and methyl tricosanoate (23:0 FAME), methanol, and *n*-hexane (HPLC grade) were obtained from J and K Scientific (Beijing, China). Other reagents were analytical grade and purchased from Sinopharm Reagent Co. Ltd. (Shanghai, China).

2.2. Human Milk Samples and Infant Formulae

Human milk samples were collected from eight healthy mothers of term infants in Wuxi, China. The study was approved by the Ethics Committee of the School of Food Science and Technology in Jiangnan University (JN No. 21212030120), and written consent was obtained from all subjects included in this study. During the lactation period from 3 to 30 days postpartum, 224 human milk samples were collected. The sample-set included colostrum (3–6 postpartum days, n = 32), transitional milk (7–14 postpartum days, n = 64), and mature milk (>15 postpartum days, n = 128). All participating mothers were non-smokers, non-medicated, and healthy. The mean age of the mothers was 28.38 ± 3.16 years, mean BMI was 21.78 ± 2.75 kg/m^2, and mean infant weight at birth was 3.35 ± 0.23 kg. The samples (5–10 mL) were collected after full expression from one breast with a breast pump between 9 and 11 am. The samples were stored at −20 °C for less than 2 h and transferred to the lab at Jiangnan University for lipid extraction.

The fatty acid composition of infant formulae is reported in a previous study [3]. A total of 181 formulae from 27 brands were collected; the tested formulae account for 75% of the Chinese infant formulae market. Three stages (infant, follow-on, and growing-up) of formulae were included. The formulae were divided into cows' milk, goats' milk, and plant oil, depending on the main fat source.

2.3. Fatty Acid Methyl Esters Preparation

Total lipids in human milk were extracted by classic Röse–Gottlieb method [26] with some modifications. Briefly, 1 mL ammonia water was added into 4 mL human milk, and then mixed in a water shaking bath at 65 °C ± 5 °C for 20 min. Then, 5 mL absolute ethanol, 10 mL absolute ether and 10 mL petroleum ether were added to extract the lipids. The samples were mixed thoroughly and stood for 2 h, and then the supernatants were collected. The lipids in the lower phase were extracted using half of the solvents as above. The solvents were removed by nitrogen and the lipids were stored in a −80 °C freezer until analysis.

The 24:1 n-9 FAME standard was prepared at a concentration of 0.5 mg/mL dissolved in *n*-hexane. The internal standard solution was prepared by weighing 10 mg of 23:0 FAME into 10 mL of *n*-hexane. Milk fat (40 mg) was suspended in 200 μL of the internal standard solution, 800 μL *n*-hexane, and 500 μL of KOH–CH_3OH (2 mol/L). After mixing for 2 min, the water in the solution was removed by adding the appropriate amount of anhydrous sodium sulfate. Then, the mixture was mixed thoroughly and left standing for half an hour. The supernatant was filtered by a 0.22 μm filter and analyzed by gas chromatography (GC).

2.4. GC Analysis

The samples were analyzed by an Agilent 7820A gas chromatograph (Agilent Technologies, Santa Clara, CA, USA) with a hydrogen flame ionization detector, and they were separated by a TRACE^{TM}-FAME capillary column (60 m × 0.25 mm × 0.25 μm, Thermo Fisher Scientific, Waltham, MA, USA) using nitrogen carrier gas [27]. The injection and detector temperature were set at 250 °C, and the injection volume was 2 μL. The temperature of the column was set at 60 °C for 3 min to start and then increased to 175 °C at a rate of 5 °C/min. The temperature was maintained at 175 °C for 15 min and then raised (at a rate of 2 °C/min) to 220 °C, which was maintained for 10 min. FAs were identified by comparing the retention times of the sample peaks with those of the FAME standards. The NA concentration was measured by the absolute detection method, with 23:0 FAME as an internal standard.

2.5. Quantitation of Nervonic Acid

In the first step, a series of standard solutions that contained varying concentrations of 24:1 n-9 FAME and an identical amount of 23:0 FAME were injected. The calibration line was constructed using Equation (1):

$$y = ax + b \tag{1}$$

where y is the ratio of the peak area of 24:1 n-9 FAME to that of 23:0 FAME, a is the slope of the calibration curve, x is the ratio of the weight of 24:1 n-9 FAME to that of 23:0 FAME and b is the intercept of the calibration curve.

The NA concentration in human milk fat was calculated using Equation (2), with 23:0 FAME as the internal standard.

$$C = (\frac{A_1}{A_0} - b) \times m_0 \times \frac{1}{a} \times \frac{1}{W} \times F_t \tag{2}$$

where C is the concentration of NA in human milk fat (mg/g fat), A_1 is the peak area of 24:1 n-9 FAME, A_0 is the peak area of 23:0 FAME, m_0 is the weight of the internal standard/mg, W is the weight of human milk fat in the test sample/g, and F_t is the transformation coefficient of 24:1 n-9 FAME to NA.

2.6. Validation of the Method

The following parameters (precision, recovery rate, and limits of detection and quantification) were used to validate this method based on the guidance of the United States Pharmacopeia (USP) [28]. For the precision test of the method, the same homogeneous sample was analyzed three times in one day to obtain the intra-day precision and in three different days to obtain the inter-day precision. The precision was described as peak area and retention time relative standard deviations (RSDs) [29]. The recovery of the methods was measured using three levels of concentration of standard solution that were added into three identical human milk samples, and no standard was added into the fourth sample. The rate was calculated by the detected concentration of NA standard divided by the actually added concentration. The limits of detection and quantitation were defined as three times and ten times of signal to noise ratio, respectively [30].

2.7. Statistical Analysis

All analyses of human milk were performed in duplicate. The results were expressed as means (%) ± standard deviations (SD) and were calculated using the SPSS 19.0 (SPSS, USA). Differences in NA concentration were tested by one-way analysis of variance (ANOVA) for continuous variables. Two-way ANOVA was used to evaluate the effect of fat sources and stages on the n-9 FA composition of infant formulae. Differences among all results were compared by use of Ducan's test at $p < 0.05$. Pearson's correlation test was used to determine the correlation coefficient between NA concentration and lactation days. Principal component analysis (PCA) was used to determine the differences in NA content in three lactation stages of human milk and three stages of infant formulae using SIMCA-P software version 13.5 (Demo Umetrics, Umea, Sweden).

3. Results

3.1. Nervonic Acid Concentration in Human Milk

In this study, to accurately quantify the NA concentration in human milk, a long GC program with an analysis time of 70 min was applied, and a FAME with a similar molecular structure (23:0) was added to the sample as an internal standard [31]. The gas chromatograms of NA in human milk are shown in Figure 1.

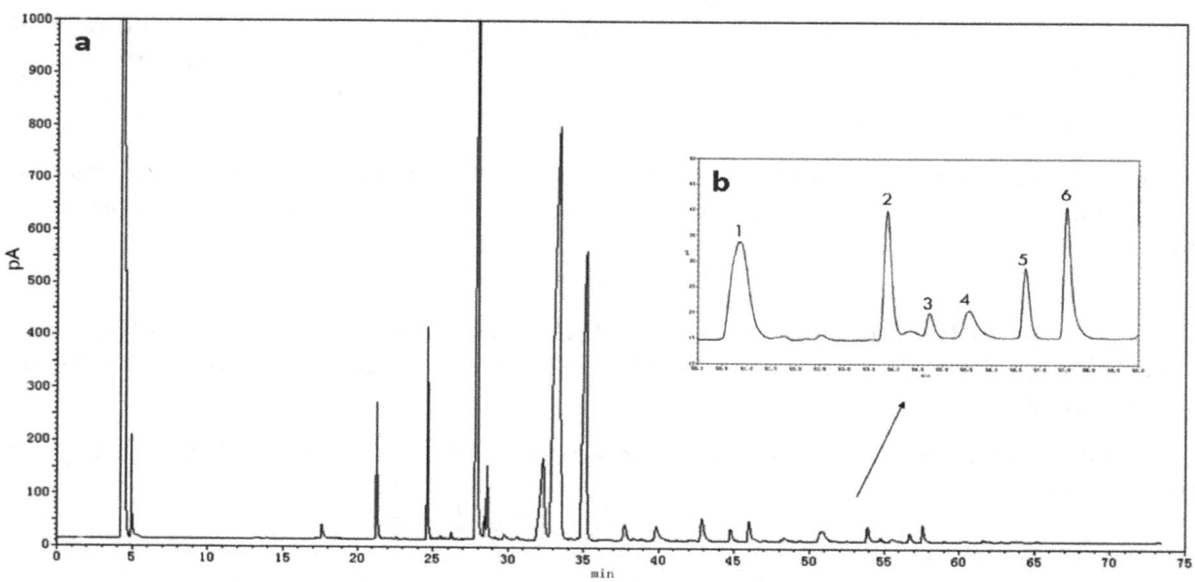

Figure 1. Gas chromatography (GC) of total fatty acids (**a**) and very-long-chain fatty acids (**b**) in one colostrum human milk. 1, tricosanoicacid (23:0); 2, docosatetraenoic acid (22:4 n-7); 3, docosapentaenoic acid (22:5 n-6); 4, nervonic acid (24:1 n-9, NA); 5, docosapentaenoic acid (22:5 n-3); 6, docosahexaenoic acid (22:6 n-3).

The calibration line of this method was defined by $y = 0.733x + 0.7417$ ($R^2 = 0.9944$) showing a good linearity [32]. The calibration lines of 24:1 n-9 and 23:0 were $y = 9.47 \times 10^6 x$ ($R^2 = 0.9938$) and $y = 9.59 \times 10^6 x$ ($R^2 = 0.9965$), respectively. The precision measured the dispersion degree between the tested results of the same sample under the same condition [29]. Both the intra-day and inter-day RSD% on the retention times were lower than 0.01%, and the intra-day and inter-day RSD% on the peak areas were lower than 0.02% and 0.18%, respectively. The recovery rate of the method ranged from 95% to 103%, which met the advisable international level of 80% to 115% [33]. The detection limits ranged from 1.34 μg/mL for NA to 3.25 μg/mL for 23:0 FAME and the quantitation limits ranged from 3.11 μg/mL to 5.36 μg/mL for NA and 23:0 FAME, respectively.

The NA concentrations in human milk are presented in Table S1. The NA concentration in all human milk samples decreased significantly ($r = -0.822$, $p < 0.001$) during the first month of lactation. The average NA concentration on day three of lactation was about five times higher than that on day 30 ($p < 0.001$), with values of 1.00 ± 0.24 mg/g and 0.18 ± 0.03 mg/g fat, respectively. No significant difference was observed in the NA concentration in human milk obtained after 15 days of lactation. The concentration of NA was highest in colostrum (0.76 ± 0.23 mg/g fat) and lowest in mature milk (0.20 ± 0.03 mg/g fat), decreasing by 82% in the first month of lactation. Figure 2 illustrates the changing trend of the mean values of NA concentration in human milk in the first month of lactation.

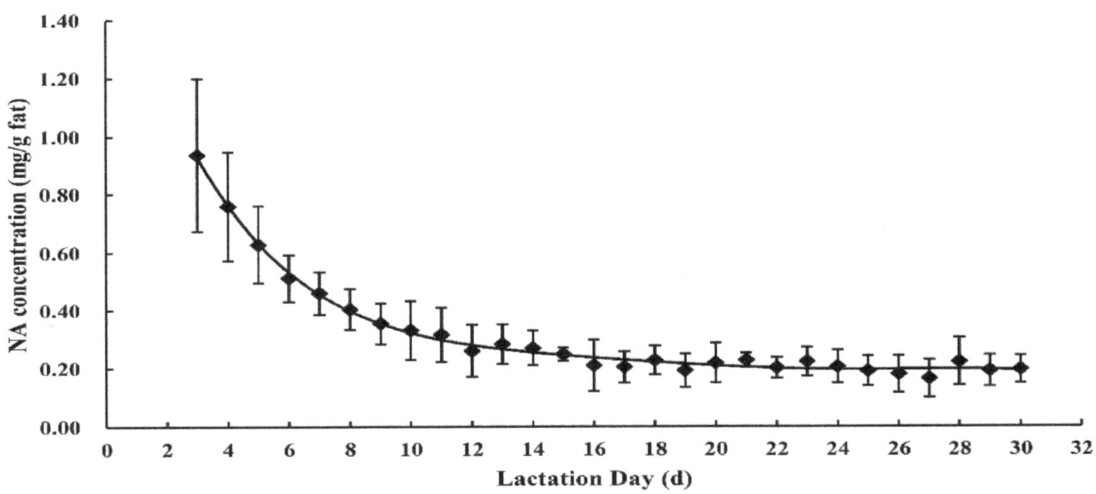

Figure 2. Nervonic acid concentrations in human milk throughout the first month of lactation.

Besides changes between lactation stages, there were significant interindividual differences in NA concentration. The differences were more pronounced from three to 15 days and marginally significant ($p > 0.05$) after day 15 of lactation. At three days postpartum, there was a two-fold variation in NA in the milk from the eight mothers, with values ranging from 0.72 to 1.44 mg/g fat. The differences between individuals decreased over time during the study period. During days 26–30 of lactation, the NA concentration varied from 0.15 mg/g fat to 0.22 mg/g fat, with a 0.07 mg/g fat difference.

3.2. *Composition of n-9 Fatty Acids in Human Milk*

In this study, four kinds of n-9 FAs (OA, EiA, EA, and NA) were detected in human milk samples. Changes in n-9 FA composition in human milk during the first month of lactation are shown in Figure 3. OA, whose percentage ranged from 30.23% to 33.86% of total FAs, was the predominant FA in human milk. During lactation, no significant difference was observed in OA content in human milk (Figure 3A). Contrary to the observed consistency of OA, there were significant changes ($p < 0.05$) in the percentage of EiA (from 0.17% to 0.06%) and NA (from 0.21% to 0.04%) as the milk progressed from colostrum to transitional milk and from transitional milk to mature milk (Figure 3b,d). Particularly, the NA percentage varied in the range of 0.18%–0.21% in colostrum and decreased to 0.12%–0.17% in transitional milk and 0.04%–0.10% in mature milk. The EA content decreased from 0.19% to 0.11% of the total FA content from the first to third lactation stage, but the discrepancies were less significant between transitional milk and mature milk (Figure 3c).

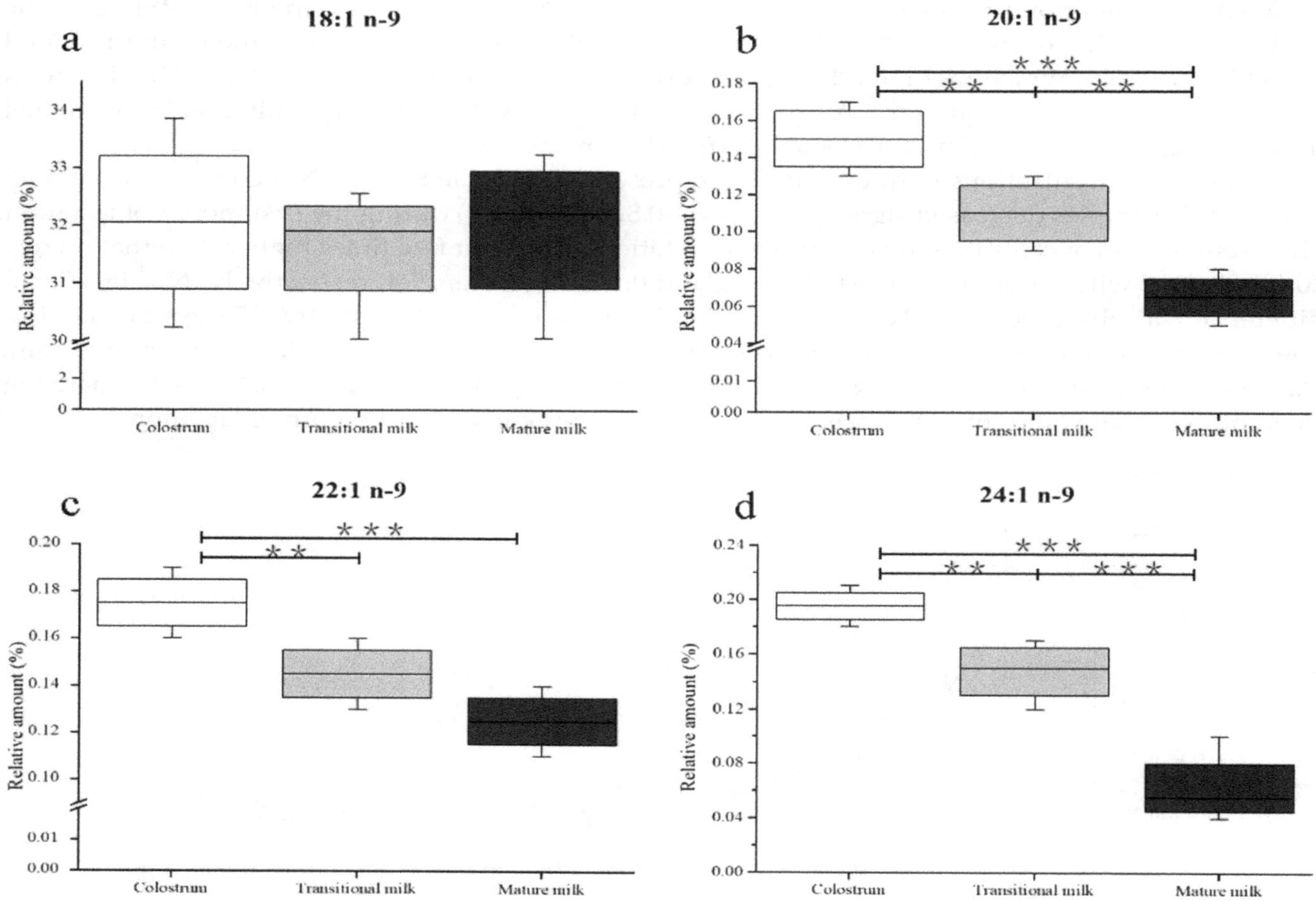

Figure 3. Changes in n-9 fatty acids including 18:1 n-9 (**a**), 20:1 n-9 (**b**), 22:1 n-9 (**c**), and 24:1 n-9 (**d**) in human milk during the first month of lactation. Significantly different from colostrum, transitional milk, and mature milk: *** $p < 0.001$; ** $p < 0.01$. No labeling indicates no significant differences.

3.3. Composition of n-9 Fatty Acids in Infant Formulae

A total of 181 infant formulae were analyzed, and 97 (53.59%) were found to contain NA. The n-9 FA composition of 97 infant formulae are presented in Table 1. The infant formulae were divided into three stages (infant formula, follow-on formula, and growing-up formula) and three sources (cows' milk formula, goats' milk formula, and plant-oil formula). There was a significant difference in fat sources of OA ($p < 0.001$), EiA ($p < 0.001$), and EA ($p < 0.01$) among different formulae. There were no significant differences in sources of NA ($p > 0.05$). The n-9 FA composition was not affected by the formulae stages or the interaction between fat sources and stages ($p > 0.05$). It is recommended that EA content in infant formulae be below 1% of the total fat content [34]. It is noteworthy that infant formulae have much lower concentrations of NA compared with human milk. The NA content of most formulae (0.02% ± 0.02%) was about <16% of that in colostrum (0.20% ± 0.04%) and less than from that found in mature milk (0.08% ± 0.04%).

Table 1. n-9 Fatty acid composition (wt%) of infant formulae.

Fatty Acids		CMF (n = 30)	GMF (n = 16)	POF (n = 51)	*p*-Value F	S	F × S
18:1 n-9	IF	32.15 ± 5.06 [a]	34.81 ± 5.66 [a,b]	40.74 ± 8.32 [b]	***	NS	NS
	FF	30.65 ± 5.95 [a]	30.15 ± 5.28 [a]	41.61 ± 6.11 [b]			
	GF	31.76 ± 5.09 [a]	29.66 ± 6.50 [a]	40.89 ± 7.31 [b]			
20:1 n-9	IF	0.23 ± 0.09	0.29 ± 0.09	0.31 ± 0.10	***	NS	NS
	FF	0.17 ± 0.10 [a]	0.24 ± 0.09 [a,b]	0.33 ± 0.09 [b]			
	GF	0.13 ± 0.04 [a]	0.21 ± 0.07 [a]	0.30 ± 0.09 [b]			
22:1 n-9	IF	0.04 ± 0.04	0.06 ± 0.04	0.04 ± 0.03	**	NS	NS
	FF	0.03 ± 0.03	0.05 ± 0.03	0.05 ± 0.03			
	GF	0.01 ± 0.01 [a]	0.04 ± 0.03 [a,b]	0.05 ± 0.04 [b]			
24:1 n-9	IF	0.03 ± 0.13	0.03 ± 0.02	0.03 ± 0.02	NS	NS	NS
	FF	0.02 ± 0.00 [a]	0.02 ± 0.01 [a]	0.03 ± 0.01 [b]			
	GF	0.02 ± 0.01	0.02 ± 0.01	0.03 ± 0.01			

CMF, cows' milk formula; GMF, goats' milk formula; POF, plant-oil formula; IF, infant formula; FF, follow-on formula; GF, growing-up formula. F, fat source; S, stage. Different superscript lowercase letters indicate significant differences ($p < 0.05$) with a row. *** $p < 0.001$; ** $p < 0.01$. NS, $p > 0.05$.

4. Discussion

NA occurs naturally in human milk; however, it has not been routinely reported in the global FA profile of human milk [18]. The main reason for its frequent omission is that the concentration of NA in human milk is low, and its retention time is similar to several polyunsaturated fatty acids (PUFAs). These factors make the quantitation of NA very difficult. In this study, 23:0 FAME was used as an internal standard to quantify NA concentration in human milk fat. In general, the validation of the method for the quantification of NA in human milk indicated that the method parameters' were well within internationally accepted limits.

The NA concentration significantly decreased ($p < 0.05$) with the progression of lactation days. Furthermore, the NA level decreased markedly during the first 10 days then decreased slowly after 15 days. The fat contents of human milk increased during lactation (Table S2). As shown in Table 2, the NA contents in human milk from mothers in different geographical regions and at different lactation stages were summarized. Most of the studies show a significantly higher NA content in colostrum compared to mature milk [11–13,19,20]. This study indicates the concentration of NA in colostrum was three times higher than that in mature milk, which is similar to Hua et al. [19] and Rueda et al. [20]. The results of the NA concentration in human milk during the three stages (colostrum, transitional milk, and mature milk), were similar to those found by Xiang [35]. Other publications show ten times higher NA content in colostrum compared to mature milk [11,12]. However, there are also a few publications that report the NA concentrations decrease from 0.35 to 0.27 mg/g of human milk, with no significant difference between colostrum and mature milk [36].

There are some discrepancies between studies, as shown in Table 2. The percentage of NA in human milk from individuals in Wuxi ranged from 0.06% to 0.20%. This result is marginally different from the values from several previous studies, which have reported values ranging from 0.19% to 0.99%. The difference could be due to analytical methods, as well as individuals from different locations and the lactation day. Further studies on the absolute detection of NA concentration from different countries and the correlation with maternal diet are needed.

Table 2. Mean value of nervonic acid (wt%) in human milk from individuals in different regions.

Regions	Colostrum	Transitional Milk	Mature Milk	References
Wuxi, China	0.20 (3–6 d)	0.15 (7–14 d)	0.06 (15–30 d)	This study
Taiwan, China	0.99 (1–6 d)	-	0.28 (2 m)	Hua et al. [19]
Switzerland	0.39 (1 week)	0.13 (2 weeks)	0.07 (3–8 weeks)	Thakkar et al. [13]
Beijing, China	0.54 (4 d)	-	0.25 (30 d)	Zhao et al. [14]
Thailand	-	-	0.06	Golfetto et al. [37]
Korean	-	0.27	-	
Bangladeshi	-	-	0.20	Yakes et al. [38]
Northern Sudanese	0.19	0.15	0.02	Nyuar et al. [11]
Wenzhou, China	0.45	-	-	Peng et al. [39]
Changzhou, China	0.25	-	-	
Shanghai, China	-	0.08	0.05	Jing et al. [40]
Guangzhou, China	-	0.06	0.06	
Nanchang, China	-	0.12	0.11	
Harbin, China	-	0.06	0.04	
Hohhot, China	-	0.21	0.19	
Granada, Spain	0.28	0.08	0.07	Sala-Vila A et al. [21]
Congolese	-	-	0.04	Rocquelin et al. [41]
Panama	0.32	0.16	0.10	Rueda et al. [20]
Spain	0.24	0.17	0.10	
Dominica	-	-	0.05	Beusekoma et al. [42]
Saint Lucia	0.41	0.11	0.04	Boersma et al. [12]
Belize	-	-	0.06	Cheristien et al. [43]
Dominica	-	-	0.02	

Dietary habits differ among regions and can cause internal physiological differences [44]. Jing and co-workers determined the NA content of transitional milk and mature milk from five regions (Shanghai, Guangzhou, Nanchang, Harbin, and Hohhot) of China, and the content in Hohhot was highest, regardless of whether the sample was transitional milk or mature milk [40]. Diets containing NA were fed to lactating rats, and the NA in the diet influenced the NA concentration in the animal's milk [45]. Although it is rare for NA to be provided by a typical diet, earlier studies have reported that dietary OA and EA influence the nervonic acid content in humans [46]. Lactating women are able to synthesize NA by carbon chain elongation with enzyme catalysts [47]. The large variation in NA concentration in the milk of human mothers from different regions may reflect differences in the mothers' diets [48].

There are differences in the diets of lactating mothers around the world that can account for the NA concentration differences between individuals. Additionally, the individual variation may also be related to maternal age [49], and Body Mass Index (BMI) [50]. However, in this study and previous studies, the NA concentration in all samples had a downward trend throughout the entire lactation period. This consistency, despite regional differences, indicates that the decline in NA content in human milk is more likely to be influenced by an endogenous factor [51] than a dietary habit.

The amounts of DHA and AA in human milk, similarly to NA, had a decreasing trend over the lactation period (Table S3). This has been attributed to the genes that encode delta (5)- and delta (6)-desaturases and their effect on the proportions of these FAs in human milk [52]. The DHA and AA precursors linolenic acid (18:3 n-3, ALA) and linoleic acid (18:2 n-6, LA) increase in parallel [53]. The hypothetical pathways of n-9 FAs metabolism are shown in Figure 4. NA is synthesized from OA by elongation. The OA content measured in this study (30.23%–33.86%) was in accordance with Qi's results (30.66%–32.71%) [27], but inconsistent with Weiss's study (43.96%–48.21%) [53]. OA content was stable in this study, which was contrary to the study by Lopez-Lopez et al., who claimed that OA content decreased as lactation progressed [54]. Additionally, the percentage of EiA, EA, and NA decreased with the progression of lactation, which agreed with the results obtained by Nyuar et al. [11]. In general, the amount of OA was stable over time, and the other precursors, EiA and EA, decreased during the same period, which differs from the precursors of DHA or AA. The mechanism by which genes regulate the metabolism of n-9 FAs remains unclear and needs further study. In human milk, OA is the richest FA and serves as a structural component. It can be assumed that the OA content might be sufficient to synthesize NA and other n-9 FAs.

Stearic acid (18:0)

↓ Δ-9 desaturase

Oleic acid (18:1 n-9)

↓ Elongase

Eicosenoic acid (20:1 n-9)

↓ Elongase

Erucic acid (22:1 n-9)

↓ Elongase

Nervonic acid (24:1 n-9)

Figure 4. Hypothetical pathway for the synthesis of nervonic acid in infants.

It has been demonstrated that infants have the capacity to convert ALA and LA to DHA and AA, respectively, and that elongases and desaturases have activity in the first week after birth [55]. However, the ability of infants to synthesis FAs is weak, and the amount of DHA formed from ALA is inadequate to support brain development [56]. For the optimal development of an infant's brain, a sufficient amount of NA, DHA, and AA is necessary for newborns.

Human milk is a rich source of NA compared with commercial infant formulae. In the 118 collected infant formulae samples, only 53.59% contained NA. The PCA revealed differences of NA content between human milk (including colostrum, transitional milk, and mature milk) and infant formulae (Figure 5). A significant distinction of NA content was observed between human milk and infant formula ($p < 0.05$). NA content in the three-stages (colostrum, transitional milk, and mature milk) of human milk differs obviously ($p < 0.05$). However, there is no significant difference of NA content in the three types (infant, follow-on, growing-up) of infant formula. Most NA-containing formulae had NA concentrations that were <16% of that measured in colostrum. NA content in formulae needs to be enhanced urgently for term newborns and especially for preterm newborns. It has been reported that the NA concentration in preterm milk is seven-fold higher compared to that in milk from mothers with full-term babies at a similar stage of lactation [9].

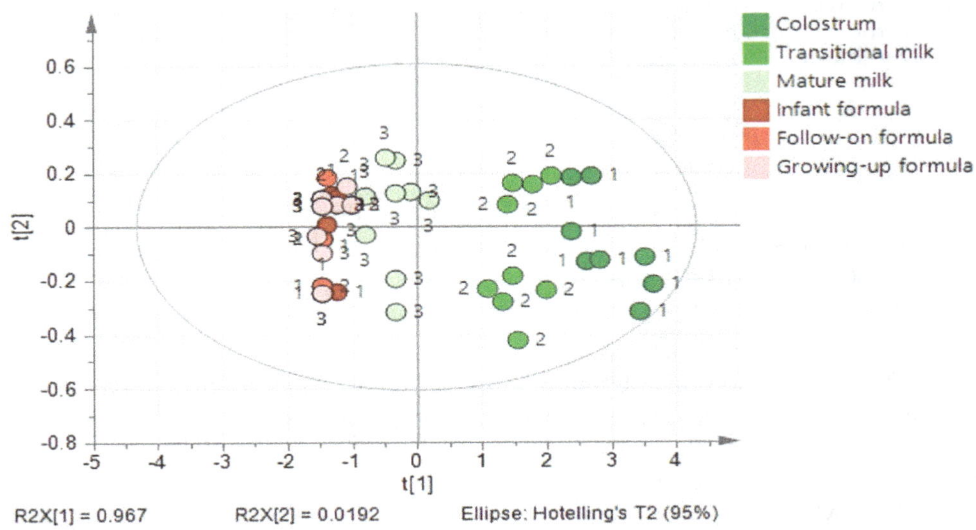

Figure 5. Principal component analysis of stage difference in the NA content in human milk (1, colostrum; 2, transitional milk; 3, mature milk) and infant formulae (1, infant formula; 2, follow-on formula; 3, growing-up formula).

The NA level is considered to reflect brain maturation, and its accumulation in the brain is a sign of the onset of myelinogenesis [57]. Newborns who cannot be breastfed fail to get sufficient levels of NA from infant formulae. Long-term NA deficiency will hamper the development of the nervous system and cause visual impairment [58]. Supplying dietary lipids to stimulate the synthesis of n-9 FAs has been advised to support myelination in newborns [23]. Thus, infant formulae need to enhance their NA content to match the NA content in human milk. This applies to formulae for full-term infants, and it is especially the case for preterm infants.

NA content in formulae was not related to fat sources or stages. However, the differences observed between other n-9 FAs in infant formulae were particularly influenced by fat sources. The current formula fat sources (generally used cow milk fat, goat milk fat, and vegetable oils) contain no or trace amount of NA. NA has been found in some plant species [59] for example *Malania oleifera* [60] and *Lunaria annua* [61]. However, oils of these plants are rarely developed and used in infant formulae because of their high EA content. It has been demonstrated that the heart may be damaged by EA, and EA is undesirable for human consumption [62]. It is necessary to explore the effect of NA as well as different forms (FA, TAG or PLs) for the optimal brain development of infants.

5. Conclusions

The NA concentration was at its highest at the onset of lactation, with an overall decrease of 82% throughout the 3–30 days postpartum study period. The concentration dropped at a faster rate in the first 10 days and then flattened out. Thus, it is crucial for infants, especially preterm infants, to get enough NA within the first ten days of lactation. The NA concentration differs between breastfeeding mothers, in part because of the regions in which they live. Further studies are needed to clarify the NA biosynthetic system in infants. Most of the 97 infant formulae in which NA was detected had less than 16% of the NA content in colostrum. There were significant differences between the fat sources of OA, EiA, and EA in the formulae, but this was not the case for NA. The effect of the stages or the interaction between sources and stages on infant formulae FA composition was not obvious. Because of the low level of NA found in infant formulae, it is suggested that the NA content in infant formulae for newborns be increased. Further work is also warranted to identify the best form of NA for infants.

Author Contributions: Data curation, X.Z.; formal analysis, Q.J.; methodology, T.Y.; project administration, W.W.; supervision, X.W.; writing—original draft, J.Y.

Acknowledgments: This work was supported by the National Natural Science Foundation of China (grant number 31701558) and the Young Elite Scientists Sponsorship Program by CAST (grant number 2017QNRC001). The authors particularly thank L. Ding from Wuxi Wanyi Infant Care and mothers who volunteered to contribute human milk.

References

1. Cheong, L.Z.; Jiang, C.Y.; He, X.Q.; Song, S.; Lai, O.M. Lipid Profiling, Particle Size Determination, and in Vitro Simulated Gastrointestinal Lipolysis of Mature Human Milk and Infant Formula. *J. Agric. Food Chem.* **2018**, *66*, 12042–12050. [CrossRef] [PubMed]
2. Wei, W.; Jin, Q.; Wang, X. Human milk fat substitutes: Past achievements and current trends. *Prog. Lipid Res.* **2019**, *74*, 69–86. [CrossRef] [PubMed]
3. Sun, C.; Zou, X.; Yao, Y.; Jin, J.; Xia, Y.; Huang, J.; Jin, Q.; Wang, X. Evaluation of fatty acid composition in commercial infant formulas on the Chinese market: A comparative study based on fat source and stage. *Int. Dairy J.* **2016**, *63*, 42–51. [CrossRef]
4. Amminger, G.P.; Schaefer, M.R.; Klier, C.M.; Slavik, J.M.; Holzer, I.; Holub, M.; Goldstone, S.; Whitford, T.J.; McGorry, P.D.; Berk, M. Decreased nervonic acid levels in erythrocyte membranes predict psychosis in help-seeking ultra-high-risk individuals. *Mol. Psychiatry* **2012**, *17*, 1150–1152. [CrossRef] [PubMed]
5. Kinney, H.C.; Brody, B.A.; Kloman, A.S.; Gilles, F.H. Sequence of central nervous system myelination in

human infancy. II. Patterns of Myelination in Autopsied Infants. *J. Neuropathol. Exp. Neurol.* **1988**, *47*, 217–234. [CrossRef] [PubMed]

6. Moser, A.B.; Jones, D.S.; Raymond, G.V.; Moser, H.W. Plasma and red blood cell fatty acids in peroxisomal disorders. *Neurochem. Res.* **1999**, *24*, 187–197. [CrossRef] [PubMed]
7. Moser, A.B.; Kreiter, N.; Bezman, L.; Lu, S.; Raymond, G.V.; Naidu, S.; Moser, H.W. Plasma very long chain fatty acids in 3000 peroxisome disease patients and 29,000 controls. *Ann. Neurol.* **1999**, *45*, 100–110. [CrossRef]
8. Yeh, Y.Y. Long chain fatty acid deficits in brain myelin sphingolipids of undernourished rat pups. *Lipids* **1988**, *23*, 1114–1118. [CrossRef]
9. Ntoumani, E.; Strandvik, B.; Sabel, K.G. Nervonic acid is much lower in donor milk than in milk from mothers delivering premature infants-Of neglected importance? *Prostaglandins Leukot. Essent. Fat. Acids* **2013**, *89*, 241–244. [CrossRef]
10. Wu, K.; Gao, R.; Tian, F.; Mao, Y.; Wang, B.; Zhou, L.; Shen, L.; Guan, Y.; Cai, M. Fatty acid positional distribution (sn-2 fatty acids) and phospholipid composition in Chinese breast milk from colostrum to mature stage. *Br. J. Nutr.* **2018**, *121*, 65–73. [CrossRef]
11. Nyuar, K.B.; Min, Y.; Ghebremeskel, K.; Khalil, A.K.H.; Elbashir, M.I.; Cawford, M.A. Milk of northern Sudanese mothers whose traditional diet is high in carbohydrate contains low docosahexaenoic acid. *Acta Pãediatr.* **2010**, *99*, 1824. [CrossRef]
12. Boersma, E.R.; Offringa, P.J.; Muskiet, F.A.; Chase, W.M.; Simmons, I.J. Vitamin E, lipid fractions, and fatty acid composition of colostrum, transitional milk, and mature milk: An international comparative study. *Am. J. Clin. Nutr.* **1991**, *53*, 1197–1204. [CrossRef]
13. Thakkar, S.K.; De Castro, C.A.; Beauport, L.; Tolsa, J.F.; Fumeaux, C.J.F.; Affolter, M.; Giuffrida, F. Temporal Progression of Fatty Acids in Preterm and Term Human Milk of Mothers from Switzerland. *Nutrients* **2019**, *11*, 12. [CrossRef]
14. Zhao, P.; Zhang, S.W.; Liu, L.; Pang, X.Y.; Yang, Y.; Lu, J.; Lv, J.P. Differences in the Triacylglycerol and Fatty Acid Compositions of Human Colostrum and Mature Milk. *J. Agric. Food Chem.* **2018**, *66*, 4571–4579. [CrossRef]
15. Jamieson, E.C.; Farquharson, J.; Logan, R.W.; Howatson, A.G.; Patrick, W.J.A.; Weaver, L.T.; Cockburn, F. Infant cerebellar gray and white matter fatty acids in relation to age and diet. *Lipids* **1999**, *34*, 1065–1071. [CrossRef]
16. Nagae, L.M.; Hoon, A.H.; Stashinko, E.; Lin, D.; Zhang, W.; Levey, E.; Wakana, S.; Jiang, H.; Leite, C.C.; Lucato, L.T. Diffusion tensor imaging in children with periventricular leukomalacia: Variability of injuries to white matter tracts. *Ajnr Am. J. Neuroradiol.* **2007**, *28*, 1213. [CrossRef]
17. De Vries, L.S.; Van Haastert, I.L.C.; Rademaker, K.J.; Corine, K.; Floris, G. Ultrasound abnormalities preceding cerebral palsy in high-risk preterm infants. *J. Pediatr.* **2004**, *144*, 815–820. [CrossRef]
18. Liu, Z.; Rochfort, S.; Cocks, B. Milk lipidomics: What we know and what we don't. *Prog. Lipid Res.* **2018**, *71*, 70–85. [CrossRef]
19. Hua, M.C.; Su, H.M.; Kuo, M.L.; Chen, C.C.; Yao, T.C.; Tsai, M.H.; Liao, S.L.; Lai, S.H.; Chiu, C.Y.; Su, K.W.; et al. Association of maternal allergy with human milk soluble CD14 and fatty acids, and early childhood atopic dermatitis. *Pediatr. Allergy Immunol.* **2019**, *30*, 204–213. [CrossRef]
20. Rueda, R.; Ramírez, M.; Garcíasalmerón, J.L.; Maldonado, J.; Gil, A. Gestational Age and Origin of Human Milk Influence Total Lipid and Fatty Acid Contents. *Ann. Nutr. Metab.* **1998**, *42*, 12–22. [CrossRef]
21. Salavila, A.; Castellote, A.I.; Rodriguezpalmero, M.; Campoy, C.; Lópezsabater, M.C. Lipid composition in human breast milk from Granada (Spain): Changes during lactation. *Nutrition* **2005**, *21*, 467–473. [CrossRef]
22. Zou, L.; Pande, G.; Akoh, C.C. Infant Formula Fat Analogs and Human Milk Fat: New Focus on Infant Developmental Needs. In *Annual Review of Food Science and Technology*; Doyle, M.P., Klaenhammer, T.R., Eds.; Annual Reviews: Palo Alto, CA, USA, 2016; Volume 7, pp. 139–165.
23. Billeaud, C.; Boue-Vaysse, C.; Couedelo, L.; Steenhout, P.; Jaeger, J.; Cruz-Hernandez, C.; Ameye, L.; Rigo, J.; Picaud, J.C.; Saliba, E.; et al. Effects on Fatty Acid Metabolism of a New Powdered Human Milk Fortifier Containing Medium-Chain Triacylglycerols and Docosahexaenoic Acid in Preterm Infants. *Nutrients* **2018**, *10*, 690. [CrossRef]
24. Dingess, K.; Valentine, C.; Davidson, B.; Peng, Y.; Guerrero, M.; Ruiz-Palacios, G.; Brenna, J.; McMahon, R.;

Morrow, A. Docosahexaenoic acid, nervonic acid and iso-20 (BCFA) concentrations in human milk from the Global Exploration of Human Milk Project. *FASEB J.* **2014**, *28*, 623.15.

25. Sala-Vila, A.; Castellote, A.I.; Campoy, C.M.; Rodriguez-Palmero, M. The source of long-chain PUFA in formula supplements does not affect the fatty acid composition of plasma lipids in full-term infants. *J. Nutr.* **2004**, *134*, 868–873. [CrossRef]
26. Jensen, R.G. *The Lipids of Human Milk*; CRC Press: Boca Raton, FL, USA, 1989.
27. Qi, C.; Sun, J.; Xia, Y.; Yu, R.Q.; Wei, W.; Xiang, J.Y.; Jin, Q.Z.; Xiao, H.; Wang, X.G. Fatty Acid Profile and the sn-2 Position Distribution in Triacylglycerols of Breast Milk during Different Lactation Stages. *J. Agric. Food Chem.* **2018**, *66*, 3118–3126. [CrossRef]
28. The United States Pharmacopeia. Validation of Compendial Procedures. In *The United States Pharmacopeia, the National. Formulary, Chapter 1225*; Stanford University: Stanford, CA, USA, 2009.
29. Quintela, M.; Báguena, J.; Gotor, G.; Blanco, M.J.; Broto, F. Estimation of the uncertainty associated with the results based on the validation of chromatographic analysis procedures: Application to the determination of chlorides by high performance liquid chromatography and of fatty acids by high resolution gas chro. *J. Chromatogr. A* **2012**, *1223*, 107–117. [CrossRef]
30. Taverniers, I.; De Loose, M.; Van Bockstaele, E. Trends in quality in the analytical laboratory. II. Analytical method validation and quality assurance. *Trac Trends Anal. Chem.* **2004**, *23*, 535–552. [CrossRef]
31. IOFI Working Group on Methods of Analysis. Guidelines for the quantitative gas chromatography of volatile flavouring substances, from the Working Group on Methods of Analysis of the International Organization of the Flavor Industry (IOFI). *Flavour Fragr. J.* **2011**, *26*, 297–299.
32. Gravador, R.S.; Harrison, S.M.; Monahan, F.J.; Gkarane, V.; Farmer, L.J.; Brunton, N.P. Validation of a Rapid Microwave-Assisted Extraction Method and GC-FID Quantification of Total Branched Chain Fatty Acids in Lamb Subcutaneous Adipose Tissue. *J. Food Sci.* **2019**, *84*, 80–85. [CrossRef]
33. AOAC. *AOAC Peer-Verified Methods Program, Manual on Policies and Procedures*; The Association of Official Analytical Chemists: Arlington, VA, USA, 1998.
34. Koletzko, B.; Baker, S.; Cleghorn, G.; Neto, U.F.; Gopalan, S.; Hernell, O.; Hock, Q.S.; Jirapinyo, P.; Lonnerdal, B.; Pencharz, P.; et al. Global standard for the composition of infant formula: Recommendations of an ESPGHAN Coordinated International Expert Group. *J. Pediatr. Gastroenterol. Nutr.* **2005**, *41*, 584–599. [CrossRef]
35. Xiang, M.; Harbige, L.S.; Zetterstrã, M.R. Long-chain polyunsaturated fatty acids in Chinese and Swedish mothers: Diet, breast milk and infant growth. *Acta Pædiatr.* **2005**, *94*, 1543–1549. [CrossRef]
36. Rydlewski, A.A.; Silva, P.D.; Manin, L.P.; Tavares, C.B.G.; Paula, M.G.; Figueiredo, I.L.; Neia, V.; Santos, O.O.; Visentainer, J.V. Lipid Profile Determination by Direct Infusion ESI-MS and Fatty Acid Composition by GC-FID in Human Milk Pools by Folch and Creamatocrit Methods. *J. Braz. Chem. Soc.* **2019**, *30*, 1063–1073. [CrossRef]
37. Golfetto, I.; Mcgready, R.; Ghebremeskel, K.; Min, Y.; Dubowitz, L.; Nosten, F.; Drury, P.; Simpson, J.A.; Arunjerdja, R.; Crawford, M.A. Fatty acid composition of milk of refugee Karen and urban Korean mothers. Is the level of DHA in breast milk of Western women compromised by high intake of saturated fat and linoleic acid? *Nutr. Health* **2007**, *18*, 319. [CrossRef]
38. Yakes, E.A.; Arsenault, J.E.; Munirul, I.M.; Hossain, M.B.; Ahmed, T.; Bruce, G.J.; Gillies, L.A.; Shafiqur, R.A.; Drake, C.; Jamil, K.M. Intakes and breast-milk concentrations of essential fatty acids are low among Bangladeshi women with 24–48-month-old children. *Br. J. Nutr.* **2011**, *105*, 1660–1670. [CrossRef]
39. Peng, Y.; Zhou, T.; Wang, Q.; Liu, P.; Zhang, T.; Zetterström, R.; Strandvik, B. Fatty acid composition of diet, cord blood and breast milk in Chinese mothers with different dietary habits. *Prostagland. Leukot. Essent. Fat. Acids* **2009**, *81*, 325–330. [CrossRef]
40. Li, J.; Fan, Y.W.; Zhang, Z.W.; Yu, H.; An, Y.; Kramer, J.K.G.; Deng, Z.Y. Evaluating the trans fatty acid, CLA, PUFA and erucic acid diversity in human milk from five regions in China. *Lipids* **2009**, *44*, 257. [CrossRef]
41. Rocquelin, G.; Tapsoba, S.; Dop, M.C.; Mbemba, F.; Traissac, P.; Martinprével, Y. Lipid content and essential fatty acid (EFA) composition of mature Congolese breast milk are influenced by mothers' nutritional status: Impact on infants' EFA supply. *Eur. J. Clin. Nutr.* **1998**, *52*, 164–171. [CrossRef]
42. van Beusekom, C.M.; Nijeboer, H.J.; Van der Veere, C.N.; Luteyn, A.J.; Offringa, P.J.; Muskiet, F.A.; Boersma, E.R. Indicators of long chain polyunsaturated fatty acid status of exclusively breastfed infants at delivery and after 20–22 days. *Early Hum. Dev.* **1993**, *32*, 207. [CrossRef]

43. Van, B.C.; Martini, I.A.; Rutgers, H.M.; Boersma, E.R.; Muskiet, F.A. A carbohydrate-rich diet not only leads to incorporation of medium-chain fatty acids (6:0–14:0) in milk triglycerides but also in each milk-phospholipid subclass. *Am. J. Clin. Nutr.* **1990**, *52*, 326.
44. Nishimura, R.Y.; Barbieiri, P.; Castro, G.S.; Jordão, A.A., Jr.; Perdoná, G.S.; Sartorelli, D.S. Dietary polyunsaturated fatty acid intake during late pregnancy affects fatty acid composition of mature breast milk. *Nutrition* **2014**, *30*, 685. [CrossRef]
45. Bettger, W.J.; DiMichelle-Ranalli, E.; Dillingham, B.; Blackadar, C.B. Nervonic acid is transferred from the maternal diet to milk and tissues of suckling rat pups. *J. Nutr. Biochem.* **2003**, *14*, 160–165. [CrossRef]
46. Bettger, W.J.; Blackadar, C.B. Dietary very long chain fatty acids directly influence the ratio of tetracosenoic (24:1) to tetracosanoic (24:0) acids of sphingomyelin in rat liver. *Lipids* **1997**, *32*, 51–55. [CrossRef]
47. Fulco, A.J.; Mead, J.F. The biosynthesis of lignoceric, cerebronic, and nervonic acids. *J. Biol. Chem.* **1961**, *236*, 2416–2420.
48. Lauritzen, L.; Jorgensen, M.H.; Hansen, H.S.; Michaelsen, K.F. Fluctuations in human milk long-chain PUFA levels in relation to dietary fish intake. *Lipids* **2002**, *37*, 237–244. [CrossRef]
49. Argov-Argaman, N.; Mandel, D.; Lubetzky, R.; Kedem, M.H.; Cohen, B.C.; Berkovitz, Z.; Reifen, R. Human milk fatty acids composition is affected by maternal age. *J. Matern. Fetal Neonatal Med.* **2017**, *30*, 34–37. [CrossRef]
50. Marín, M.C.; Sanjurjo, A.; Rodrigo, M.A.; de Alaniz, M.J. Long-chain polyunsaturated fatty acids in breast milk in La Plata, Argentina: Relationship with maternal nutritional status. *Prostagland. Leukot. Essent. Fat. Acids* **2005**, *73*, 355–360. [CrossRef]
51. Muskiet, F.A.; Hutter, N.H.; Martini, I.A.; Jonxis, J.H.; Offringa, P.J.; Boersma, E.R. Comparison of the fatty acid composition of human milk from mothers in Tanzania, Curacao and Surinam. *Hum. Nutr. Clin. Nutr.* **1987**, *41*, 149–159.
52. Molto-Puigmarti, C.; Plat, J.; Mensink, R.P.; Muller, A.; Jansen, E.; Zeegers, M.P.; Thijs, C. FADS1 FADS2 gene variants modify the association between fish intake and the docosahexaenoic acid proportions in human milk. *Am. J. Clin. Nutr.* **2010**, *91*, 1368–1376. [CrossRef]
53. Weiss, G.A.; Troxler, H.; Klinke, G.; Rogler, D.; Braegger, C.; Hersberger, M. High levels of anti-inflammatory and pro-resolving lipid mediators lipoxins and resolvins and declining docosahexaenoic acid levels in human milk during the first month of lactation. *Lipids Health Dis.* **2013**, *12*, 89. [CrossRef]
54. Lópezlópez, A.; Lópezsabater, M.C.; Campoyfolgoso, C.; Riverourgell, M.; Castellotebargalló, A.I. Fatty acid and sn-2 fatty acid composition in human milk from Granada (Spain) and in infant formulas. *Eur. J. Clin. Nutr.* **2002**, *56*, 1242–1254. [CrossRef]
55. Salem, N.; Wegher, B.; Mena, P.; Uauy, R. Arachidonic and docosahexaenoic acids are biosynthesized from their 18-carbon precursors in human infants. *Proc. Natl. Acad. Sci. USA* **1996**, *93*, 49–54. [CrossRef]
56. Gibson, R.A.; Makrides, M.; Neumann, M.A.; Simmer, K.; Mantzioris, E.; James, M.J. Ratios of linoleic acid to alpha-linolenic acid in formulas for term infants. *J. Pediatr.* **1994**, *125*, 48–55. [CrossRef]
57. Martinez, M. Tissue levels of polyunsaturated fatty acids during early human development. *J. Pediatr.* **1992**, *120*, S129. [CrossRef]
58. Uzman, L.L.; Rumley, M.K. Changes in the composition of the developing mouse brain during early myelination. *J. Neurochem.* **2010**, *3*, 170–184. [CrossRef]
59. Fan, Y.; Meng, H.-M.; Hu, G.-R.; Li, F. Biosynthesis of nervonic acid and perspectives for its production by microalgae and other microorganisms. *Appl. Microbiol. Biotechnol.* **2018**, *102*, 3027–3035. [CrossRef]
60. Wang, X.Y.; Fan, J.S.; Wang, S.Q. Development situation and outlook of nervonic acid plants in China. *China Oils Fats* **2006**, *31*, 69–71.
61. Yiming, G.; Elzbieta, M.; Tammy, F.; Vesna, K.; Brost, J.M.; Michael, G.; Barton, D.L.; Taylor, D.C. Increase in nervonic acid content in transformed yeast and transgenic plants by introduction of a *Lunaria annua* L. 3-ketoacyl-CoA synthase (KCS) gene. *Plant Mol. Biol.* **2009**, *69*, 565–575.
62. Das, S.; Roscoe, T.J.; Delseny, M.; Srivastava, P.S.; Lakshmikumaran, M. Cloning and molecular characterization of the Fatty Acid Elongase 1 (FAE 1) gene from high and low erucic acid lines of *Brassica campestris* and *Brassica oleracea*. *Plant Sci.* **2002**, *162*, 245–250. [CrossRef]

10

A Moderated Mediation Model of Maternal Perinatal Stress, Anxiety, Infant Perceptions and Breastfeeding

Jessica P. Riedstra * and Nicki L. Aubuchon-Endsley

Department of Psychology, Idaho State University, Pocatello, ID 83209, USA; aubunick@isu.edu
* Correspondence: riedjess@isu.edu

Abstract: This study examined a moderated mediation model of relations among maternal perinatal stress/anxiety, breastfeeding difficulties (mediator), misperceptions of infant crying (moderator), and maternal breastfeeding duration to understand risk factors for early breastfeeding termination. It was hypothesized that more breastfeeding difficulties would mediate the relation between greater prenatal stress/anxiety and shorter breastfeeding duration, and that perceptions of response to infant crying as spoiling would moderate the relation between more breastfeeding difficulties and reduced breastfeeding duration. Additionally, it was hypothesized that participants who breastfed through 6 months would demonstrate less postnatal stress/anxiety and there would be a positive relation between fewer breastfeeding difficulties and less postnatal stress/anxiety through 6 months. Participants included 94 expectant mothers at 33–37 weeks gestation and 6 months (±2 weeks) postpartum. Greater prenatal anxiety was associated with shorter breastfeeding duration. Results presented are the first to document negative relations between prenatal (as opposed to postnatal) anxiety and breastfeeding duration (as opposed to frequency or other indicators) in a U.S. sample. Future studies should seek to replicate findings in a more diverse sample and compare findings from clinical and non-clinical samples. Studies may also wish to explore the effects of anxiety prevention/intervention on breastfeeding duration.

Keywords: perinatal; maternal stress; maternal anxiety; infant crying; breastfeeding

---

1. Introduction

Despite efforts to improve breastfeeding rates, about half of mothers discontinue breastfeeding by 6 months, and two-thirds by 12 months [1]. Breastfed children and mothers who breastfeed benefit from improved physical and psychological health and maternal perinatal stress and anxiety may impact breastfeeding behaviors [2–11]. About 10% of pregnant women and 13% of women who recently gave birth have a mental disorder (most commonly depression and anxiety) [12]. While perinatal depression is heavily researched, stress and anxiety receive considerably less attention and remain less understood [13–17]. Furthermore, limited research has examined these psychological experiences among medically underserved perinatal women (e.g., those with limited access to physical and mental health services).

Feelings of stress (i.e., reaction to a stressor) and anxiety (i.e., emotion not necessarily tied to a specific event or stressor) can be defined as two separate, though similar, constructs [18]. Literature suggests that women may experience perinatal stress and/or anxiety; therefore, it is important to measure them separately. For this project, subjective measures of stress and anxiety were utilized given the practical utility for perinatal health providers. Regarding anxiety, worldwide estimates suggest 7%–60% of women experience high levels of general anxiety during pregnancy and 5%–33% in the postpartum period. Furthermore, 3%–39% of women experience an anxiety disorder, as do 4%–20% of postpartum women [15]. In addition, 17% of Idaho women experience some form of anxiety 3 months prior to pregnancy [19]. Research regarding the prevalence of psychosocial stress during pregnancy is limited, and suggests that during the antenatal period, 6% of women reported high stress, 78% low to moderate stress, and 16% no stress [20]. In 2010, 70% of women reported a stressful life event within the year prior to their infant's birth [21]. With regard to Idaho, 21% of women described experiencing high prenatal stress (i.e., three or more stressful life events in the 12 months prior to delivery) [19]. Therefore, women in this region may experience more pregnancy stressful life events than the national average, making perinatal samples from these understudied regions important to consider. Many of these women also have poorer access to healthcare, thereby enhancing the potential impact and outcomes of stress-related difficulties during pregnancy [22].

1.1. *Breastfeeding Difficulties*

Numerous research findings support relations between stress or anxiety and lower breastfeeding rates [23–31]. Breastfeeding difficulties also may play a role (e.g., mediation) in breastfeeding behaviors. Early in the postpartum period, breastfeeding concerns or perceptions, like difficulty latching or low milk supply, are a significant source of maternal stress [32]. The Centers for Disease Control (CDC) Pregnancy Risk Assessment Monitoring System (PRAMS) is perhaps the most comprehensive and widely used assessment of U.S. women's experiences during and 2–6 months after pregnancy, including breastfeeding. It is utilized to examine difficulties initiating and continuing breastfeeding, including: Difficulties for mother, infant, and with time management, among others [33]. Women discontinue breastfeeding due to physical pain and discomfort (e.g., cracked nipples, biting, and scratching); uncertainty of milk supply and latching issues; personal, professional, social, and physical difficulties; beliefs regarding infant preferences; and lack of confidence [9,11,34,35]. Several breastfeeding difficulties may influence breastfeeding initiation, frequency, and duration, however, the relation between stress and anxiety and breastfeeding difficulties remains unexplored.

1.2. *Infant Crying*

Considering the potential relation between breastfeeding difficulties and behaviors, perceptions of infant crying may serve as a moderating factor. Crying can be disruptive and challenging for families, including experiencing guilt, stress, frustration, social isolation, and strained relationships [36]. Many mothers use breastfeeding as a method to console crying infants, and breastfeeding to comfort is a strong predictor of longer partial breastfeeding duration [37]. However, women who perceive responding to their infant's crying cues with breastfeeding as spoiling may experience a more robust relation between increased breastfeeding difficulties and decreased breastfeeding behaviors [38,39]. The compounded effect of breastfeeding difficulties and a decreased response to infant crying with breastfeeding may serve to decrease breastfeeding duration, such that women may avoid difficulties and the risk of spoiling their infants by removing feeding to console. Therefore, maternal perceptions of spoiling an infant via breastfeeding to console crying behavior were investigated in the present study.

Taken together, little, if any, research has focused on women from medically underserved, U.S. samples wherein breastfeeding resources and support may be limited. Few studies have examined both anxiety and stress, and their impact on specific breastfeeding behaviors during the prenatal and postpartum periods. To our knowledge, no research has evaluated mechanisms by which perinatal stress, anxiety, breastfeeding difficulties, perceptions of responding to infant crying, and breastfeeding behaviors may be related. Additionally, research to date has demonstrated variability in when and how peripartum stress and/or anxiety is measured. Thus, the present study used psychometrically sound measures at two time points to explore whether prenatal (i.e., during third trimester) or postnatal (i.e., up to 6 months postpartum) stress or anxiety is more predictive of breastfeeding behavior. The study also sought to examine the role of breastfeeding difficulties as a potential mediator of relations between prenatal stress and anxiety and breastfeeding duration, and perceptions of infant crying as a moderator between breastfeeding difficulties and duration. Additionally, the study sought to examine univariate relations between postnatal maternal stress, anxiety, and breastfeeding difficulties, relevant covariates, and breastfeeding duration. Understanding risk factors that contribute to decreased breastfeeding behavior may prove beneficial for infants and mothers, which may assist in prevention/intervention research. The following models and hypotheses were used to fill these gaps in the extant literature.

1.3. Proposed Models and Hypotheses

Given the relation between breastfeeding difficulties and duration, it is plausible that breastfeeding difficulties mediate the relation between stress and anxiety and breastfeeding duration [34,35]. Furthermore, a mother's perception of responding to infant crying with breastfeeding as spoiling may interact with breastfeeding difficulties to further negatively impact breastfeeding duration. Therefore, high scores on measures of maternal misperceptions of infant crying may moderate, or strengthen, the mediated relation between anxiety and stress, breastfeeding difficulties, and breastfeeding duration. Given these predicted relations, two moderated mediation models were proposed: Hypothesis 1 consisted of a moderated mediation model with prenatal stress as the predictor, breastfeeding difficulties as the mediator, perceptions of infant crying as spoiling as the moderator along the b path, and breastfeeding duration through 6 months as the outcome variable. Hypothesis 2 proposed the same model, however the predictor was prenatal anxiety. To examine the impact of breastfeeding experiences on postnatal stress and anxiety, two further relations were hypothesized. Specifically, it was hypothesized that participants who breastfed through 6 months postpartum would demonstrate lower levels of postnatal stress (Hypothesis 3) and anxiety (Hypothesis 4) than those who discontinued prior to 6 months. We also hypothesized that among women who breastfeed through 6 months, there would be a positive relation between fewer breastfeeding difficulties and lower levels of postnatal stress (Hypothesis 5) and anxiety (Hypothesis 6). As breastfeeding difficulties appear related to shorter breastfeeding duration, women who continue breastfeeding at 6 months may experience fewer difficulties and report lower levels of stress and anxiety.

2. Methods

2.1. Participants

Data were collected as part of a larger longitudinal research project examining maternal health and infant development. The project was approved by the Idaho State University Human Subjects Committee (protocol 4191, entitled "Infant Development and Healthy Outcomes in Mothers Study"). Data were collected for 125 prenatal participants and 96 participants at 6 months postpartum (See Figure 1).

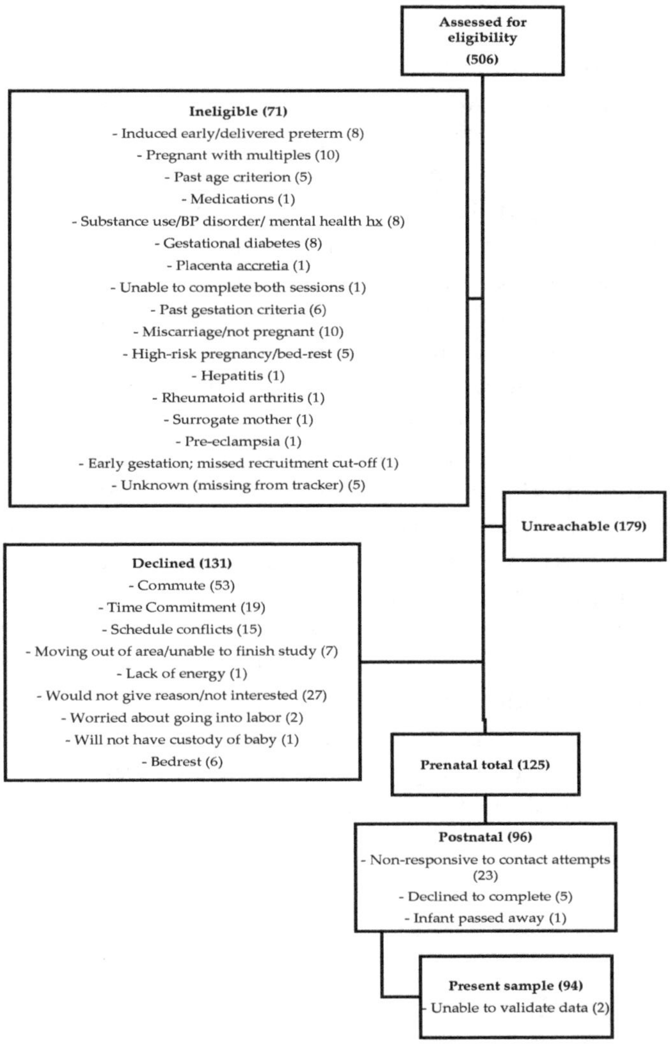

Figure 1. Response rate throughout recruitment and each data collection time point. Bolded numbers in parentheses indicate total sample size at each stage and non-bolded numbers in parentheses indicate the number of participants who withdrew for the reason listed.

2.2. Recruitment

Participants were recruited throughout southeastern Idaho and screened for eligibility via brief phone calls. During the third trimester, prospective participants met individually with a trained research assistant (RA) and completed written informed consent, if eligible. Exclusion criteria included mothers with: More than one baby; certain health conditions (e.g., gestational diabetes, pre-eclampsia, and toxemia) that could impact endocrine functioning; certain behavioral or physical health diagnoses/symptoms (e.g., Schizophrenia, Bipolar Disorder, HIV, and AIDS); or chronic use of recreational substances (e.g., marijuana, or cocaine), medications from FDA categories D and X with documented detrimental fetal effects, or alcohol (>40 drinks) during pregnancy. Mothers had to be at least 18 years of age to provide consent, and 35 years of age or younger given that infertility, chromosomal abnormalities, miscarriage, stillbirth, and multiple pregnancies occur at greater rates after age 35 and all of these factors are related to other exclusion criteria [40]. Participants were recruited from medical centers (e.g., hospitals, clinics), family programs and service centers, childcare facilities, local businesses, schools/university, libraries, recreational centers, the local tribal reservation, community organizations and professionals (e.g., doulas, La Leche League, midwives), and through a variety of mediums (e.g., newsletters, social media).

2.3. Quantitative Analyses

Based on Fritz and MacKinnon's mediation model simulations, a sample size of 71 is required to achieve a power of 0.80 in a mediation model assessed via bias-corrected bootstrapping with medium effect sizes ($d = 0.39$) for a and b paths [41]. Similarly, a priori power analyses utilizing *GPower* suggest that a sample size of 85 is sufficient for the most complex analyses tested in Hypothesis 1 and 2 [41,42]. In *GPower*, a least squares linear multiple regression with three predictors and one outcome variable and up to three covariates was used. This included a medium effect size ($f^2 = 0.15$) for R squared change in steps 1 and 2 after covariates then predictors are added into the model. Analyses also included a two-tailed p-value of 0.05 and power of 0.80. Medium effects size parameters were used based upon prior research findings on maternal affect and breastfeeding behaviors [14]. Two participants' data on the Perinatal Anxiety Screening Scale (PASS) were deemed to be likely inaccurate due to extremely low scores, which indicated that participants did not attend to measure items. Therefore, they were removed from the dataset, resulting in a final sample size of 94. The PROCESS macro v2.16, Model 14 was used to test moderated mediation Hypotheses 1 and 2 [43]. The macro uses bias-corrected bootstrapping to assess statistical significance of direct and indirect effects, which maximizes power and is robust against Type II error and violations of normality. These methods require a smaller sample size to attain sufficient power for the conditional indirect effect with recent simulation studies supporting that sample sizes <100 have power ≥0.80 with a and b paths of medium effect size [44]. The macro quantifies the effect of V on the indirect effect of X on Y through M, with significance determined via bias-corrected confidence intervals [43]. Independent samples t-tests were used to test Hypotheses 3 and 4, and Pearson's product–moment correlations for Hypotheses 5 and 6. Power analyses utilizing *GPower* suggested a sample size of 82 to achieve a medium effect (i.e., 0.3) and a power of 0.80 [42]. Prenatal and postnatal PASS scores were positively skewed and transformed using a natural log function.

2.4. Measures

2.4.1. Stress

The Perceived Stress Scale (PSS) is a 14-item self-report measure developed to assess the degree to which respondents find their lives "unpredictable, uncontrollable, and overloading," or components central to experiencing stress [45] (p. 387). In two college and one smoking cessation sample, the PSS demonstrated Cronbach's $\alpha = 0.84–0.86$, test-retest reliability after 2 days of 0.85, and test-retest reliability after 6 days of 0.55. The College Student Life-Event Schedule and PSS correlated between 0.17–0.49 in all samples [46]. The PSS-10 ($\alpha = 0.74$) and PSS-4 ($\alpha = 0.79$) have demonstrated good reliability in pregnancy samples [47] and a recent, large ($n = 2847$) validation study suggested that the PSS-14 has similar factor structure, internal consistency, and convergent and divergent validity than the PSS-10 in two prenatal samples [48]. The PSS demonstrated good reliability at prenatal and 6-month postnatal time points in the current sample (Cronbach's $a = 0.80$ and 0.78, respectively).

2.4.2. Anxiety

The PASS is a 31-item self-report questionnaire developed to screen for a broad range of anxiety symptoms in perinatal women [49]. The PASS total score is statistically significantly correlated with the Depression Anxiety Stress Scale anxiety (Pearson's product–moment $r = 0.78$, $p < 0.01$) and stress (Pearson's product–moment $r = 0.81$, $p < 0.01$) scales, anxiety scale of the Edinburg Postnatal Depression Scale (Pearson's product–moment $r = 0.74$, $p < 0.01$) and the State–Trait Anxiety Inventory (STAI; State Pearson's product–moment $r = 0.75$, $p < 0.01$; Trait Pearson's product–moment $r = 0.83$, $p < 0.01$)), which support the measure's convergent validity [50,51]. A correlation between PASS scores in subsamples of antenatal and postnatal women ($n = 35$) was 0.74. Internal consistency of the total PASS score in the present sample was high at prenatal ($a = 0.95$) and postnatal ($a = 0.93$) time points.

2.4.3. Breastfeeding difficulties

Breastfeeding difficulties were measured as part of the 6-Month Infant Dietary Questionnaire, a measure created utilizing similar item content from the PRAMS. The 7-item self-report questionnaire measures infant feeding behaviors since birth, including formula feeding, breastfeeding, consuming solid foods, and difficulties breastfeeding. Breastfeeding difficulties were measured with a yes/no question asking whether difficulties have been present, at any time and with any frequency, during breastfeeding. Mothers answering "yes" were asked to specify which difficulties they experienced including maternal-related difficulties (i.e., expressing milk, soreness, or fatigue), difficulties an infant may experience (i.e., latching, sucking, not obtaining enough milk, or not interested in feeding), difficulties with time management (i.e., returning to work and unable to pump), difficulties with insufficient environment (i.e., discomfort feeding in public or around others at home), or others (e.g., open-ended question). Difficulties were quantified as the number endorsed (ranging from 0 to 10 or more). Frequency of difficulties were provided as percentages (See Results).

2.4.4. Infant crying behavior

The Infant Crying Questionnaire-Revised (ICQ-R) is a 43-item self-report measure of maternal perceptions of infant crying [52]. The postnatal version includes 20 items that assess mothers' perceptions of their babies' crying behavior. The ICQ-R consists of five scales, and the present study utilized the Spoiling scale as an index of maternal perceptions of response to infant crying as spoiling. The Spoiling scale has demonstrated internal consistency of Cronbach's $\alpha = 0.70$ [52]. Scores for the three items related to infant spoiling are totaled. The Spoiling scale in the present sample demonstrated Cronbach's $a = 0.76$.

2.4.5. Breastfeeding duration

Breastfeeding duration was measured as part of the 6-Month Infant Dietary Questionnaire [53] via a single open-ended item asking participant how many months, weeks, or days they breastfed. All data were quantified as days.

2.5. Procedures

The prenatal visit included an interview regarding participants' current and past pregnancy-related information, brief health history, and sociodemographic characteristics (socioeconomic status, ethnicity, race, age), and electronic self-report questionnaires including the PSS and PASS. Participants were reimbursed $30 for completing the prenatal session. A mental health resource list was provided if participants endorsed any critical items or reported experiencing distress. RAs scheduled participant's 6-month postnatal session 1 month after their due date and sent reminders to ensure sessions occurred as scheduled. During the 6-month session, mothers completed interviews regarding their and their baby's health, the 6-Month Infant Dietary Questionnaire, and the following electronic self-report measures: PSS, PASS, and ICQ-R postpartum version.

3. Results

3.1. Sample Characteristics

Data were collected from adult mothers ($M_{AGE} = 27.29$ years, $SD_{AGE} = 4.02$ years) during the third trimester ($M_{GESTATION} = 34.25$ weeks, $SD_{GESTATION} = 1.22$ weeks), and 6 months postpartum ($M_{AGE} = 6.05$ months, $SD_{AGE} = 2.13$ months). The largest percentage of participants identified as White/Caucasian (94%), married (84%), and members of the Church of Jesus Christ of Latter-day Saints (LDS; 62%), with annual household incomes between $50,000–$74,999 (29%), having completed a standard college or university degree (i.e., BS/BA; 38%), employed (60%), and having birthed one other child (30%; see Table 1). Additionally, 14% qualified as living in a rural area [22]. Chi-square tests of independence revealed that there were no significant differences in race ($\chi^2(2) = 3.119$, $p = 0.210$), marital status ($\chi^2(1) = 1.407$, $p = 0.236$), employment status ($\chi^2(1) = 3.185$, $p = 0.074$) or education status ($\chi^2(20) = 12.951$, $p = 0.879$) between participants who chose to return for the 6 month session and those who did not. Independent samples t-tests also revealed no differences in income ($t(217) = -0.289$, $p = 0.773$), prenatal stress ($t(123) = -0.924$, $p = 0.358$), prenatal anxiety ($t(123) = -1.289$, $p = 0.200$), and parity ($t(123) = 0.187$, $p = 0.187$) between time points. Religious preference data were only collected at 6 months.

Table 1. Sample sociodemographic description.

Race (Categories Not Mutually Exclusive)	*n*	%
White/Caucasian	88	94
Black/African American	2	2
Native Hawaiian or other Pacific Islander	2	2
American Indian/Alaska Native	1	1
Hispanic/Latino	13	14
Asian	1	1
Other	5	5
Relationship Status		
Single/never married	9	10
Married	79	84
Divorced	1	1
Committed relationship	3	3
Engaged	2	2
Employment Status		
Employed	56	60
Not currently working	38	40
Highest Degree of Education		
Partial high school	2	2
High school	13	14
Partial college	33	35
Standard college or university	36	38
Graduate training with a degree	10	11
Income ($)		
<5000	1	1
5000–9000	2	2
10,000–19,000	14	15
20,000–29,000	16	17
30,000–39,000	12	13
40,000–49,000	9	10
50,000–74,999	27	29
75,000–99,999	7	7
≥100,000	6	6
Religious Preference		
Agnostic	3	3
Assembly of God	2	2
Atheist	2	2
Baptist	2	2
Catholic	4	4

Table 1. *Cont.*

Race (Categories Not Mutually Exclusive)	*n*	%
Lutheran	2	2
Methodist	1	1
Church of Jesus Christ of Latter-day Saints	58	62
Non-denominational	10	11
Pentecostal	1	1
Presbyterian	1	1
Other	12	13
Prefer not to answer	9	10
Parity		
No other child	39	41
One other child	28	30
Two other children	12	13
Three other children	6	6
Four other children	3	3
5 other children	5	5
6 other children	1	1

Note. $n = 94$. Categories for race and religious preference were not mutually exclusive.

3.2. Correlations

Pearson correlations between primary predictor and outcome variables (See Table 2) supported significant relations between stress and anxiety at both time points. None of the potential covariates (number of maternal prenatal, labor/delivery, or postnatal health conditions, infant physical health conditions through 6 months of age, socioeconomic status (SES) measured by the Hollingshead Four Factor Index of Social Status, and parity) significantly correlated with predictor and outcome variables and were not included in moderated mediation models [54]. SES was related to postnatal stress ($r = -0.312$, $p = 0.002$) and anxiety ($r = -0.275$, $p = 0.007$), colic was related to postnatal stress ($r = 0.215$, $p = 0.04$), and postnatal maternal illness was related to postnatal anxiety ($r = 0.257$, $p = 0.05$). Therefore, these variables were controlled for in follow-up analyses for Hypotheses 3 and 4.

Table 2. Correlations among primary study variables.

	PASS (Prenatal)	PSS (Prenatal)	PASS (6 M)	PSS (6 M)	Bf diff.	Spoiling	Duration
PASS (prenatal)	1						
PSS (prenatal)	0.686 **	1					
PASS (6 M)	0.608 **	0.506 **	1				
PSS (6 M)	0.483 **	0.578 **	0.487 **	1			
Bf difficulties	0.036	0.019	0.109	0.027	1		
Spoiling	0.218 *	0.178	0.222 *	0.169	−0.028	1	
Duration	−0.258 *	−0.121	−0.155	−0.130	−0.105	−0.102	1

Note. PASS = Perinatal Anxiety Screening Scale; PSS = Perceived Stress Scale; 6 M = postnatal 6-month time point; Bf = breastfeeding; Spoiling = response to infant crying with breastfeeding as spoiling; Duration = breastfeeding duration. * $p < 0.05$. ** $p < 0.01$.

3.3. Descriptive Statistics

Sixty five percent of participants reported breastfeeding at 6 months postpartum, with 86% having initiated breastfeeding since giving birth. The average PSS score was 19.59 (SD = 6.65) prenatally and 20.23 (SD = 5.96) at the 6-month postnatal visit, out of 56 points. Participants' average PASS score was 16.73 (SD = 11.99) prenatally and 14.46 (SD = 9.45) postnatally out of 93 points. Both PASS average scores fall in the minimal anxiety range. On average, participants ICQ-R Spoiling score was 5.62 (SD = 2.10) out of 15. Participants reported an average of 0.52 (SD = 0.96) difficulties with breastfeeding.

Specifically, 19% endorsed difficulties for themselves, 17% endorsed difficulties for their babies, 11% endorsed difficulties with time management, 2% endorsed an insufficient environment, and 3% noted other difficulties, although their responses were found to be iterations of the previously mentioned answer choices. Participants reported an average of 0.83 (SD = 0.94) prenatal maternal illnesses, 0.64 (SD = 0.80) postnatal maternal illnesses, 1.62 (SD = 0.49) complications during labor or delivery, and 4.83 (SD = 2.09) infant illnesses from birth to 6 months postpartum. The average duration of breastfeeding through 6 months was 138 days (SD = 69.13 days) or 4.4 months.

Hypothesis 1. *The moderated mediation model proposed in Hypothesis 1 was not statistically significant (See Table 3).*

Hypothesis 2. *The moderated mediation model proposed in Hypothesis 2 was also not statistically significant (See Table 3). However, the model with prenatal anxiety as the predictor revealed that prenatal anxiety significantly predicted breastfeeding duration (b = −25.253, t(93) = −2.325, SE = 10.860, p = 0.022).*

Table 3. Prenatal moderated mediation findings.

	F	R^2	S/A → bf diff	Bf Difficulties → Duration	S/A → Duration	Interaction (Bf Difficulties × Spoiling)
			b/SE	*b/SE*	*b/SE*	*b/SE*
Stress	0.747	0.033	0.003/0.015	−10.416/24.829	−1.068/1.103	0.503/4.201
Anxiety	1.889	0.078	0.052/0.149	−6.633/24.299	−25.253 */10.860	0.069/4.109

Note. Bf = breastfeeding; Spoiling = response to infant crying with breastfeeding as spoiling; Duration = breastfeeding duration; SE = standard error; S/A = stress/anxiety. Arrows indicate direction of prediction. * $p < 0.05$.

An independent samples *t*-test was conducted to determine the difference in breastfeeding duration between the 14 participants (approximately 15% of mothers) who were at or above the prenatal PASS cut-off of 26 and those below. All 96 participants were used, as natural log transformations were only necessary for postnatal PASS scores. The two groups were statistically significantly different (t(94) = −3.90, $p < 0.001$, $d = 1.044$), with mothers who were above the clinical cut score for prenatal anxiety breastfeeding 72.58 days or 2.5 months less in duration. Of the mothers with clinically elevated prenatal anxiety, only 4 (29%) breastfed through 6 months, while 56 of the 82 (68%) mothers who did not have clinically elevated prenatal anxiety continued breastfeeding at 6 months. Due to small sample sizes, results should be replicated before drawing strong conclusions.

Hypothesis 3. *We conducted an independent samples t-test to compare women who breastfed through 6 months to women who did not on postnatal stress (Hypothesis 3). Results suggests no significant differences in postnatal stress (t(92) = −0.711, p = 0.479). As follow-up analyses, we examined the relation between breastfeeding duration as a continuous variable, and postnatal stress and anxiety, while controlling for covariates. An analysis of covariance (ANCOVA) suggested that the relationship between stress and breastfeeding duration was not statistically significant (F(13) = 0.753, p = 0.706), though SES was significantly related to postnatal stress (F(1) = 7.865, p = 0.006).*

Hypothesis 4. *We conducted an independent samples t-test to compare women who breastfed through 6 months to women who did not on postnatal anxiety (Hypothesis 4). Results suggests no significant differences in postnatal anxiety (t(92) = −1.369, p = 0.174). An additional ANCOVA suggested that the relationship between greater postnatal anxiety and longer breastfeeding duration was statistically significant (F(13) = 2.385, p = 0.009), even after controlling for postnatal maternal illness and SES.*

Hypothesis 5. *Utilizing a two-tailed Pearson correlation among women who continued to breastfeed through 6 months postpartum, breastfeeding difficulties were not significantly related to postnatal stress (Hypothesis 5, $r = -0.156$, $p = 0.114$).*

Hypothesis 6. *An additional two-tailed Pearson correlation also suggested that breastfeeding difficulties were not significantly related to postnatal anxiety among women who continued to breastfeed through 6 months postpartum, (Hypothesis 6, $r = -0.137$, $p = 0.144$).*

4. Discussion

The purpose of the present project was to investigate a novel mediator and moderator in the relation between prenatal and postnatal anxiety and stress and breastfeeding duration among a medically underserved sample. While none of the moderated mediation models were significant, results indicated that greater prenatal anxiety was significantly related to shorter breastfeeding duration. This finding replicates previous literature in non-U.S. samples suggesting that high levels of trait anxiety in early and mid-pregnancy were associated with decreased breastfeeding rates [25]. Furthermore, many women who experience anxiety during pregnancy breastfeed for less than 6 months [26]. Researchers speculate that poor psychosocial health during pregnancy may be an indicator of poorer overall health, which may influence breastfeeding behaviors [25,26].

Prior literature suggests that prenatal anxiety predicts shorter exclusive breastfeeding at 1 month postpartum, but only prenatal depression is related to breastfeeding duration [55]. A literature review revealed mixed findings regarding prenatal anxiety and breastfeeding behaviors [56]. While there are no associations between prenatal anxiety and breastfeeding initiation, a relation does exist between high levels of prenatal anxiety and a decrease in breastfeeding intention and exclusivity. The relation between prenatal anxiety and breastfeeding is still poorly understood and necessitates further research [56]. Researchers report possible explanations for this relation, including that trait anxiety may interfere with oxytocin release, which stimulates the milk-ejection reflex [56]. State anxiety may result in heightened levels of cortisol and glucose, potentially decreasing milk volume and resulting in decreased breastfeeding duration. Additionally, mothers who experience prenatal anxiety about parenting may avoid challenging parenting behaviors, such as breastfeeding, leading to decreased maternal-infant interaction and decreased breastfeeding.

Few, if any studies have examined and found that various forms of prenatal anxiety, including state, trait, and perinatal, influence breastfeeding duration. Thus, the present project provides novel and important findings regarding correlates of breastfeeding duration. Future research should investigate whether prenatal state, strait, or perinatal anxiety is most related to breastfeeding duration. While the present study provides further support for the relation between heightened prenatal anxiety and decreased breastfeeding duration, the interactive biopsychosocial mechanisms by which this relation exists remains elusive and should be further explored (e.g., stress hormone systems, immune functioning, maternal-infant bonding, and sociocultural understanding and support for breastfeeding). Our analyses also suggest a positive relation between postnatal anxiety and breastfeeding duration, which further indicates the importance of continuing to examine mechanisms of action (e.g., mediating role of breastfeeding difficulties) for these complex and poorly understood relations. Additionally, the positive relation between increased SES and increased postnatal stress may be due to factors like occupation, which warrants investigation.

Correlation analyses suggest that stress and anxiety are related within and over time. Moreover, prenatal and postnatal anxiety were also significantly related to perceptions of infant spoiling. As previous literature suggests, excessive infant crying can be challenging for mothers, and this may lead to heightened feelings of stress and anxiety [36]. If mothers misperceive their response to infant cries with breastfeeding as spoiling, they may decrease breastfeeding behaviors [38,39]. Subsequently, mothers' stress and anxiety may increase if they notice a decrease in their milk supply due to decreased feeding behavior, or due to infant crying behavior that they are not addressing. Additional studies are needed to further investigate these relations.

Our study variables were grounded in strong theory and largely assessed by psychometrically sound measures, and conditional process analysis allowed for a robust and multivariate examination of prenatal stress and anxiety. However, the present study also included limitations, including the way in which we measured breastfeeding difficulties/duration and perinatal stress, homogenous sample demographics (e.g., White), relatively lower power for Hypotheses 5 and 6, and a correlational design. Possible future directions include creating comprehensive and well-validated measures of breastfeeding behaviors, difficulties, and psychosocial experiences, tracking breastfeeding duration and anxiety at multiple time points and beyond 6 months postpartum, examining other breastfeeding outcomes (e.g., initiation or frequency), studying more heterogeneous samples, exploring additional risk and reliance factors, and examining perceptions of infant crying more broadly. Future research should continue to explore possible explanations for decreased breastfeeding duration among women with psychological distress, as these relations are still not fully understood. Focus in each of these areas will lead to a richer understanding of maternal experiences in the perinatal period, informing future intervention and policy.

Practical Implications

The current study's findings hold important implications. Although our sample was a relatively low-risk, healthy community sample, we still found a significant relation between greater prenatal anxiety and shorter breastfeeding duration. Furthermore, even minimal levels of prenatal anxiety are related to breastfeeding duration, thus pregnant women with low levels of anxiety may benefit from screening and intervention. Future prevention and intervention research should focus on the nature of maternal prenatal anxiety, including women who experience relatively low levels of anxiety as well as clinical samples. Understanding the characteristics of prenatal anxiety may help inform more specific targets for psychosocial prevention, intervention, and support.

Follow-up analysis using the PASS cut-off score of 26, demonstrated that mothers who experienced clinically significant levels of prenatal anxiety on average breastfed for 72.58 days, approximately 2.5 months, less than mothers without clinically significant levels of prenatal anxiety (i.e., 148 days or almost 5 months). The magnitude of this effect was quantified by a large Cohen's d effect size as well, indicating a strong statistical effect ($d = 1.044$). A review of the literature suggests that even a 2.5-month difference in breastfeeding duration is clinically meaningful, including numerous implications in maternal and infant physical health (e.g., infant risk of infectious diseases) [57,58]. Of note, only 4 of the 14 mothers who were elevated on the prenatal PASS breastfed through 6 months, while 56 of the 82 mothers who did not have clinically elevated prenatal anxiety continued breastfeeding at 6 months. This suggests that the effects of prenatal anxiety on breastfeeding duration may play a robust and critical role within the first few months, such that this is a time period when breastfeeding difficulties should be assessed in greater detail and breastfeeding resources, support, and interventions may be most efficacious. As the two groups in the present analyses were not proportional (i.e., only 14 mothers met the threshold for clinically significant prenatal anxiety), findings should be replicated with larger sample sizes. Nonetheless, these findings indicate that maternal prenatal anxiety may be clinically significantly related to breastfeeding duration, and subsequently, health outcomes for mother-infant dyads. While the present study examined several possible covariates in relation to these variables, breastfeeding duration and PASS scores were related even after controlling for maternal illness and SES. Future studies should consider examining the role of social support among other factors that may influence broad relations between maternal affect and breastfeeding outcomes.

5. Conclusions

The present project sought to better understand the relations among perinatal stress, anxiety, breastfeeding difficulties, perceptions of responding to infant crying, and breastfeeding duration in an underserved sample. Previous cross-cultural research has demonstrated some relations among these variables, however there is inconsistency in these findings. Furthermore, this is the first study to our knowledge to examine these variables collectively through moderated mediation models. The present project also fills a gap in the literature by exploring the unique experiences of U.S. women, specifically in Idaho. Study results revealed a statistically and clinically significant relation between clinical levels of prenatal anxiety and decreased breastfeeding duration, highlighting that even low levels of prenatal anxiety should not be overlooked in research or clinical settings.

Author Contributions: J.P.R., the first and corresponding author contributed to the present project in conceptualization, data curation, formal analysis, investigation, visualization, and writing. N.L.A.-E. contributed in conceptualization, data curation, formal analysis, funding acquisition, methodology, project administration, resources, supervision, visualization, and writing.

Acknowledgments: We would like to thank Idaho State University for their assistance in funding this project. Additionally, we would like to acknowledge the research assistants in the Perinatal Psychobiology Lab who assisted with data collection, and thank our many participants for their contribution to science.

References

1. U.S. Department of Health and Human Services. Centers for Disease Control and Prevention, National Center for Chronic Disease Prevention and Health Promotion. Available online: https://www.cdc.gov/breastfeeding/data/reportcard.htm (accessed on 6 June 2017).
2. Cook, C. Oxytocin and prolactin suppress cortisol responses to acute stress in both lactating and non-lactating sheep. *J. Dairy Res.* **1997**, *64*, 327–339. [CrossRef] [PubMed]
3. Freeman, M.E.; Kanyicska, B.; Lerant, A.; Nagy, G. Prolactin: Structure, function, and regulation of secretion. *Physiol Rev.* **2000**, *80*, 1523–1631. [CrossRef] [PubMed]
4. Heinrichs, M.; Neumann, I.; Ehlert, U. Lactation and stress: Protective effects of breast-feeding in humans. *Stress* **2002**, *5*, 195–203. [CrossRef] [PubMed]
5. Mezzacappa, E.S. Breastfeeding and maternal stress response and health. *Nutr. Rev.* **2004**, *62*, 261–268. [CrossRef]
6. Tu, M.T.; Lupien, S.J.; Walker, C. Multiparity reveals the blunting effect of breastfeeding on physiological reactivity to psychological stress. *J. Neuroendocrinol.* **2006**, *18*, 494–503. [CrossRef]
7. Uvnäs Moberg, K.; Prime, D.K. Oxytocin effects in mothers and infants during breastfeeding. *Infant* **2013**, *9*, 201–206.
8. Johnson, K. Maternal-infant bonding: A Review of literature. *Int. J. Childbirth Educ.* **2013**, *28*, 17–22.
9. Phillips, K.F. First-time breastfeeding mothers: Perceptions and lived experiences with breastfeeding. *Int. J. Childbirth Educ* **2011**, *26*, 17–20.
10. Prendergast, E.; James, J. Engaging mothers: Breastfeeding experiences recounted (EMBER). A pilot study. *Breastfeed. Rev.* **2016**, *24*, 11–19.
11. Schmied, V.; Barclay, L. Connection and pleasure, disruption and distress: Women's experience of breastfeeding. *J. Hum. Lact.* **1999**, *15*, 325–334. [CrossRef]
12. World Health Organization. Available online: http://www.who.int/mental_health/maternal-child/maternal_mental_health/en/ (accessed on 5 May 2017).
13. Dunkel Schetter, C.; Tanner, L. Anxiety, depression and stress in pregnancy: Implications for mothers, children, research, and practice. *Curr. Opin. Psychiatry* **2012**, *25*, 141–148. [CrossRef]
14. Fallon, V.; Groves, R.; Halford, J.G.; Bennett, K.M.; Harrold, J.A. Postpartum anxiety and infant-feeding outcomes. *J. Hum. Lact.* **2016**, *32*, 740–758. [CrossRef] [PubMed]
15. Leach, L.S.; Poyser, C.; Fairweather-Schmidt, K. Maternal perinatal anxiety: A Review of Prevalence and correlates. *Br. J. Clin. Psychol.* **2017**, *21*, 4–19. [CrossRef]
16. Leight, K.L.; Fitelson, E.M.; Weston, C.A.; Wisner, K.L. Childbirth and mental disorders. *Int. Rev. Psychiatry* **2010**, *22*, 453–471. [CrossRef]
17. O'Hara, M.; Wisner, K. Perinatal mental illness: Definition, description and aetiology. *Best Pract. Res. Clin. Obstet Gynaecol.* **2013**, *28*, 3–12. [CrossRef]

18. American Psychiatric Association. *Diagnostic and Statistical Manual of Mental Disorders*, 5th ed.; American Psychiatric Association: Washington, DC, USA, 2013.
19. Idaho Department of Health and Welfare. Available online: http://healthandwelfare.idaho.gov/Health/VitalRecordsandHealthStatistics/HealthStatistics/PregnancyRiskAssessmentTrackingSystem/tabid/915/Default.aspx (accessed on 5 May 2017).
20. Woods, S.; Melville, J.; Guo, Y.; Fan, M.; Gavin, A.; Woods, S.M.; Gavin, A. Psychosocial stress during pregnancy. *Am. J. Obstet. Gynecol.* **2010**, *202*, 61. [CrossRef]
21. Burns, E.R.; Farr, S.L.; Howards, P.P. Stressful life events experienced by women in the year before their infants' births–United States, 2000–2010. *Morb. Mortality Weekly Report* **2015**, *64*, 247–251.
22. Rural Health Information Hub. Available online: https://www.ruralhealthinfo.org/data-explorer?id=209&state=ID (accessed on 1 September 2019).
23. Britton, J.R. Postpartum anxiety and breastfeeding. *J. Reprod. Med.* **2007**, *52*, 689–695.
24. Doulougeri, K.; Panagopoulou, E.; Montgomery, A. The impact of maternal stress on initiation and establishment of breastfeeding. *J. Nanosci. Nanotechnol.* **2013**, *19*, 162–167. [CrossRef]
25. Insaf, T.Z.; Fortner, R.T.; Pekow, P.; Dole, N.; Markenson, G.; Chasan-Taber, L. Prenatal stress, anxiety and depressive symptoms as predictors of intention to breastfeed among Hispanic women. *J. Women's Health* **2011**, *20*, 1183–1192. [CrossRef]
26. Kehler, H.L.; Chaput, K.H.; Tough, S.C. Risk factors for cessation of breastfeeding prior to six months postpartum among a community sample of women in Calgary, Alberta. *Can J Public Health* **2009**, *100*, 376–380. [CrossRef] [PubMed]
27. Li, J.; Kendall, G.E.; Henderson, S.; Downie, J.; Landsborough, L.; Oddy, W.H. Maternal psychosocial well-being in pregnancy and breastfeeding duration. *Acta Paediatr.* **2008**, *97*, 221–225. [CrossRef] [PubMed]
28. O'Brien, M.; Buikstra, E.; Hegney, D. The influence of psychological factors on breastfeeding duration. *J. Adv. Nurs.* **2008**, *63*, 397–408. [CrossRef]
29. Papinczak, T.A.; Turner, C.T. An analysis of personal and social factors influencing initiation and duration of breastfeeding in a large Queensland maternity hospital. *Breastfeed. Rev.* **2000**, *8*, 25–33. [PubMed]
30. Ystrom, E. Breastfeeding cessation and symptoms of anxiety and depression: A longitudinal cohort study. *BMC Pregnancy Childbirth* **2012**, *12*, 36–41. [CrossRef]
31. Zhu, P.; Hao, J.; Jiang, X.; Huang, K.; Tao, F. New insight into onset of lactation: Mediating the negative effect of multiple perinatal biopsychosocial stress on breastfeeding duration. *Breastfeed. Med.* **2013**, *8*, 151–158. [CrossRef]
32. Henshaw, E.J.; Fried, R.; Siskind, E.; Newhouse, L.; Cooper, M. Breastfeeding self- efficacy, mood, and breastfeeding outcomes among primiparous women. *J. Hum. Lact.* **2015**, *31*, 511. [CrossRef]
33. Centers for Disease Control and Prevention. Available online: https://www.cdc.gov/prAm.s/pdf/questionnaire/phase-7-standard-questions-508.pdf (accessed on 5 May 2017).
34. Purdy, I.B. Social, cultural, and medical factors that influence maternal breastfeeding. *Issues Ment Health Nurs.* **2010**, *31*, 365–367. [CrossRef]
35. Ertem, I.O.; Votto, N.; Leventhal, J.M. The timing and predictors of the early termination of breastfeeding. *Pediatrics* **2001**, *107*, 543. [CrossRef]
36. Long, T.; Johnson, M. Living and coping with excessive infantile crying. *J. Adv. Nurs.* **2001**, *34*, 155–162. [CrossRef]
37. Howard, C.R.; Lanphear, N.; Lanphear, B.P.; Eberly, S.; Lawrence, R.A. Parental responses to infant crying and colic: The effect on breastfeeding duration. *Breastfeed. Med.* **2006**, *1*, 146–155. [CrossRef] [PubMed]
38. Bell, S.M.; Ainsworth, M.S. Infant crying and maternal responsiveness. *Child Dev.* **1972**, *43*, 1171–1190. [CrossRef] [PubMed]
39. Mathews, M.; Leerkes, E.; Lovelady, C.; Labban, J. Psychosocial predictors of primiparous breastfeeding initiation and duration. *J. Hum. Lact.* **2014**, *30*, 480–487. [CrossRef] [PubMed]
40. The American College of Obstetrics and Gynecology. Available online: https://www.acog.org/Patients/FAQs/Having-a-Baby-After-Age-35-How-Aging-Affects-Fertility-and-Pregnancy?IsMobileSet=false (accessed on 2 November 2019).
41. Fritz, M.S.; Mackinnon, D.P. Required sample size to detect the mediated effect. *Psychol. Sci.* **2007**, *18*, 233–239. [CrossRef] [PubMed]
42. Faul, F.; Erdfelder, E.; Lang, A.-G.; Buchner, A. G *Power 3: A flexible statistical power analysis program. for

the social, behavioral, and biomedical sciences. *Behav. Res. Methods* **2007**, *39*, 175–191. [CrossRef] [PubMed]
43. Hayes, A.F. *Introduction to Mediation, Moderation, and Conditional Process Analysis: A Regression-Based Approach*, 2nd ed.; The Guilford Press: New York, NY, USA, 2013.
44. Yzerbyt, V.; Muller, D.; Batailler, C.; Judd, C. New recommendations for testing indirect effects in the mediational models: The need to report and test component paths. *J. Personal. Soc. Psychol.* **2018**, *115*, 929–943. [CrossRef] [PubMed]
45. Cohen, S.; Kamarck, T.; Mermelstein, R. A global measure of perceived stress. *J. Health Soc. Behav.* **1983**, *4*, 385. [CrossRef]
46. Levine, M.; Perkins, D.V. Tailor making life events scale. In Proceedings of the 88th Annual Convention of the American Psychological Association, Montreal, QC, Canada, 1–5 September 1980.
47. Lee, E. Review of the psychometric evidence of the perceived stress scale. *Asian Nurs. Res.* **2012**, *6*, 121–127. [CrossRef]
48. Yokokura, A.; Silva, A.; Fernandes, J.; Del-Ben, C.; Figueiredo, F.; Barbieri, M.; Bettiol, H. Perceived Stress Scale: Confirmatory factor analysis of the PSS14 and PSS10 versions in two samples of pregnant women from the BRISA cohort. *Cad. Saude Pub.* **2017**, *33*, e00184615. [CrossRef]
49. Somerville, S.; Dedman, K.; Hagan, R.; Oxnam, E.; Wettinger, M.; Byrne, S.; Page, A. The Perinatal Anxiety Screening Scale: Development and preliminary validation. *Arch. Women's Ment. Health* **2014**, *17*, 443–454. [CrossRef]
50. Cox, J.L.; Holden, J.M.; Sagovsky, R. Detection of postnatal depression: Development of the 10-item Edinburgh Postnatal Depression Scale. *Br. J. Psychiatry* **1987**, *150*, 782–786. [CrossRef] [PubMed]
51. Spielberger, C.D.; Gorsuch, R.L.; Lushene, R.; Vagg, P.R.; Jacobs, G.A. *Manual for the State-Trait. Anxiety Inventory*; Consulting Psychologists Press: Palo Alto, CA, USA, 1983.
52. Haltigan, J.; Leerkes, E.; Burney, R.; O'Brien, M.; Supple, A.; Calkins, S. The Infant Crying Questionnaire: Initial factor structure and validation. *Infant Behav. Dev.* **2012**, *35*, 876–883. [CrossRef] [PubMed]
53. Fein, S.B.; Labiner-Wolfe, J.; Shealy, K.; Li, R.; Chen, J.; Grummer-Strawn, L.M. Infant feeding practices study II: Study methods. *Pediatrics* **2008**, *122* (Suppl. 2), S28–S35. [CrossRef] [PubMed]
54. Hollingshead, A.B. *Four-Factor Index of Social Status*; Yale University: New Haven, CT, USA, 1975.
55. Mehta, U.J.; Siega-Riz, A.M.; Herring, A.H.; Adair, L.S.; Bentley, M.E. Pregravid body mass index, psychological factors during pregnancy and breastfeeding duration: Is there a link? *Matern. Child Nutr.* **2012**, *8*, 423–433. [CrossRef]
56. Fallon, V.; Bennett, K.M.; Harrold, J.A. Prenatal anxiety and infant feeding outcomes. *J. Hum. Lact.* **2016**, *32*, 53. [CrossRef]
57. Dieterich, C.; Felice, J.; O'Sullivan, E.; Rasmussen, K. Breastfeeding and health outcomes for the mother-infant dyad. *Pediatr. Clin. N. Am.* **2013**, *60*, 31–48. [CrossRef]
58. Duijts, L.; Jaddoe, V.V.; Moll, H.A.; Hofman, A. Prolonged and exclusive breastfeeding reduces the risk of infectious diseases in infancy. *Pediatrics* **2010**, *126*, E18–E25. [CrossRef]

Formula Milk Supplementation on the Postnatal Ward

Kirsty V. Biggs [1], Katherine Hurrell [2], Eleanor Matthews [3], Ekaterina Khaleva [4,5], Daniel Munblit [3,5,6,†] and Robert J. Boyle [3,5,*,†]

1 Brighton and Sussex Medical School, Brighton BN2 5BE, UK; K.Biggs1@uni.bsms.ac.uk
2 Royal United Hospital, Combe Park, Bath BA1 3NG, UK; Katherine.hurrell@nhs.net
3 Department of Paediatrics, Imperial College Healthcare NHS Trust, London W2 1NY, UK; ellie.matthews@imperial.nhs.uk (E.M.); daniel.munblit08@imperial.ac.uk (D.M.)
4 Department of Paediatrics, Saint-Petersburg State Paediatric Medical University, 194353 Saint-Petersburg, Russia; doctor.khaleva@gmail.com
5 inVIVO Planetary Health, Group of the Worldwide Universities Network (WUN), 6010 Park Ave, West New York, NJ 07093, USA
6 Faculty of Pediatrics, I. M. Sechenov First Moscow State Medical University, 119991 Moscow, Russia
* Correspondence: r.boyle@nhs.net
† Authors contributed equally to this work.

Abstract: Breastfeeding rates are low in the UK, where approximately one quarter of infants receive a breastmilk substitute (BMS) in the first week of life. We investigated the reasons for early BMS use in two large maternity units in the UK, in order to understand the reasons for the high rate of early BMS use in this setting. Data were collected through infant feeding records, as well as maternal and midwife surveys in 2016. During 2016, 28% of infants received a BMS supplement prior to discharge from the hospital maternity units with only 10% supplementation being clinically indicated. There was wide variation in BMS initiation rates between different midwives, which was associated with ward environment and midwife educational level. Specific management factors associated with non-clinically indicated initiation of BMS were the absence of skin-to-skin contact within an hour of delivery ($p = 0.01$), and no attendance at an antenatal breastfeeding discussion ($p = 0.01$). These findings suggest that risk of initiating a BMS during postnatal hospital stay is largely modifiable. Concordance with UNICEF Baby Friendly 10 steps, attention to specific features of the postnatal ward working environment, and the targeting of midwives and mothers with poor educational status may all lead to improved exclusive breastfeeding rates at hospital discharge.

Keywords: breastfeeding; attitudes; knowledge; midwifery; formula supplementation; justification of supplementation

---

1. Introduction

Breastfeeding has long been regarded as the preferred infant feeding choice with established long- and short-term benefits for mothers, infants, and society [1,2]. Many high-quality studies from developed countries similar and applicable to the United Kingdom (UK) show that breastfed babies are less likely to develop infections than babies fed with breastmilk substitutes (BMS), specifically those of the lower respiratory tract, gastrointestinal system, and otitis media [3–9]. Indeed, a meta-analysis of 33 studies in developed counties concluded formula-fed infants had three times more severe infections compared to infants exclusively breastfed to four months [10].

Studies have found other beneficial health associations of breastfed infants compared to infants fed with BMS, including lower rates of Sudden Infant Death Syndrome, necrotizing enterocolitis, atopic diseases, childhood obesity, and enhanced neurocognitive function [11–20].

Breastfeeding not only confers health benefits to the infant, but also to the mother, for example by incurring faster weight loss and as a natural contraceptive [21,22]. The longer the duration of breastfeeding, the increased protection against breast and ovarian cancer, and reduced post-menopausal hip fractures [23–27]. Emerging evidence suggests that breastfeeding positively impacts mother-baby relationships, bonding, and post-natal depression [28–30]. From an economic perspective, the improvements in child and maternal morbidity and mortality, plus reduced workforce productivity loss are estimated to be substantial [1].

Exclusive breastfeeding (EBF) is defined as an infant who receives only breastmilk, or expressed breastmilk, but no other solids or liquids except prescribed medicines, vitamins, or mineral supplements [31].

The World Health Organisation (WHO) recommends all infants to be breastfed exclusively for the first six months of life, and for breastfeeding to continue until age 2 years or beyond [31]. Despite this, data from the National Infant Feeding survey 2010 demonstrates <1% of mothers in the UK reach this target. The greatest decline in exclusive breastfeeding (23%) occurred within the infant's first week of life, with infants who exclusively breastfed for the first two days having a greater chance of achieving the six-month target, with greater self-efficacy [32–34]. This demonstrates the importance of providing adequate in-hospital support.

The literature has highlighted associations between the use of BMS and negative impacts on breastfeeding. In a prospective cohort study of mothers with the intention to exclusively breastfeed, the introduction of BMS on post-natal wards, alongside intrapartum opiate-use, were the only modifiable predictors of non-exclusivity at three months [35]. Chantry et al. found a three-fold increase in the risk of breastfeeding cessation by day 60 for those receiving in-hospital BMS supplementation, regardless of the mother's intention [36]. There are also concerns about BMS use and its impact on the neonatal gut microbiota, with long-term health implications [37]. Current evidence has demonstrated that early in-hospital supplementation is commonplace in developed countries [34].

The use of BMS supplementation within the early hospital environment is a multifactorial practice. The most commonly cited reason for BMS supplementation was due to breastfeeding difficulties, demonstrating that a high proportion of supplementation occurs without medical explanation [38]. Significant variation in BMS supplementation of breastfed infants was also reported in concordance with maternal education and ethnicity [39]. Within the early postnatal environment, midwives are responsible for the initial administration of supplementary BMS. Previous work has identified a lack of time, poor staffing levels, and a resistance to change as key contributing factors to non-compliance of a breastfeeding support intervention on UK postnatal wards [40].

The training a midwife receives has also been suggested to be clinically relevant to infant feeding practices in the hospital, with those demonstrating higher breastfeeding knowledge reporting best clinical practice [41]. A UK comparative study identified negative staff attitudes as a contributing factor to the early cessation of breastfeeding [42]. However, qualitative research suggests that midwives underestimate the influence they have on maternal feeding choices [43,44]. Overall, these studies highlight the need to investigate the influence of maternal and midwife factors on rates of neonatal infant-formula supplementation in the absence of medical indication (NIFS-AMI).

2. Materials and Methods

2.1. Study Design

A cross-sectional analytic study evaluated features of mothers, midwives, and postnatal care which are associated with NIFS-AMI on the postnatal ward (Figure 1). Data were routinely collected over one year about feeding method at discharge at Queen Charlotte's and Chelsea Hospital (QCCH) and St Mary's Hospital (SMH), UK to determine the recorded supplementation rate within the

Trust. A detailed analysis of one month's data from the hospital's patient records determined infant feeding method and further categorisation of supplementation into either medical or non-medical reasons (NIFS-AMI). Bedside interviews of mothers were conducted to determine maternally reported supplementation rate and explore the relationship between features of birth, mother, and family and risk of NIFS-AMI. Interviews of midwives were used to determine the range and values of midwife NIFS-AMI rate and explore midwife characteristics associated with this rate.

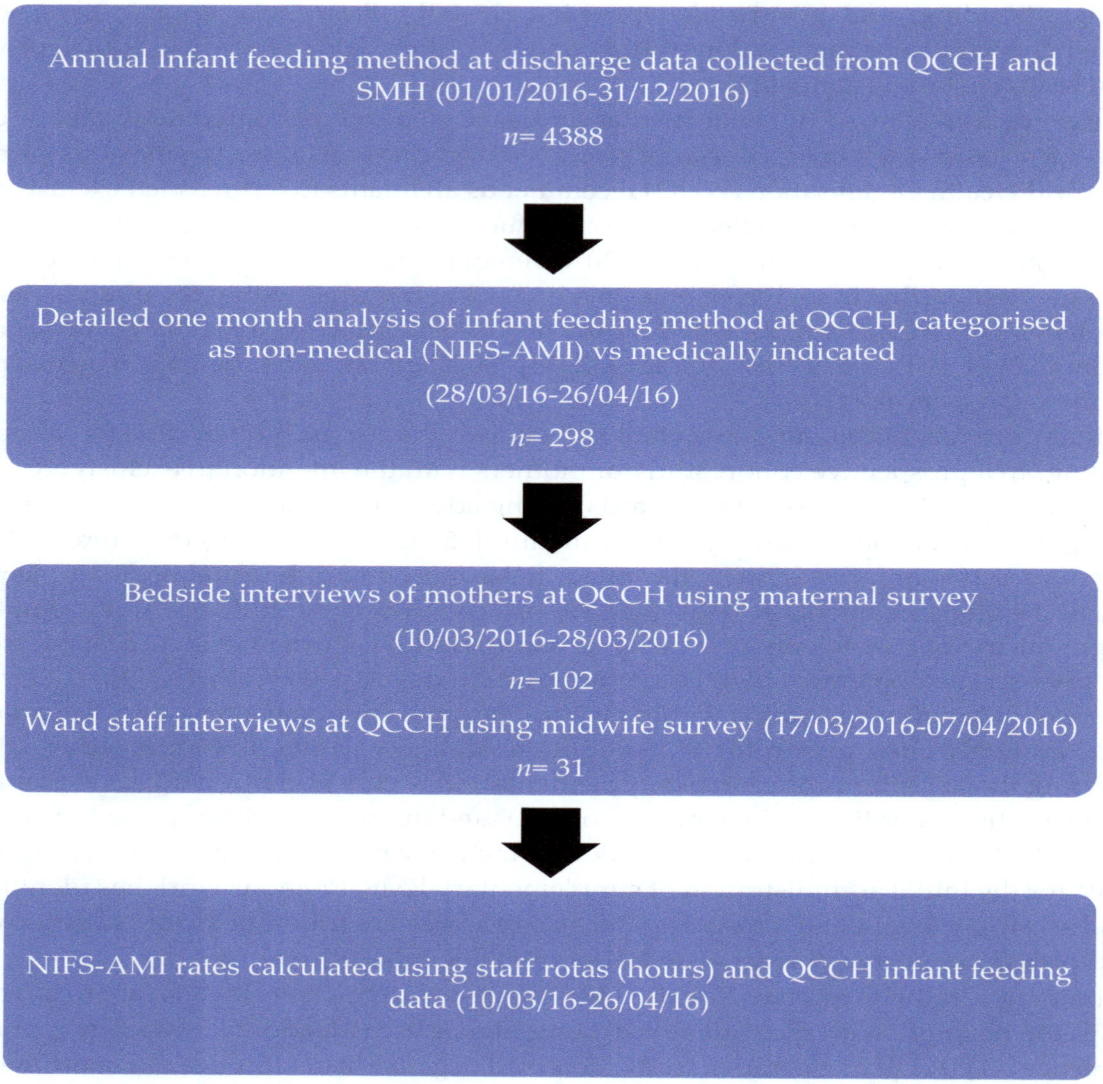

Figure 1. Study design. QCCH: Queen Charlotte's and Chelsea Hospital; SMH: Saint Mary's Hospital; NIFS-AMI: neonatal infant-formula supplementation in the absence of medical indication.

2.2. *Study Participants*

We undertook two separate cross-sectional surveys. In the maternal survey, mothers of newborn infants were surveyed at the bedside between 10 March 2016 and 28 March 2016. Women with conditions or medications that prevented breastfeeding, who had multiple pregnancies, or whose infants were inpatients on the neonatal intensive care unit were excluded. All participating mothers gave informed consent.

In the midwife survey, midwives working on the postnatal wards between 17 March 2016 and 7 April 2016 were assessed. Royal College of Midwifery registered midwives working at least one shift during this period, either as agency, temporary, or permanent staff members, were included. The postnatal department is divided into three distinct wards; the public National Health Service (NHS) facility (43 beds), the self-pay (private) ward (eight private rooms), and the NHS birth centre (eight birthing rooms). Care is primarily delivered by midwives and maternal support workers. At the study site, BMS cannot be initially administered without the involvement and approval of a registered midwife. An obstetrician may be present on the private and NHS postnatal wards; however, the birth centre is an entirely midwife-led provision for labour and post-natal care. As part of the NHS screening programme, an in-hospital newborn and infant physical examination (NIPE) is conducted on all neonates by a paediatrician prior to discharge. Typically in the UK, mother-infant dyads are discharged to the community midwifery team once assessed as healthy, having established feeding and having received appropriate education on caring for their infant. Home visits are provided by community midwives for the first 10 days until care transitions to the responsibility of the health visitor. A general practitioner will provide a six-week postnatal check.

All participating midwives provided verbal consent and were assured that their responses would remain anonymous. They were informed of the purpose of the study—to examine behaviours associated with formula supplementation. The project was conducted as a clinical audit, as part of the requirements of the Baby Friendly Initiative. Formal review by an ethics committee was therefore not required, but the audit was approved by the clinical department and was approved by the Queen Charlotte's and Chelsea Hospital, London, UK audit office (March 2016).

2.3. Data Collection

Data were collected through infant feeding records, as well as maternal and midwife surveys. Annual infant feeding data were retrieved from CERNER electronic patient records, demonstrating the feeding method at discharge for 4388 mother-infant dyads at QCCH and SMH during the study period (1 January 2016 to 31 December 2016). Data from SMH were included to better assess the generalisability of the participants recruited from QCCH. Length of admission, ethnicity, delivery methods, parity, birth weight, gestation, and ward type were compared between the two hospital sites. To determine infant feeding method at inpatient discharge, data from ward records on the postnatal unit were collected from 298 patients between 28 March 2016 and 26 April 2016. CERNER medical and nursing notes for both mother and infant were accessed to assess any recorded medical reasons for supplementation. Reasons for supplementation were categorised as either medical or non-medical (NIFS-AMI), according to WHO criteria. Accepted clinical reasons for using BMS included the following infant conditions: classic galactosemia, maple syrup urine disease, and phenylkenonuria. Infants who may require BMS in addition to breastmilk for a limited period include very low birth weight (<1500 g), very pre-term (<32 weeks gestation), and newborn infants who are at risk of hypoglycaemia if their blood glucose fails to respond to optimal breastmilk feeding. Maternal conditions that justify the temporary avoidance of breastfeeding included severe illness that prevents a mother from caring for her infant (e.g., sepsis), herpes simplex virus type 1 lesions on the mother's breasts, and certain maternal medications. HIV infection was the only named justification for permanent avoidance of breastfeeding [45].

2.3.1. Maternal Survey

All participating women were interviewed with the UNICEF Baby Friendly Hospital Initiative (BFHI) accredited audit tool [46]. Data were collected with regard to the education received on breastfeeding and relationship building from a healthcare professional, their birth experience, and the antenatal and postnatal support received. Original additional questions were included regarding maternal demographic data, infant feeding methods, durations of breastfeeding both as a mother and as an infant, and general attitudes of their close friends and relatives. Maternal levels of breastfeeding (BF) confidence were assessed using a Likert scale (1–10) for both before and after the birth of their infant. Maternal demographic data, gestation at delivery, and infant birth weight were obtained from patient electronic records. Ethnicity was categorised according to Office of National Statistics England [47].

2.3.2. Midwife Survey

Quantitative and qualitative data were obtained through staff questionnaires to assess attitudes as well as personal and professional experiences of infant feeding. The survey instrument was developed based on expert opinion and previously published literature [40–44]. Within the questionnaire, staff were asked to describe three scenarios in which they had supplemented a breastfed infant and to discuss the barriers they encountered with regard to supporting breastfeeding.

We also obtained data on the frequency of initiated NIFS-AMI across the three wards and for each midwife. Infants supplemented for medical reasons were excluded from analysis. To control for the inevitable influence of working hours, a supplementation rate was calculated. Staff rotas from the corresponding seven-week period were reviewed to total the number of hours each midwife worked, which was divided by the supplementation frequency to produce an hourly percentage rate. The hourly rate was used to estimate a monthly rate; the hourly rate was multiplied by 37.5 and divided by 7 before multiplying the value by 30.

2.4. Data Analysis

Data were tested for normality to determine the choice of statistical methods using a visual inspection of histograms and the Shapiro-Wilk test. For univariate analysis, the Mann-Whitney U test for non-parametric data was employed. For categorical data, Pearson's Chi-squared test was used to determine statistically significant differences between groups. Fisher's Exact Test was used if cells had an expected count of less than 5. A p-value of <0.05 was considered significant. The Spearman Correlation coefficient was used to test associations between variables with a non-parametric distribution.

Due to the relatively small sample size, the private ward and birth centre were grouped due to similarities in size, facilities, staff to patient ratios, and working environment when using 'postnatal ward type' as a variable in analyses.

Analysis of covariance (ANCOVA) was used for multivariate analysis, considering cofounding variables that had been identified through correlation coefficients and a review of the literature, to produce the final model.

IBM SPSS 23 statistical software (IBM, Armonk, NC, USA) was used for all statistical analysis.

3. Results

3.1. Maternal Descriptive Characteristics

Table 1 presents the clinical and demographic characteristics of mothers and infants surveyed, in comparison to QCCH and SMH electronic records during April 2016. Of the 102 women included in the study, 55 were exclusively breastfeeding (EBF) their baby (54%), 41 were supplementing with BMS (40%), and six were exclusively receiving BMS (6%). The monthly rates of exclusive breastfeeding at discharge for 2016 are displayed in Figure S1. The median maternal age was 32 years (28, 36 IQR) and infant age was 1 day (1, 2). Primiparous women were overrepresented in our study sample (58%); however, other characteristics were illustrative of the wider cohort.

Table 1. Clinical and demographic characteristics of mothers and infants.

	Survey	QCCH	SMH	Both Sites
	n = 102	n = 486	n = 329	n = 815
Maternal age (years)	32 (28, 36)	32 (29, 36)	33 (28, 36)	33 (29, 36)
Feeding status		n = 220 *	n = 117 *	n = 337 *
Exclusively BF	55 (54)	138 (63)	75 (64)	213 (63)
Supplemented with medical justification	3 (3)	67 (30)	28 (24)	95 (28)

Table 1. *Cont.*

	Survey	QCCH	SMH	Both Sites
Supplemented without medical justification				
NIFS-AMI	38 (37)			
Exclusive BMS	6 (6)	15 (7)	14 (12)	29 (9)
Baby age (days)	1 (1, 2)			
Length of admission (days)		2 (1, 3)	2 (1, 4)	2 (1, 3)
Age left education (years)	23 (21, 24)			
Highest level of education: University degree	66 (65)			
Ethnicity: White Caucasian	53/88 (60)	149/295 (51)	106/182 (58)	255/477 (53)
Vaginal delivery	64 (63)	357 (73)	201 (61)	558 (68)
Laboured <2 h	82 (80)	410 (84)	280 (85)	690 (85)
Primiparous	59 (58)	83 (17)	42 (13)	125 (15)
Weight of infant	3.2 (2.9, 3.6)	3.2 (2.9, 3.5)	3.3 (3.0, 3.6)	3.3 (2.9, 3.6)
Low (<2.5 kg)	8 (8)	41 (8)	20 (7)	61 (8)
Gestational age (weeks)	39 (38, 40)	39 (38, 40)	39 (39, 40)	39 (38, 40)
If multiparous, EBF previous infants	26/43 (61)			
Ward type				
Postnatal	82 (80)	406 (84)	216 (66)	622 (76)
Private Ward	9 (9)	0 (0)	70 (21)	70 (9)
Birth Centre	11 (11)	80 (16)	43 (13)	123 (15)
Private room	25 (25)			
Infant remained with mother in hospital	92 (90)			
Partner present at night	42 (41)			
Any skin-to-skin after birth	84 (82)			
Skin-to-skin for 1 h after birth	50 (49)			
Supported to BF after birth	68 (67)			
Assisted with positioning and attachment	82 (80)			
Reports having received education about signs that infant is receiving enough milk	50 (49)			
Reports having received education about hand expression	39 (38)			
Reports having antenatal BF discussion with HCP	39 (38)			

All data are displayed as number (% or IQR) as shown. Single numerical values (*n*) in brackets indicate %, double numerical values (*n*, *n*) indicate IQR. Ethnic groups represented in the non-Caucasian sample were categorised according to National Statistics recommended criteria and were represented as follows; surveyed mothers: Black 13 (15), Asian 22 (25), Mixed 0 (0); QCCH: Black 50 (17), Asian 80 (27), Mixed 16 (5); SMH: Black 25 (14), Asian 37 (20), Mixed 14 (8). BF—breastfeeding; BMS—breastmilk substitute; EBF—exclusive breastfeeding; HCP—healthcare professional; NIFS-AMI—neonatal infant-formula supplementation in the absence of medical indication; QCCH—Queen Charlotte's and Chelsea Hospital; SMH—Saint Mary's Hospital. * percentages in the corresponding columns were calculated on the available data for statistical analysis.

3.2. Maternal Characteristics and NIFS-AMI

Univariate analysis was conducted to determine which variables of maternal characteristics were associated with NIFS-AMI (Table 2). Skin-to-skin contact for at least one hour ($p = 0.01$), higher education ($p < 0.01$), and antenatal discussions regarding breastfeeding ($p = 0.01$) were all inversely associated with non-clinical supplementation behaviour on the postnatal ward.

Table 2. Association between maternal characteristics and NIFS-AMI: univariate analysis ($n = 96$).

	Number of Infants Receiving NIFS-AMI	Number of Infants EBF + Medically Justified Supplementation	*p* Value
	$n = 38$	$n = 55 + 3$	
Maternal age (years)	29 (25, 37)	34 (29, 36)	0.13
Baby age (days)	2 (1, 3)	1 (1, 1)	**0.01**
Age left education (years)	22 (19, 24)	23 (21, 24)	0.19
Highest level of education: University degree	18 (47)	44 (76)	**<0.01**
Employed prior to pregnancy	21 (55)	43 (74)	0.08
Ethnicity: White Caucasian	23 (61)	33 (57)	0.29
Vaginal delivery	23 (61)	38 (66)	0.62
Laboured >2 h	31 (82)	45 (78)	0.64
Primiparous	24 (63)	32 (55)	0.44

Table 2. *Cont.*

	Number of Infants Receiving NIFS-AMI	Number of Infants EBF + Medically Justified Supplementation	*p* Value
Weight of infant	3.3 (2.8, 3.6)	3.3 (3.0, 3.5)	
Gestational age (weeks)	39 (38, 40)	40 (39, 41)	0.07
If multiparous, EBF previous infants	6/14 (43)	19/26 (73)	0.06
BF duration with previous infants	12 (5, 24)	7 (6, 9)	0.39
Ward type			**0.04**
Postnatal	34 (45)	42 (55)	
Birth Centre/Private Ward	4 (25)	16 (75)	
Private room	7 (18)	18 (31)	0.17
Infant remained with mother in hospital	36 (95)	52 (90)	0.47
Partner present at night	18 (47)	20 (35)	0.13
Any skin-to-skin after birth	26 (68)	54 (93)	**<0.01**
Skin-to-skin for 1 h after birth	13 (34)	36 (62)	**0.01**
Supported to BF after birth	27 (71)	41 (71)	0.97
Assisted with positioning and attachment	33 (87)	47 (81)	0.46
Mother reported antenatal education about signs that infant is receiving enough milk	22 (58)	25 (43)	0.16
Mother reported antenatal education on responsive feeding	10 (26)	33 (57)	0.10
Mother reported antenatal education about hand expression	23 (61)	15 (26)	**<0.01**
Mother reported antenatal education on benefits of developing relationship with infant	14 (37)	32 (55)	**0.01**
Informed of support available within the community	17 (45)	24 (41)	0.75
Attended BF antenatal class at QCCH	3 (8)	7 (12)	0.74
Attended BF antenatal class at another site	7 (18)	16 (28)	0.30
Antenatal BF discussion	9 (24)	29 (50)	**0.01**
Mother reports having been EBF as infant	16 (43)	23 (40)	0.99
Duration EBF as infant	12 (12, 24)	7 (6, 12)	**0.05**
BF confidence on ward (1–10)	7 (6, 8)	7 (6, 9)	0.28
BF confidence before birth (1–10)	8 (6, 10)	6 (5, 9)	0.09
BMS first introduced (hours)	6 (4, 24)	5 (3, 39)	0.94
Positive attitude to BF in social/cultural background	29 (76)	46 (79)	0.73

All data are displayed as number (% or IQR) as shown. Single numerical values (*n*) in brackets indicate %, double numerical values (*n*, *n*) indicate IQR. Mothers exclusively feeding their infants with BMS have been excluded from the multivariate analysis ($n = 6$). Significant results are indicated by the bold text. BF—breastfeeding; BMS—breastmilk substitute; EBF—exclusively breastfed; NIFS-AMI—neonatal infant-formula supplementation in the absence of medical indication; QCCH—Queen Charlotte's and Chelsea Hospital.

3.3. Midwife Descriptive Characteristics

The demographics of the participating midwives are detailed in Table S1. The median age was 38 years (28–50 IQR) with the majority having studied midwifery at the university level (87%). The median years' experience as a midwife was 7 years (4–18). All the participating staff members had received mandatory breastfeeding training provided by Imperial College London NHS Hospital Trust (100%). Of the 31 midwives available for interview, 20 had initiated NIFS-AMI within the seven-week study period (65%), with a median hourly rate of 0.62% (0–2.8).

3.4. Midwife Attitudes and Recalled Infant Feeding Behaviour

Twenty-four midwives reported their cultural and social backgrounds to have a positive attitude towards breastfeeding (77%) (Table 3). The mean perceived impact of BMS supplementation was 8/10 (6–10), with 1 being lowest impact and 10 greatest. Of all the supplementation scenarios described by staff, 62% ($n = 111$) violated WHO criteria, with only a third able to describe three scenarios appropriately and 13% unable to provide any acceptable answers. Inappropriate reasons cited for BMS supplementation are shown as number (%); hungry infant 15 (21.7); medical recommendation 13 (18.8); jaundice 12 (17.4); latching problems 10 (14.5); low birth weight or weight loss 8 (11.6); prematurity 7 (10.1); reluctant feeders 1 (1.5); nasogastric tube-use 1 (1.5); transitional care 1 (1.5); 12 h without feeding 1 (1.5).

Table 3. Midwife attitude and knowledge of breastfeeding.

Midwife Attitude and Knowledge of Breastfeeding	*n* (IQR)
Perceived importance of role in BF (1–10) *	10 (10, 10)
Perceived impact of BMS supplements (1–10) *	8 (6, 10)
Perceived time satisfaction (1–10) *	5 (1, 8)
Confidence in FF (1–10) *	8 (4, 10)
	***n* (%)**
Positive attitudes to BF in social/cultural background	24 (77)
Staff satisfied with time for FF	10 (32)
Received training on FF	19 (61)
Supplementation practice violates WHO criteria	20 (65)
One of three examples violated criteria	6 (19)
Two of three examples violated criteria	10 (32)
All examples described violated criteria	4 (13)
Percentage of time allocation to feeding support versus other tasks during a typical day	**% (IQR)**
Specific feeding support	12 (10, 20)
General patient care	25 (20, 40)
Computer/paperwork	50 (30, 60)
Taking bedside observations	10 (10, 15)

BF—breastfeeding; BMS—breastmilk substitute; FF—finger feeding; WHO—World Health Organisation. *—Likert scale was used to assess these items.

3.5. Assessment of Real-Life BMS Prescription

Figure 2 illustrates the frequency of supplementation behaviour of midwives on the postnatal unit at QCCH. The vast majority of supplements administered during the study period were for non-medically indicated reasons (90%), which was consistent with current literature [48]. Fifty-nine percent of NIFS-AMI instances occurred during between the hours of 22.00–06.00. Medical reasons to supplement included infant hypoglycaemia and very low birth weight (<1500 g). The most commonly recorded reason for NIFS-AMI was maternal request.

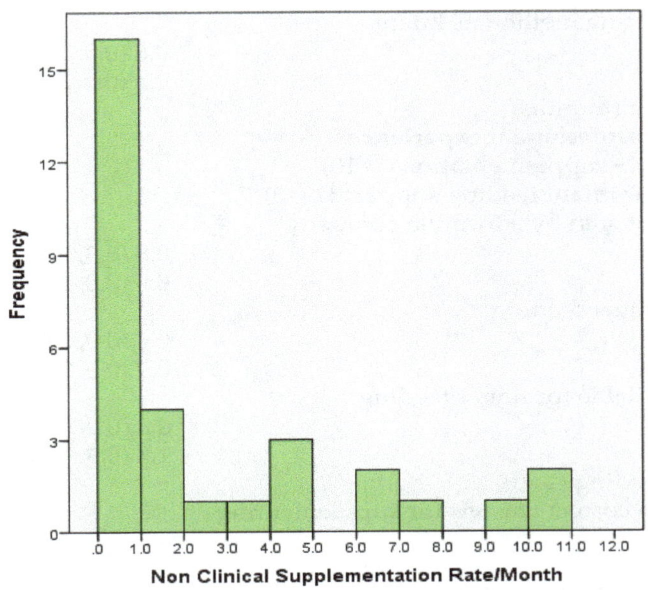

Figure 2. Midwives' estimated monthly rates of neonatal infant-formula supplementation in the absence of medical indication (NIFS-AMI) as defined by WHO ($n = 31$). Monthly rates were extrapolated from hourly rates. Midwives worked for a median of 212.5 (161.3, 248) hours during the seven-week study period (9 March 2016–26 April 2016).

3.6. What Influences NIFS-AMI?

Table 4 illustrates the univariate analysis of midwife variables in relation to rates of NIFS-AMI. Statistical differences in hourly rates were observed according to ward types ($p < 0.01$), time satisfaction with breastfeeding ($p = 0.01$), and finger feeding support ($p = 0.02$), alongside finger feeding confidence ($p = 0.03$). Borderline significant values were found regarding level of education, perceived impact of BMS supplementation ($p = 0.07$), and the ability to correctly describe three appropriate scenarios ($p = 0.07$).

Table 4. Hourly rates of NIFS-AMI (%) according to midwife variables ($n = 31$).

Descriptive Characteristics	**Median/IQR**	**r**	***p* Value**
Staff age		0.2	0.28
Years' experience as a midwife		0.03	0.89
Ward Type			
Postnatal	1.9 (0.7, 4.2)		**<0.01**
Birth Centre/Private Ward	0.0 (0.0, 0.4)		
Ethnic Background			
White Caucasian	0.4 (0.0, 0.7)		0.26
Non-Caucasian	1.9 (0.6, 3.0)		
Highest level of education			
Degree	0.4 (0.0, 1.9)		0.07
Non-degree	3.4 (2.2, 4.7)		
Personal experiences			
Attitudes to BF in social/cultural background			
Positive	0.7 (0.0, 2.7)		0.84
Negative or mixed	0.4 (0.0, 2.7)		
Parity			
Primiparous/multiparous	0.7 (0.4, 4.2)		0.22
Nulliparous	0.4 (0.0, 1.8)		
Infant feeding method			
EBF	0.6 (0.0, 1.9)		0.57
Non-EBF	2.5 (0.5, 4.2)		
Longest BF duration (months)		−0.29	0.32
Earliest age child received non-breastmilk (months)		−0.79	0.58
Midwife's reported feeding method as infant			0.62
EBF	0.6 (0.0, 1.8)		
Mon-EBF	0.8 (0.0, 2.7)		
Duration of BF as infant (months)		0.43	0.11
Staff perceptions and professional experiences			
Perceived impact of BMS supplementation (1–10)		−0.33	0.07
Happiness with time for infant feeding support (1–10)		−0.47	**0.01**
Attended training sponsored by a formula company			
Yes	0.8 (0.3, 2.7)		0.62
No	0.5 (0.0, 2.6)		
Received training on finger feeding			
Yes	0.4 (0.0, 3.0)		0.86
No	0.9 (0.0, 2.7)		
Satisfied with time available for finger feeding			
Yes	0.0 (0.0, 0.6)	0.43	**0.02**
No	1.2 (0.3, 4.2)		
Confidence in finger feeding (1–10)		−0.40	**0.03**
Correctly identify three correct reasons for supplementing			
Yes	0.6 (0.0, 4.6)		0.07
No	0.6 (0.0, 2.1)		

Table 4. *Cont.*

Descriptive Characteristics	Median/IQR	r	p Value
Percentage of time allocation to feeding support versus other tasks during a typical day (%)			
Infant feeding support		0.56	0.77
General patient care		−0.01	0.96
Computer/paperwork		−0.01	0.95
Taking bedside observations		0.14	0.47

r—Spearman Rho or Pearson's correlation coefficient. Mann-Whitney U, Spearman Rho, and Pearson's coefficient were used for categorical, non-parametric, and parametric correlations, respectively. Significant results are indicated by the bold text. BF—breastfeeding; BMS—breastmilk substitute; EBF—exclusively breastfed; NIFS-AMI—neonatal infant-formula supplementation in the absence of medical indication.

Univariate analysis according to supplementation categorisation is displayed in Table S2. As a recurring theme, time satisfaction and ward type were significantly associated.

To assess the association between the midwives' rate of NIFS-AMI and most important exposures, a bootstrapping regression model was used in the multivariate analysis (Table 5). Ward type ($p = 0.01$) and midwife education ($p = 0.01$) were statistically significant.

Table 5. Multivariate analysis of factors influencing midwives' decision for NIFS-AMI.

Parameter	B	p Value	95% Confidence Interval	
			Lower Bound	Upper Bound
Education	2.53	**0.01**	0.95	4.12
Breastmilk substitute impact (1–10)	−0.19	0.22	−0.48	0.07
Ability to provide three correct scenarios (100%)	1.01	0.18	−2.47	0.23
Ward	−1.63	**0.01**	−2.50	−0.66

Dependent variable; rate of NIFS-AMI (%), a; this parameter is set to zero because it is redundant. Significant results are indicated by the bold text.

3.7. Perceived Barriers to Supporting Breastfeeding

When asked about barriers encountered on the wards, 78% of the 31 staff members reported time constraints as a key factor affecting breastfeeding support (Figure S2). According to self-reported time allocation, midwives allocated a median of only 12% of their shift to supporting infant feeding, with the largest proportion of their time allocated to computer and paperwork (50%). This was consistent across wards and NIFS-AMI categories.

As a key theme, many midwives expressed emotive responses relating to their perceived lack of time:

> "*Sometimes I get depressed, it is a terrible thing not being able to help*". Midwife 4

> "*The training courses are pointless if you don't have the time to use it*". Midwife 12

> "*It's never them, the mothers want the support; it's the time*". Midwife 30

> "*It has repercussions on our own health, not being able to help, as well as of course the baby and the mothers. The mothers get so depressed*". Midwife 23

There were also several members of staff expressing the mothers' poor antenatal preparation as an interfering factor (27.5%). This was expressed in relation to a lack of knowledge and exposure to breastfeeding videos:

> "*They [the mothers] genuinely don't know how good it is! They underestimate the difference between breast and formula, it is such a shame*". Midwife 24

"The videos they show in antenatal classes give women unrealistic expectations of breastfeeding, it is harder than they make it look". Midwife 7

Additionally, workload and staff shortage related issues were common complaints, as reported by 55% of staff. Alongside this, the requirement for more specific staff with dedicated roles to infant feeding and one-to-one opportunities was expressed by 38.5%:

"You cave in sometimes due to the workload, giving the bottle is so easy and that is why it is so sad". Midwife 23

"I tell the women breastfeeding is hard and needs perseverance. One-to-one support is so important and 30 min isn't enough". Midwife 31

"It is exhausting helping women one-to-one to breastfeed all the time, especially when the ward is busy, it takes a lot of effort". Midwife 18

Although finger feeding was included in the compulsory training day, 38.7% of midwives regarded themselves to have not received training, which was relatively constant across the groups. Time satisfaction and confidence for this technique varied significantly according to ward type. In addition, six staff members (15%) expressed negative attitudes towards finger feeding, describing the practice as *"unhygienic"*, *"dangerous"*, and *"a waste of time"*.

4. Discussion

With significant evidence that NIFS-AMI has detrimental consequences on breastfeeding, the factors influencing early BMS use by staff in the post-natal environment is highly relevant. In this study, maternal and midwife factors were sought to determine possible impacts upon NIFS-AMI activity on the postnatal ward.

4.1. The Use of BMS Supplementation on the Postnatal Ward

Our data demonstrates that a significant proportion of BMS supplementation occurs for no defined medical reason. In nine out of 10 cases of BMS supplementation, breastmilk substitute was provided by the staff without appropriate medical indication. Local statistics from 2015 Good Food for London Report show a good level of community breastfeeding support, achieving full BFHI accreditation, which further highlights the need to change the current infant feeding practice in the postnatal unit [49]. This recommendation was supported further in the report from the National Maternity and Perinatal Audit 2017, which advised that "Commissioners, together with clinicians, services, and policymakers should strongly prioritise the provision of resources to support breastfeeding, both in maternity units and in the community, to reduce the variation in the proportion of babies receiving breastmilk at their first feed and at discharge from the maternity unit" [50].

4.2. Maternal Factors

Maternal characteristics protective against NIFS-AMI were associated with higher educational status, one hour of uninterrupted skin-to-skin after delivery, and breastfeeding discussions during pregnancy with a healthcare professional. These findings are reflective of previous work [51]. The evidence for skin-to-skin as an intervention to improve breastfeeding outcomes is particularly well studied. A 2016 Cochrane review concluded with good evidence that skin-to-skin was beneficial to healthy infants [52]. Our results are supportive of the UNICEF recommendations, which is in agreement with the BFHI 10 steps to successful breastfeeding.

4.3. Midwife Factors

Our findings suggest that the staff at QCCH experience many barriers to supporting breastfeeding. One key theme arising from this exploration regards the lack of suitable antenatal preparation. Previous research shows that under-preparation and the availability of BMS are key reasons why mothers requested artificial supplements [53]. In addition, prior expectations, formed from healthcare staff and the media, influence maternal breastfeeding confidence to a major extent [54].

As described by the midwives at QCCH, antenatal classes have been named as partly responsible for these unrealistic expectations [55,56]. This is consistent with the available evidence worldwide, demonstrating antenatal education to have negative or inconclusive impact on breastfeeding rates [57–59]. Consequently, a lack of concordance between a mother's expectations and the reality of breastfeeding can lead to feelings of guilt, failure, and a lack of confidence in breastfeeding and motherhood [60,61].

There have been several studies investigating the factors likely to affect midwives' behaviour in relation to infant feeding. Lack of time, poor staffing levels, and a resistance to change were all identified as contributing factors to non-compliance of a breastfeeding support intervention on UK postnatal wards [40]. Our data support previous findings in the UK, as the barriers most commonly reported by QCCH maternity staff were a lack of time alongside workload issues and the need for more specific feeding support with one-to-one care. The number of hospitals applying the BFHI policy is on the rise, but the real-life effectiveness of this strategy is somehow limited due to the increasing issue of staff shortages [62,63].

The views of inadequate availability of staff support appear to be consistent across cultural and ethnic backgrounds, with evidence that one-to-one feeding support is effective at significantly reducing supplementation rates [64–66]. The perception of active support from midwives postnatally in England was predictive of lower odds of breastfeeding cessation as assessed by maternal questionnaires at day 10 [67]. In this study, many midwives reported computer work, particularly discharges, to take up a considerable percentage of their day. Bowers et al. revealed that very little staff time is spent educating and supporting mothers with infant feeding; this was concordant with the midwives' time allocation at QCCH. Recent literature has demonstrated a reduction in the duration of postnatal admissions with proportionate reductions in staffing, resulting in an increased workload which negatively impacted quality of care and staff morale [68].

In our study, the most-cited reason for NIFS-AMI was maternal request for BMS. In the literature, reasons for parents requesting BMS supplementation included a lack of preparation for breastfeeding and viewing infant-formula as the answer to breastfeeding problems [24,53].

The UNICEF Maternity Standards document states that clear documentation of the mother's reason, alternative options, and information provided by midwife must be recorded when BMS supplementation is initiated for maternal requests. The recommended care includes hand expression education, support with positioning, and plans made for future feeding to maximise breastfeeding (or the use of breastmilk) [69]. In reality, this was rarely the case at QCCH; documented notes provided very little details around the initiation of NIFS-AMI. Of the 102 mothers surveyed, only 38% could recall a discussion on hand expressing. The reported midwife dissatisfaction in the workplace appears to be a significant driver in the promotion of breastfeeding and time allocation for appropriate counselling.

As time and workload appear to have significant impacts on patients' postnatal support, the different working environments may explain the differences reported across ward types [70]. With a lower staff/patient ratio on the NHS postnatal ward, the perceived time satisfaction unsurprisingly differs to those working on private wards or at birth centres. Our study reveals that finger feeding confidence and time satisfaction were negatively associated with higher supplementation rates, which staff attributed to their lack of time. Although time availability appears to play a role in the interference of infant feeding support, a multivariate analysis identified staff perceptions of BMS to be the most influential factor upon rates of NIFS-AMI. This is supported by the inconsistencies identified across shift type and BMS use. For example, many staff reported having more time to support mothers during the night shift; however, a higher frequency of NIFS-AMI instances were reported, suggesting the current practice to be a complex, multifactorial issue.

The next section of the survey was concerned with midwives' perceptions in relation to supplementation behaviour. Existing evidence suggests that midwives' behaviour is influential upon a mother's feeding decisions, with regard to their perceived attitudes and the support offered [71–73]. However, the current literature into midwives' supplementation perceptions and behaviour has not been thoroughly explored. An association between support offered by staff and their attitudes has been shown, with evidence of midwives with poor breastfeeding attitudes failing to support mothers [74]. Mothers usually perceiving maternity staff to have 'no preference' with regard to breastfeeding were less likely to breastfeed beyond six weeks [75]. Midwife characteristics associated with greater breastfeeding knowledge in other studies included midwives over 30 years old, with higher qualifications, as well as more clinical and personal experience of breastfeeding for over three months [76,77]. The training a midwife receives has also been suggested to be clinically relevant to breastfeeding practices in the hospital, with those demonstrating higher breastfeeding knowledge reporting best clinical practice [41].

Despite the fact that all maternity staff at QCCH had attended the Trust's breastfeeding training, only a third of them were able to successfully describe three valid scenarios in which they had supplemented a breastfed infant. This data is in agreement with the outcomes of an American study, reporting high rates of non-medically indicated supplementation, with staff often providing inaccurate information and failing to correct mothers who possessed incorrect information [48]. Although this may indicate that staff lack the knowledge to best advise mothers, there is evidence of non-adherence to the BFHI standards with deviant behaviour described such as undercover supplementation and concealing their actions by recording the supplementation as a 'maternal choice' rather than a 'midwife suggestion' [78]. This would suggest that midwives may be aware that their behaviour is not the best clinical practice.

4.4. Application of BFHI Policy into Clinical Practice

In order to explain the gap between evidence-based knowledge and clinical practice, the knowledge translation theory can be applied to the BFHI policy implementation using five stages from acceptance to adherence [79,80]. Our data demonstrate lack of knowledge as a crucial factor in real-life decision-making on whether to supplement an infant with BMS. In addition, emotional responses expressed by several staff members reflecting personal beliefs on breastfeeding support are consistent with previous qualitative studies in the UK and is thought to have a negative impact on clinical reasoning and adherence to BFHI criteria [81]. It has therefore been suggested that for midwives to develop new behaviour, their attitudes and belief systems need to be reframed [82,83]. This can be particularly difficult to achieve for those who have had positive experiences of supplementing, as beliefs associated with personal involvement most strongly predict forthcoming behaviour [84].

It is evident that for hospital practice modification, active participation and planning for change, alongside establishing targets, are necessary [85]. The midwife-identified barriers, such as those relating to the workplace, require consideration from the establishment to address issues surrounding infant feeding. Making BFHI an organisational priority, reducing the accessibility of BMS, and establishing financial support dedicated to the initiative are all suggestions to overcome barriers from an integrative review [86]. Enforcing the requirement for all parents to read and complete paperwork before BMS is permitted may also be successful at reducing both staff suggested and maternally requested supplementation with greater knowledge communication to ensure that parents give informed consent [87]. This also agrees with earlier results, which shows that support and encouragement from other midwives and managerial staff can promote adherence to BFHI practices, and indicates that involving staff in processes such as mentoring schemes can help promote positive attitudes towards the BFHI [79,87]. Conversely, midwives reverting back to outdated protocols have been demonstrated to influence the behaviour of newly qualified midwives and mothers, highlighting the potential for a cascade of incorrect conduct and the vital requirement for a committed workforce [83,88].

4.5. Study Limitations

The main limitations of this study surround the cross-sectional design, with data collection only occurring within a defined point in time. It is therefore impossible to infer causality between outcomes and exposures [89]. A prospective study assessing the attitudes of newly qualified midwives before starting work may therefore provide better insight into the temporal relationship. With limited time available for the interview period, it was not possible to survey all postnatal staff at the QCCH, which could therefore increase the risk of a non-representative sample. Additionally, due to the sample size, only a limited number of confounders could be accounted for in the multivariate analysis. However, the statistically significant correlation between midwives' education and work placement and the use of NIFS-AMI is worth further investigation. As the survey was presented in English and staff in a single hospital were approached, results cannot be generalised to all medical professionals across the globe. However, we believe that our results are closer to a best-case interpretation and therefore are even more concerning.

5. Conclusions

Known modifiable maternal factors confirmed in this study included the protective value of skin-to-skin and antenatal discussions against unnecessary BMS supplementation. A striking number of midwives failing to name medically appropriate scenarios for BMS introduction, which highlights failure in the education system, even when provided in accordance with the latest BFHI guidelines. Available evidence on BFHI effectiveness is somehow conflicting and cannot fully support existing training in its present form. The main outcome of BFHI efficiency is normally limited to breastfeeding initiation rates, which has been continuously critisised as an inappropriate measure to measure the success of the BFHI [90,91].

With an association between the lack of knowledge and greater rates of NIFS-AMI, this study confirms the necessary requirement to reduce in-hospital supplementary feeds, through the development of a better model of breastfeeding support, which may include an extensive use of cell phone-based applications, educational programme development, and postnatal staff training improvement. Midwife interviews in this study suggested a need for more one-to-one support of women in the immediate postnatal period. Maternal request for BMS is a major factor influencing non-clinical supplementation and this should be tackled by developing strategies to train staff to respond constructively to such requests as well as by a more effective education of pregnant women, using online resources and distance learning tools. If changes could be successfully implemented, a reduction in non-clinical supplementation, with regard to both staff suggestion and maternal requests, could be achieved with predicted benefits in breastfeeding outcomes.

Key Messages:

- The use of in-hospital breastmilk substitute supplementation for breastfed infants is commonplace in the study hospital, as 95 (28%) of infants received a BMS supplement prior to discharge from maternity unit and 90% of BMS supplementation was given without medical indication.
- Maternal factors protective of neonatal infant-formula supplementation in the absence of medical indication included skin-to-skin and antenatal breastfeeding discussions.
- Although midwives were appropriately trained in accordance with BFHI protocols, they identified a number of workplace barriers in breastfeeding support, with lack of time and heavy workload being the major contributors.
- We found significant associations between the midwives' decisions on non-medical infant-formula supplementation and educational status, which suggests a need to focus the existing BFHI training programme.
- In order to reduce unnecessary supplementation as well as address attitudes and perceived barriers, additional educational programmes should be developed, with a focus on one-to-one support for establishing lactation in the postnatal environment.

Author Contributions: K.B., K.H., E.M., R.J.B., and D.M. conceived and designed the study; K.B. designed the survey tool; K.B. and K.H. collected the data, K.B. and D.M. analysed the data and interpreted results; K.B. wrote the paper; E.K., D.M., and R.J.B. formatted and edited the manuscript.

Acknowledgments: All authors critically reviewed and approved the final manuscript. Many thanks are extended to all of the mothers and midwives who participated in this study.

References

1. Rollins, N.C.; Bhandari, N.; Hajeebhoy, N.; Horton, S.; Lutter, C.K.; Martines, J.C.; Piwoz, E.G.; Richter, L.M.; Victora, C.G. Why invest, and what it will take to improve breastfeeding practices? *Lancet* **2016**, *387*, 491–504. [CrossRef]
2. Victora, C.G.; Bahl, R.; Barros, A.J.; França, G.V.; Horton, S.; Krasevec, J.; Murch, S.; Sankar, M.J.; Walker, N.; Rollins, N.C. Breastfeeding in the 21st century: Epidemiology, mechanisms, and lifelong effect. *Lancet* **2016**, *387*, 475–490. [CrossRef]
3. Kramer, M.S.; Kakuma, R. Optimal duration of exclusive breastfeeding. *Cochrane Database Syst. Rev.* **2012**, *15*, CD003517. [CrossRef] [PubMed]
4. Duijts, L.; Jaddoe, V.W.; Hofman, A.; Moll, H.A. Prolonged and exclusive breastfeeding reduces the risk of infectious diseases in infancy. *Pediatrics* **2010**, *126*, e18–e25. [CrossRef] [PubMed]
5. Quigley, M.A.; Kelly, Y.J.; Sacker, A. Breastfeeding and hospitalization for diarrheal and respiratoryinfection in the United Kingdom Millennium Cohort Study. *Pediatrics* **2007**, *119*, e837–e842. [CrossRef] [PubMed]
6. Klement, E.; Cohen, R.V.; Boxman, J.; Joseph, A.; Reif, S. Breastfeeding and risk of inflammatory bowel disease: A systematic review with meta-analysis. *Am. J. Clin. Nutr.* **2004**, *80*, 1342–1352. [CrossRef] [PubMed]
7. Akobeng, A.K.; Ramanan, A.V.; Buchan, I.; Heller, R.F. Effect of breast-feeding on risk of coeliac disease: A systematic review and meta-analysis of observational studies. *Arch. Dis. Child.* **2006**, *91*, 39–43. [CrossRef] [PubMed]
8. World Health Organisation. Evidence on the Long-Term Effects of Breastfeeding, Systematic Reviews and Meta-Analysis, Department of Child and Adolescent Health and Development (CAH). 2007. Available online: http://apps.who.int/iris/bitstream/10665/43623/1/9789241595230_eng.pdf (accessed on 20 April 2018).
9. WHO Collaborative Study Team on the Role of Breastfeeding on the Prevention of Infant Mortality. Effect of breastfeeding on infant and child mortality due to infectious diseases in less developed countries: A pooled analysis. *Lancet* **2000**, *355*, 451–455.
10. Bachrach, V.R.; Schwarz, E.; Bachrach, L.R. Breastfeeding and the risk of hospitalization for respiratory disease in infancy: A meta-analysis. *Arch. Pediatr. Adolesc. Med.* **2003**, *157*, 237–243. [CrossRef] [PubMed]
11. Hauck, F.R.; Thompson, J.M.; Tanabe, K.O.; Moon, R.Y.; Vennemann, M.M. Breastfeeding and reduced risk of sudden infant death syndrome: A meta-analysis. *Pediatrics* **2011**, *128*, 103–110. [CrossRef] [PubMed]
12. Rothenbacher, D.; Weyermann, M.; Beermann, C.; Brenner, H. Breastfeeding, soluble CD14 concentration in breast milk and risk of atopic dermatitis and asthma in early childhood: Birth cohort study. *Clin. Exp. Allergy* **2005**, *35*, 1014–1021. [CrossRef] [PubMed]
13. Greer, F.R.; Sicherer, S.H.; Burks, A.W.; American Academy of Pediatrics Committee on Nutrition; American Academy of Pediatrics Section on Allergy and Immunology. Effects of early nutritional interventions on the development of atopic disease in infants and children: The role of maternal dietary restriction, breastfeeding, timing of introduction of complementary foods, and hydrolyzed formulas. *Pediatrics* **2008**, *121*, 183–191. [CrossRef] [PubMed]
14. Horta, B.L.; Bahl, R.; Martines, J.C.; Victora, C.G. Evidence on the Long-Term Effects of Breastfeeding. Geneva: World Health Organization. 2007. Available online: http://apps.who.int/iris/bitstream/handle/10665/43623/9789241595230_eng.pdf;jsessionid=96C96746137B09E506E1051FAAA5CDDC?sequence=1 (accessed on 23 April 2018).
15. Harder, T.; Bergmann, R.; Kallischnigg, G.; Plagemann, A. Duration of breastfeeding and risk of overweight: A meta-analysis. *Am. J. Epidemiol.* **2005**, *162*, 397–403. [CrossRef] [PubMed]
16. Arenz, S.; Ruckeri, R.; Koletzko, B.; von Kries, R. Breastfeeding and Childhood obesity: A systematic review. *Int. J. Obes. Relat. Metab. Disord.* **2004**, *28*, 1247–1256. [CrossRef] [PubMed]

17. Kramer, M.S.; Aboud, F.; Mironova, E.; Vanilovich, I.; Platt, R.W.; Matush, L.; Igumnov, S.; Fombonne, E.; Bogdanovich, N.; Ducruet, T.; et al. Breastfeeding and child cognitive development: New evidence from a large randomized trial. *Arch. Gen. Psychiatry* **2008**, *65*, 578–584. [CrossRef] [PubMed]
18. Heikkilä, K.; Sacker, A.; Kelly, Y.; Renfrew, M.J.; Quigley, M.A. Breastfeeding and child behaviour in the Millennium Cohort Study. *Arch. Dis. Child.* **2011**, *96*, 635–642. [CrossRef] [PubMed]
19. Quigley, M.A.; Hockley, C.; Carson, C.; Kelly, Y.; Renfrew, M.J.; Sacker, A. Breastfeeding is Associated with Improved Child Cognitive Development: A Population-Based Cohort Study. *J. Pediatr.* **2012**, *160*, 25–32. [CrossRef] [PubMed]
20. Kramer, M.S.; Chalmers, B.; Hodnett, E.D.; Sevkovskaya, Z.; Dzikovich, I.; Shapiro, S.; Collet, J.P.; Vanilovich, I.; Mezen, I.; Ducruet, T.; et al. Promotion of Breastfeeding Intervention Trial (PROBIT). A randomized trial in the Republic of Belarus. *JAMA* **2001**, *285*, 413–420. [CrossRef] [PubMed]
21. Dewey, K.G.; Heinig, M.J.; Nommsen, L.A. Maternal weight-loss patterns during prolonged lactation. *Am. J. Clin. Nutr.* **1993**, *58*, 162–166. [CrossRef] [PubMed]
22. Short, R.V. Lactational infertility in family planning. *Ann. Med.* **1993**, *25*, 175–180. [CrossRef] [PubMed]
23. Collaborative Group on Hormonal Factors in Breast Cancer. Breast cancer and breastfeeding: Collaborative reanalysis of individual data from 47 epidemiological studies in 30 countries, including 50302 women with breast cancer and 96973 women without the disease. *Lancet* **2002**, *360*, 187–195.
24. Islami, F.; Liu, Y.; Jemal, A.; Zhou, J.; Weiderpass, E.; Colditz, G.; Boffetta, P.; Weiss, M. Breastfeeding and breast cancer risk by receptor status—A systematic review and meta-analysis. *Ann. Oncol.* **2015**, *26*, 2398–2407. [CrossRef] [PubMed]
25. Tung, K.H.; Goodman, M.T.; Wu, A.H.; McDuffie, K.; Wilkens, L.R.; Kolonel, L.N.; Nomura, A.M.; Terada, K.Y.; Carney, M.E.; Sobin, L.H. Reproductive factors and epithelial ovarian cancer risk by histologic type:a multiethnic case-control study. *Am. J. Epidemiol.* **2003**, *158*, 629–638. [CrossRef] [PubMed]
26. Rosenblatt, K.A.; Thomas, D.B. Lactation and the risk of epithelial ovarian cancer—The WHO Collaborative Study of Neoplasia and Steroid Contraceptives. *Int. J. Epidemiol.* **1993**, *22*, 192–197. [CrossRef] [PubMed]
27. Bjornerem, A.; Ahmed, L.A.; Jorgensen, L.; Stormer, J.; Joakimsen, R.M. Breastfeeding protects against hip fracture in postmenopausal women: The Tromso study. *J. Bone Miner. Res.* **2011**, *26*, 2843–2850. [CrossRef] [PubMed]
28. Stafford, M.; Kuh, D.L.; Gale, C.R.; Mishra, G.; Richards, M. Parent-child relationships and offspring's positive mental wellbeing from adolescence to early older age. *J. Posit. Psychol.* **2016**, *11*, 326–337. [CrossRef] [PubMed]
29. Puckering, C.; Allely, C.S.; Doolin, O.; Purves, D.; McConnachie, A.; Johnson, P.C.; Marwick, H.; Heron, J.; Golding, J.; Gillberg, C.; et al. Association between parent-infant interactions in infancy and disruptive behaviour disorders at age seven: A nested, case–control ALSPAC study. *BMC Pediatr.* **2014**, *14*, 223. [CrossRef] [PubMed]
30. Brown, A.; Rance, J.; Bennett, P. Understanding the relationship between breastfeeding and postnatal depression: The role of pain and physical difficulties. *J. Adv. Nurs.* **2016**, *72*, 273–282. [CrossRef] [PubMed]
31. World Health Organisation. Up to What Age Can a Baby Stay Well Nourished by Just Being Breastfed? 2015. Available online: http://www.who.int/features/qa/21/en/ (accessed on 24 April 2018).
32. Kılcı, H.; Çoban, A. The correlation between breastfeeding success in the early postpartum period and the perception of self-efficacy in breastfeeding and breast problems in the late postpartum. *Breastfeed. Med.* **2016**, *11*, 188–195. [CrossRef] [PubMed]
33. Forster, D.A.; Johns, H.M.; McLachlan, H.L.; Moorhead, A.M.; McEgan, K.M.; Amir, L.H. Feeding infants directly at the breast during the postpartum hospital stay is associated with increased breastfeeding at 6 months postpartum: A prospective cohort study. *BMJ Open* **2015**, *5*, e007512. [CrossRef] [PubMed]
34. National Infant Feeding Survey 2010. Chapter 2: Incidence Prevalence and Duration of Breastfeeding. 2012. Available online: http://www.hscic.gov.uk/catalogue/PUB08694/ifs-uk-2010-chap2-inc-prev-dur.pdf (accessed on 6 May 2016).
35. O'Connor, M.; Allen, J.; Kelly, J.; Gao, Y.; Kildea, S. Predictors of breastfeeding exclusivity and duration in a hospital without Baby Friendly Hospital Initiative accreditation: A prospective cohort study. *Women Birth* **2017**. [CrossRef] [PubMed]

36. Chantry, C.J.; Dewey, K.G.; Peerson, J.M.; Wagner, E.A.; Nommsen-Rivers, L.A. In-hospital formula use increases early breastfeeding cessation among first-time mothers intending to exclusively breastfeed. *J. Pediatr.* **2014**, *164*, 1339–1345. [CrossRef] [PubMed]
37. Gaufin, T.; Tobin, N.H.; Aldrovandi, G.M. The importance of the microbiome in pediatrics and pediatric infectious diseases. *Curr. Opin. Pediatr.* **2018**, *30*, 117–124. [CrossRef] [PubMed]
38. Bentley, J.P.; Nassar, N.; Porter, M.; de Vroome, M.; Yip, E.; Ampt, A.J. Formula supplementation in hospital and subsequent feeding at discharge among women who intended to exclusively breastfeed: An administrative data retrospective cohort study. *Birth* **2017**, *44*, 352–362. [CrossRef] [PubMed]
39. Nguyen, T.; Dennison, B.A.; Fan, W.; Xu, C.; Birkhead, G.S. Variation in Formula Supplementation of Breastfed Newborn Infants in New York Hospitals. *Pediatrics* **2017**, *140*, E20170142. [CrossRef] [PubMed]
40. Hunter, L.; Magill-Cuerden, J.; McCourt, C. 'Oh no, no, no, we haven't got time to be doing that': Challenges encountered introducing a breast-feeding support intervention on a postnatal ward. *Midwifery* **2015**, *31*, 798–804. [CrossRef] [PubMed]
41. Cantrill, R.; Creedy, D.; Cooke, M. Midwives' knowledge of newborn feeding ability and reported practice managing the first breastfeed. *Breastfeed. Rev.* **2004**, *12*, 25–33. [PubMed]
42. Darwent, K.L.; Kempenaar, L.E. A comparison of breastfeeding women's, peer supporters' and student midwives' breastfeeding knowledge and attitudes. *Nurse Educ. Pract.* **2014**, *14*, 319–325. [CrossRef] [PubMed]
43. Marks, D.; O'Connor, R. Breastfeeding support and promotion: The health professional's perspective. *J. Health Visit.* **2015**, *3*, 38–46. [CrossRef]
44. Marks, D.; O'Connor, R. Health professionals' attitudes towards the promotion of breastfeeding. *Br. J. Midwifery* **2015**, *23*, 50–58. [CrossRef]
45. World Health Organization. *Acceptable Medical Reasons for Use of Breast Milk Substitutes*; WHO: Geneva, Switzerland, 2009. Available online: http://apps.who.int/iris/bitstream/10665/69938/1/WHO_FCH_CAH_09.01_eng.pdf (accessed on 4 May 2016).
46. UNICEF. Tools and Forms to Help Support Baby Friendly. Available online: https://www.unicef.org.uk/babyfriendly/baby-friendly-resources/guidance-for-health-professionals/tools-and-forms-for-health-professionals/ (accessed on 4 May 2016).
47. Office of National Statistics-Ethnicity Groups. Available online: https://www.google.co.uk/url?sa=t&rct=j&q=&esrc=s&source=web&cd=6&cad=rja&uact=8&ved=0ahUKEwjxqNqfxfzWAhXBPBoKHXa3AVQQFgg0MAU&url=https%3A%2F%2Fwww.ons.gov.uk%2Fons%2Fguide-method%2Fharmonisation%2Fprimary-set-of-harmonised-concepts-and-questions%2Fethnic-group.pdf&usg=AOvVaw3O-S-j3HqaDLWP0_wT-jhs (accessed on 4 May 2016).
48. Tender, J.A.; Janakiram, J.; Arce, E.; Mason, R.; Jordan, T.; Marsh, J.; Kin, S.; He, J.; Moon, R.Y. Reasons for in-hospital formula supplementation of breastfed infants from low-income families. *J. Hum. Lact.* **2009**, *25*, 11–17. [CrossRef] [PubMed]
49. Good Food for London. 2015. Available online: http://www.sustainweb.org/londonfoodlink/goodfoodforlondon2015/ (accessed on 6 May 2016).
50. National Maternity and Perinatal Audit 2017. Available online: http://www.maternityaudit.org.uk/downloads/RCOG%20NMPA%20Clinical%20Report(web).pdf (accessed on 13 February 2018).
51. Flacking, R.; Nyqvist, K.H.; Ewald, U. Effects of socioeconomic status on breastfeeding duration in mothers of preterm and term infants. *Eur. J. Public Health* **2007**, *17*, 579–584. [CrossRef] [PubMed]
52. Moore, E.R.; Bergman, N.; Anderson, G.C.; Medley, N. Early skin-to-skin contact for mothers and their healthy newborn infants. *Cochrane Database Syst. Rev.* **2016**, *11*, CD003519. [CrossRef] [PubMed]
53. DaMota, K.; Bañuelos, J.; Goldbronn, J.; Vera-Beccera, L.E.; Heinig, M.J. Maternal request for in-hospital supplementation of healthy breastfed infants among low-income women. *J. Hum. Lact.* **2012**, *28*, 476–482. [CrossRef] [PubMed]
54. Larsen, J.S.; Hall, E.O.; Aagaard, H. Shattered expectations: When mothers' confidence in breastfeeding is undermined–a metasynthesis. *Scand. J. Caring Sci.* **2008**, *22*, 653–661. [CrossRef] [PubMed]
55. Bailey, C.; Pain, R.H.; Aarvold, J.E. A 'give it a go' breast-feeding culture and early cessation among low-income mothers. *Midwifery* **2004**, *20*, 240–250. [CrossRef] [PubMed]

56. Trickey, H.; Newburn, M. Goals, dilemmas and assumptions in infant feeding education and support. Applying theory of constraints thinking tools to develop new priorities for action. *Matern. Child Nutr.* **2014**, *10*, 72–91. [CrossRef] [PubMed]
57. Lumbiganon, P.; Martis, R.; Laopaiboon, M.; Festin, M.R.; Ho, J.J.; Hakimi, M. Antenatal breastfeeding education for increasing breastfeeding duration. *Cochrane Database Syst. Rev.* **2012**, *9*, CD006425. [CrossRef]
58. Wong, K.L.; Fong, D.Y.; Lee, I.L.; Chu, S.; Tarrant, M. Antenatal education to increase exclusive breastfeeding: A randomized controlled trial. *Obstet. Gynecol.* **2014**, *124*, 961–968. [CrossRef] [PubMed]
59. Lavender, T.; Baker, L.; Smyth, R.; Collins, S.; Spofforth, A.; Dey, P. Breastfeeding expectations versus reality: A cluster randomised controlled trial. *BJOG* **2005**, *112*, 1047–1053. [CrossRef] [PubMed]
60. Hauck, Y.L.; Irurita, V.F. Incompatible expectations: The dilemma of breastfeeding mothers. *Health Care Women Int.* **2003**, *24*, 62–78. [CrossRef] [PubMed]
61. Fox, R.; McMullen, S.; Newburn, M. UK women's experiences of breastfeeding and additional breastfeeding support: A qualitative study of Baby Café services. *BMC Pregnancy Childbirth* **2015**, *15*, 147. [CrossRef] [PubMed]
62. Kmietowicz, Z. Staff shortages and lack of data continue to blight England's NHS and care regulator. *BMJ* **2015**, *351*, h4000. [CrossRef] [PubMed]
63. Triggle, N. Staff shortage puts neonatal services under strain. *Nurs. Child. Young People* **2015**, *27*, 7. [CrossRef] [PubMed]
64. Furber, C.M.; Thomson, A.M. Midwives in the UK: An exploratory study of providing newborn feeding support for postpartum mothers in the hospital. *J. Midwifery Womens Health* **2007**, *52*, 142–147. [CrossRef] [PubMed]
65. Ockleford, E.M.; Berryman, J.C.; Hsu, R. Postnatal care: What new mothers say. *Br. J. Midwifery* **2004**, *12*, 166–170. [CrossRef]
66. Sharp, D.; Entwistle, F. Why women stop breastfeeding in the early days. *Pract. Midwife* **2015**, *18*, 30–33. [PubMed]
67. Oakley, L.L.; Henderson, J.; Redshaw, M.; Quigley, M.A. The role of support and other factors in early breastfeeding cessation: An analysis of data from a maternity survey in England. *BMC Pregnancy Childbirth* **2014**, *14*, 88. [CrossRef] [PubMed]
68. Bowers, J.; Cheyne, H. Reducing the length of postnatal hospital stay: Implications for cost and quality of care. *BMC Health Serv. Res.* **2016**, *16*, 16. [CrossRef] [PubMed]
69. UNICEF/BFI Supplementation Guidance: Maternity Standard 4. March 2016. Available online: https://www.unicef.org.uk/babyfriendly/wp-content/uploads/sites/2/2016/10/Supplementation-guidance.pdf (accessed on 17 April 2018).
70. Forster, D.A.; McLachlan, H.L.; Yelland, J.; Rayner, J.; Lumley, J.; Davey, M.A. Staffing in postnatal units: Is it adequate for the provision of quality care? Staff perspectives from a state-widereview of postnatal care in Victoria, Australia. *BMC Health Serv. Res.* **2006**, *6*, 83. [CrossRef] [PubMed]
71. Odom, E.C.; Li, R.; Scanlon, K.S.; Perrine, C.G.; Grummer-Strawn, L. Association of family and health care provider opinion on infant feeding with mother's breastfeeding decision. *J. Acad. Nutr. Diet.* **2014**, *114*, 1203–1207. [CrossRef] [PubMed]
72. Swanson, V.; Power, K.G. Initiation and continuation of breastfeeding: Theory of planned behaviour. *J. Adv. Nurs.* **2005**, *50*, 272–282. [CrossRef] [PubMed]
73. Radzyminski, S.; Callister, L.C. Mother's beliefs, attitudes, and decision making related to infant feeding choices. *J. Perinat. Educ.* **2016**, *25*, 18–28. [CrossRef] [PubMed]
74. Taylor, A.M.; Hutchings, M. Using video narratives of women's lived experience of breastfeeding in midwifery education: Exploring its impact on midwives' attitudes to breastfeeding. *Matern. Child Nutr.* **2012**, *8*, 88–102. [CrossRef] [PubMed]
75. DiGirolamo, A.M.; Grummer-Strawn, L.M.; Fein, S.B. Do perceived attitudes of physicians and hospital staff affect breastfeeding decisions? *Birth* **2003**, *30*, 94–100. [CrossRef] [PubMed]
76. Creedy, D.K.; Cantrill, R.M.; Cooke, M. Assessing midwives' breastfeeding knowledge: Properties of the Newborn Feeding Ability questionnaire and Breastfeeding Initiation Practices scale. *Int. Breastfeed. J.* **2008**, *3*, 7. [CrossRef] [PubMed]

77. Cantrill, R.M.; Creedy, D.K.; Cooke, M. An Australian study of midwives' breast-feeding knowledge. *Midwifery* **2003**, *19*, 310–317. [CrossRef]
78. Pierro, J.; Abulaimoun, B.; Roth, P.; Blau, J. Factors associated with supplemental formula feeding of breastfeeding infants during postpartum hospital stay. *Breastfeed. Med.* **2016**, *11*, 196–202. [CrossRef] [PubMed]
79. Atchan, M.; Davis, D.; Foureur, M. Applying a knowledge translation model to the uptake of the Baby Friendly Health Initiative in the Australian health care system. *Women Birth.* **2014**, *27*, 79–85. [CrossRef] [PubMed]
80. Glasziou, P.; Haynes, B. The paths from research to improved health outcomes. *Evid. Based Nurs.* **2005**, *8*, 36–38. [CrossRef] [PubMed]
81. Furber, C.M.; Thomson, A.M. The emotions of integrating breastfeeding knowledge into practice for English midwives: A qualitative study. *Int. J. Nurs. Stud.* **2008**, *45*, 286–297. [CrossRef] [PubMed]
82. Crano, W.D.; Prislin, R. (Eds.) *Attitudes and Attitude Change*; Psychology Press, Taylor and Francis Group: New York, NY, USA, 2008; p. 11. Available online: https://books.google.co.uk/books?hl=en&lr=&id=HpF5AgAAQBAJ&oi=fnd&pg=PP1&dq=change+attitudes+&ots=dyeEeCvkgp&sig=6rxaq_rrILyrOBbwYRkpRw4izOs#v=onepage&q=behavior&f=false (accessed on 14 May 2016).
83. Schwarz, J.; Gaito, P.; Lennick, D. That's the way we (used to) do things around here. *Strateg. Bus.* **2011**, *62*, 45–53.
84. Fazio, R.H.; Zanna, M.P.; Cooper, J. Direct experience and attitude-behavior consistency: An information processing analysis. *Pers. Soc. Psychol. Bull.* **1978**, *4*, 48–51. [CrossRef]
85. Russell, K.; Walsh, D. Can the use of behavioural intervention studies support change in professional practice behaviours? *Evid. Based Midwifery* **2009**, *7*, 54–59.
86. Salvador, A.; Dumas, L.; Davies, B.; Emard, M.J.; Lortie, K. A dozen strategies along the ten steps Baby-Friendly Initiative journey. *Healthc. Q.* **2016**, *18*, 80–86. [CrossRef] [PubMed]
87. Rogers, M. Baby Friendly: A way to accreditation. Part 2. *Br. J. Midwifery* **2003**, *11*, 657–662. [CrossRef]
88. Reddin, E.; Pincombe, J.; Darbyshire, P. Passive resistance: Early experiences of midwifery students/graduates and the Baby Friendly Health Initiative 10 steps to successful breastfeeding. *Women Birth* **2007**, *20*, 71–76. [CrossRef] [PubMed]
89. Levin, K.A. Study design III: Cross-sectional studies. *Evid. Based Dent.* **2006**, *7*, 24–25. [CrossRef] [PubMed]
90. Gomez-Pomar, E.; Blubaugh, R. The Baby Friendly Hospital Initiative and the ten steps for successful breastfeeding. A critical review of the literature. *J. Perinatol.* **2018**, *7*. [CrossRef] [PubMed]
91. Howe-Heyman, A.; Lutenbacher, M. The Baby-Friendly Hospital Initiative as an Intervention to Improve Breastfeeding Rates: A Review of the Literature. *J. Midwifery Womens Health* **2016**, *61*, 77–102. [CrossRef] [PubMed]

12

Breast Milk Content of Vitamin A and E from Early- to Mid-Lactation is Affected by Inadequate Dietary Intake in Brazilian Adult Women

Michele R. Machado [1,2], Fernanda Kamp [1,3,*], Juliana C. Nunes [1,4], Tatiana El-Bacha [1,5,6] and Alexandre G. Torres [1,*]

1 Laboratory of Food Science and Nutritional Biochemistry, Institute of Chemistry, Federal University of Rio de Janeiro, Rio de Janeiro 21941-909, Brazil
2 School of Nutrition, Faculdade Arthur Sa Earp Neto (FMP/FASE), Petropolis, Rio de Janeiro 25680-120, Brazil
3 Biochemistry Core, Federal Institute of Education, Science and Technology of Rio de Janeiro, Rio de Janeiro 20270-021, Brazil
4 School of Nutrition, Federal University of the State of Rio de Janeiro, Rio de Janeiro 22290-250, Brazil
5 Institute of Nutrition, Federal University of Rio de Janeiro, Rio de Janeiro 21941-902, Brazil
6 Department of Physiology, Development and Neuroscience, University of Cambridge, Cambridge CB2 3EL, UK
* Correspondence: fernanda.kamp@ifrj.edu.br (F.K.); torres@iq.ufrj.br (A.G.T.)

Abstract: Our aims were to investigate vitamin A and E status during lactation and the determinants of breast milk content for the appropriate nutrition of the infant in a study with nursing Brazilian women. We hypothesized that both inadequate intake and the lipoprotein distribution of vitamin A and E during lactation could have an impact on their breast milk levels from early- to mid-lactation. Nineteen adult lactating women participated in this longitudinal observational study, in which dietary records, blood and mature breast milk samples were collected for the analysis of vitamin A and E, and carotenoids in early- (2nd to 4th week) and mid-lactation (12th to 14th week). Nutrient intake was balanced by the Multiple Source Method (MSM), and the intake of vitamin A and E was inadequate in 74 and 100% of the women, respectively. However, these results were not reflected in low serum concentrations of retinol and only 37% of the volunteers were vitamin E deficient according to the blood biomarker. As lactation progressed, vitamin A and E status worsened, and this was clearly observed by the decrease in their content in breast milk. The reduced content of vitamin A and E in the breast milk was not related to their distribution in lipoproteins. Taken together, the contents of vitamin A and E in breast milk seemed to be more sensitive markers of maternal nutrition status than respective blood concentrations, and dietary assessment by the MSM in early lactation was sensitive to indicate later risks of deficiency and should support maternal dietary guidance to improve the infant's nutrition.

Keywords: retinol; α-tocopherol; inadequate intake; nutritional status; breast milk; undernourishment; dietary assessment; multiple source method

1. Introduction

Vitamin A and E are essential to newborns, and their transfer to breast milk is key for the nutrition of infants. Vitamin A is crucial for newborn development, epithelial function and protection against infections. Vitamin A deficiency affects millions of preschool-age children, especially in developing countries, and it increases the susceptibility to infection and infant mortality rate, especially before the age of 2 [1]. Vitamin A nutritional requirements are met by the intake of retinoids, such as retinyl esters, and provitamin A carotenoids, especially β-carotene and less prominently by α-carotene and β-cryptoxanthin. In addition to serving as retinoid precursors, these carotenoids are transferred to breast milk and, together with lycopene and lutein, might contribute to breastfed infant health, as they present potential bioactivity. The primary function of vitamin E is related to its activity as a potent free radical scavenger and, although overt signs of deficiency are rare, pre-term infants might be more susceptible to associated illnesses [2].

Essential nutrients, such as vitamins, are provided to the breastfed infant via transfer from the maternal circulation into the milk by the mammary gland. The contents of retinol and α-tocopherol in the breast milk are mainly determined by maternal diet and nutritional status [3,4]. However, to what extent changes in the maternal nutritional status throughout lactation might affect the transfer of vitamin A and E to the breast milk is not entirely known. Interactions between vitamin A and E seem to influence their contents in breast milk as it has been shown that postpartum retinyl-ester supplementation decreased vitamin E content in the colostrum [5]. On the other hand, the mechanisms underlying this biochemical interaction are not known and are possibly related to serum transport in lipoproteins and uptake by the mammary gland [3]. Vitamin A and E distribution in major lipoprotein fractions might fluctuate throughout lactation, which would impact their transfer to breast milk.

Our aim was to investigate vitamin A and E status, and carotenoids during lactation, and the determinants of breast milk levels for the appropriate nutrition of breastfed infants. We hypothesized that both inadequate intake and the lipoprotein distribution of vitamin A and E during lactation could have an impact on their breast milk levels from early- to mid-lactation. By taking advantage of a longitudinal study with adult nursing women in Rio de Janeiro, Brazil, we used multiple regression models to explain the impact of maternal diet and serum concentration of vitamin A and E on their breast milk content during early- and mid-lactation.

2. Materials and Methods

2.1. Experimental Design and Recruitment of Volunteers

This is a longitudinal observational study, approved by the Research Ethics Committee of the Pedro Ernesto University Hospital, Rio de Janeiro State University (CEP/HUPE-UERJ:3043/2011–CAAE:0186.0.228.228-11). Data and sample collection were conducted after signing written informed consent. The volunteers were recruited at Policlínica Américo Piquet Carneiro (UERJ) and at health facilities in the city of Rio de Janeiro. Recruitment occurred in the last month of gestation, when the first visit of the study was scheduled according to the probable delivery date. Of the 22 recruited women, three refused to participate during mid-lactation and their data were excluded. Thus, 19 pregnant women (age 20–40 years) participated in the study, exclusively or predominantly breastfeeding. They did not have any chronic or acute diseases, were not using prescribed medicines or dietary supplements, and were non-smokers and non-alcoholic who had completed single and full-term gestations. In the present study, mature breast milk was collected, because in full lactation, when mature milk is produced, tight junctions between mammary epithelial cells are fully functional, and, therefore, paracellular transport (between cells) is virtually absent. Therefore, one can expect that there are no major changes in the mammary epithelial cells transport systems during the time span assessed in this study.

2.2. Data Collection and Qualification of Lactation Practices

Demographics and medical history were obtained in early lactation (2nd to 4th week postpartum; mean 24.7 days). In mid-lactation (12th to 14th week postpartum; mean 94 days), volunteers answered a questionnaire concerning lactation practices. All women reported adopting practices consistent with exclusive or predominant breastfeeding. Total body mass (kg) and height (meters) were obtained in an anthropometric scale (Filizola, Brazil) to calculate body mass index (BMI, in kg/m^2) [6].

2.3. *Assessment of Dietary Intake*

Dietary intake throughout lactation was estimated using the Multiple Source Method (MSM). The MSM is a statistical method to estimate usual food intake and uses at least two different dietary inputs (e.g., dietary recalls and/or food frequency questionnaires) [7] and it has been shown to be adequate to estimate usual intake during pregnancy [8]. Using this method, 24-h dietary recalls (24hRs) were applied in early- and mid-lactation (one in each period) to evaluate possible changes in eating habits and to estimate recent intake of energy and nutrients. The nutrient composition of the 24hRs was analyzed with the NutriSurvey® software v. 2007 (Dr. Juergen Erhardt; Germany; available at www.nutrisurvey.de/nutrisurvey2007.exe) using the food composition database from the US Department of Agriculture release 22 [9] adapted for common fat sources in the Brazilian diet [10]. A semi-quantitative food frequency questionnaire (SQ-FFQ) was applied in the first lactation period to assess food sources of the nutrients of interest in the present investigation and to confirm the feasibility of the 24hR to evaluate usual dietary intake.

The prevalence of inadequate nutrient intake was estimated using Estimated Average Requirements (EARs), as set by the Institute of Medicine [11–14] as cut-off points. The prevalence of the inadequate intake of each nutrient was estimated by the proportion of individuals with intake below the EAR value. Since the EAR cut-off point method is not suitable for assessing energy adequacy, the proportion of the group with BMIs below, within, and above the desirable range was used to classify inadequate, adequate, and excessive energy intakes [11].

2.4. *Collection and Processing of Biological Samples*

Blood and milk samples were collected in the morning after fasting overnight, were immediately processed for the separation of plasma, serum and erythrocytes, and frozen at −80 °C until analysis. Whole blood aliquots were used for the immediate determination of hematocrit and hemoglobin concentrations. Milk samples (10 mL) were manually expressed in the morning from the breast which the baby last suckled and transferred into sterile plastic bottles. An aliquot was taken for analysis of the crematocrit. For the analysis of lactose and protein, aliquots were stored at −20 °C and for retinol, carotenoids and tocopherols analyses, at −80 °C and tubes were protected with aluminum foil.

2.5. *Determination of Hematocrit and Hemoglobin, and Triglycerides and Cholesterol in Blood*

Hematocrit was determined in a microhematocrit centrifuge (Hemospin, Incibrás; São Paulo, Brazil) and hemoglobin concentration was determined by the cyanmethemoglobin method by a commercial kit (BioClin; Belo Horizonte, Brazil). Triglyceride, total cholesterol and HDL-c (total serum and HDL-c fraction after LDL-c+VLDL-c precipitation) were determined by the enzymatic colorimetric method using commercial kits (BioClin, Brazil), using sodium phosphotungstate and Mg^{2+} for precipitation of LDL and VLDL particles, as described [15]. The clear supernatant, containing the HDL fraction, was used for the analysis of HDL-c (and vitamins by HPLC, described in Section 2.7), and the concentration of LDL-c+VLDL-c was determined by the difference between the concentration of HDL-c and total cholesterol. All analyses were performed in duplicate and the automatic reading was performed in triplicate.

2.6. *Breast Milk Macronutrient Composition*

Total fat was determined by the crematocrit method, in a microhematocrit centrifuge (Hemospin, Incibrás) [16]. Lactose was determined by a colorimetric assay [17] adapted by [18], based on the reaction with picric acid. Total protein content was determined by the Lowry method [19], after eliminating interference of fat and lactose, by precipitating the proteins with 20% trichloroacetic acid and 2.5% sodium deoxycholate, and centrifugation. The supernatant with interfering substances was discarded and precipitated milk proteins were suspended in Folin–Ciocalteu's reagent and analyzed [20]. The standard curve was prepared with casein in concentrations ranging from 20.0 to 100.0 μg/mL. All these analyses, as well as standard curves, were performed in triplicates.

2.7. Determination of Retinol, Carotenoids and Tocopherols by HPLC in Breast Milk, Whole Blood Serum, and Lipoprotein Fractions

Serum samples were prepared and extracted as described by [21], adapted from [22]. Retinol, tocopherols, and carotenoids were analyzed by HPLC in serum and in the HDL fraction, in duplicate. The concentration of these vitamins in the LDL+VLDL fraction was calculated by the difference between contents in whole serum and in the HDL fraction. Milk samples were prepared as described [21], adapted from [23], and care was taken to avoid direct light to avoid vitamin losses during sample extraction and analysis.

HPLC analysis was performed in a Shimadzu chromatographic system (Shimadzu, Kyoto, Japan), composed of a LC-20AT pump, a Shimadzu SPD-M20AV UV-Vis detector, and a CBM-20A system controller. A total of 20 μL of sample extracts and standards solutions were injected through a Rheodyne injection valve with a volumetric loop, onto a C18 reversed-phase column (Kromasil; 150 × 4.6 mm), and compounds were eluted isocratically with a ternary solvent composed of acetonitrile, tetrahydrofuran, and 15 mM methanolic ammonium acetate (65:25:10, v/v/v), at 0.9 mL/min. Each sample extract was injected twice, one run monitored at λ (nm) 450, for the analysis of carotenoids, and the other run monitored at 325 and 292 for the analysis of retinol and tocopherols, respectively. All analyses were performed in duplicate.

Identities of chromatographic peaks corresponding to the fat-soluble vitamins in samples chromatograms were determined based on standards retention times, and by exact co-elution with standards spiking in representative samples. Vitamin concentrations in samples were determined by external calibration, with linear calibration curves and direct extrapolation. Commercial standards of retinol, α-tocopherol and γ-tocopherol were from Sigma-Aldrich (São Paulo, Brazil), and carotenoid standards (purity > 95%) were isolated from foods naturally rich in these pigments, as previously described [24], by the open column method [25]. Representative chromatograms from HPLC standards are shown in Supplementary Figure S1.

2.8. Statistical Analyses

Paired *t*-tests were used to investigate differences between early- and mid-lactation on the variables studied. Variable frequency distribution was assessed by standardized coefficients of skewness and kurtosis, and those with values < -2.0 or $> +2.0$ were characterized as having a non-normal distribution, which were presented as median and minimum and maximum levels, in contrast to normally distributed variables that were presented as the mean ± standard deviation (SD). Non-normally distributed variables were log-transformed before running Pearson's correlation analysis, which was used to investigate associations between continuous variables. Stepwise multiple regression analyses (backward) were used to investigate the effect of independent factors on the composition of vitamins in serum and in breast milk. The criteria for the inclusion of independent variables in the multiple regression models were based on results from Pearson correlations and on data from the literature. In the final model, only significant variables that improved the model were kept (p-to-remove ≥ 0.05; p-to-persist < 0.05). The multiple regression models were further assessed by analysis of residual plots that were checked to determine if they were randomly distributed. Data analyses were performed with the Multiple Source Method (MSM) software for dietary data analysis, GraphPad Prism 7.0 (GraphPad Software, San Diego, CA, USA) and Statgraphics Centurion 18 (Statgraphics Technologies, Inc.; The Plains, VA, USA) for statistics. Values of $p < 0.05$ were considered significant.

3. Results

3.1. General Characteristics of Lactating Women

The nursing women who participated in the present study were adults (31.9 ± 5.9 years of age), primiparous and had term pregnancies (gestational age of 39.8 ± 1.1 weeks), from which 58% had vaginal delivery (Table 1). According to the BMI, 58% of women were overweight (25–30 kg/m^2 [6]) in early lactation (2nd to 4th lactation week). In mid-lactation (12th to 14th lactation week), 42% of the lactating mothers were overweight. Most of the volunteers (63%) were anemic at the beginning of the study and after 10 weeks, there was a significant 11% increase in the mean blood hemoglobin concentration and a decrease in anemia frequency to 26% in mid-lactation (Table 1).

Table 1. General characteristics of adult Brazilian lactating women in early- (2nd to 4th week) and mid-lactation (12th to 14th week) (n = 19).

Characteristics	Lactation Period		p	Recommended Value or Range [1]
	Early Lactation 2nd–4th Week	Mid-Lactation 12th–14th Week		
Body mass index (kg/m^2)	25.9 ± 4.0	25.3 ± 4.2	0.068 *	18–24.9 [6]
Hemoglobin (g/dL)	11.6 ± 1.7	12.5± 1.6	0.029 *	≥12.0 [26]
Hematocrit (%)	39.2 ± 3.5	37.8 ± 3.5	0.131	≥36 [26]
Triglycerides (mg/dL)	74.7 ± 21.4	57.0 ± 21.2	0.007 *	<150 [27]
Total cholesterol (mg/dL)	190.2 ± 41.9	182.2 ± 41.0	0.219	<200 [27]
LDL-c (mg/dL)	156.0 ± 44.1	146.6 ± 35.9	0.164	100–129 [27]
HDL-c (mg/dL)	34.2 ± 6.2	35.6 ± 9.4	0.601	>60 [27]

Data presented as the mean ± standard deviation; * Significant differences between lactation periods, paired t-test.
[1] Shown in the same respective units as the first column.

Serum triglyceride concentration was adequate in all volunteers and reduced significantly by 24% from early- to mid-lactation. Serum HDL concentrations, on the other hand, were below the minimum value in all volunteers and 74% of the nursing women presented LDL concentrations above the desirable range, irrespective of the lactation period [27]. Regarding total cholesterol in the serum, 47 and 31% of the volunteers presented concentrations above the desirable value, in early- and mid-lactation, respectively.

3.2. Dietary Intake of Vitamin A and E Were Inadequate throughout Lactation

Dietary data assessment indicated that nutrient intake did not vary significantly between the two lactation periods, considering both recent and usual dietary consumption. Therefore, these data were presented combined, as estimated by the MSM, which assesses habitual intake considering data from two or more 24hRs and one FFQ (Table 2). The frequency of volunteers with sub-adequate nutrient intake was estimated as proposed [12,13] using EAR whenever available (Table 2). The very high prevalence of inadequate intake of vitamin A and E (Table 2) may set these lactating mothers and their offspring's health at increased risk. Although the median intake of β-carotene (Table 2) was within the range considered prudent, 47% of the volunteers presented β-carotene intake below this range. In contrast, the average intake of lycopene was lower than the level established as prudent [12], and intake was sub-adequate in 89% of the volunteers.

Table 2. Intake of energy and nutrients by Brazilian nursing women from the 2nd to the 14th week of lactation.

Energy and Nutrients	Intake (24hR-MSM)	Inadequacy (%) [3]	Nutrient Intake Adequacy	
			Reference Value (Daily Intake) [4]	Method [Ref.]
Energy (kcal)	1577 ± 164 [1]	53	—	BMI distribution [14]
Carbohydrate (en%)	51.2 ± 7.7 [1]	21	160 g [5]	EAR cut-off [14]
Protein (en%)	17.7 ± 3.1 [1]	47	1.05 g/kg [5]	EAR cut-off [14]
Total lipids (en%)	31.1 ± 0.52 [1]	26	20 to 35	AMDR [14]
Vitamin A (μg RE)	824.7 ± 21.8 [1]	74	900	EAR cut-off [13]
β-Carotene (μg)	3249 (1408–6707) [2]	—	3000–6000 [12]	—
α-Carotene (μg)	1053 (56–3712) [2]	—	—	—
Lycopene (μg)	1854 (302–6472) [2]	—	≥5000 [12]	—
Lutein + zeaxanthin (μg)	2446 (872–4873) [2]	—	—	—
Vitamin E (mg)	4.4 ± 0.9 [1]	100	16	EAR cut-off [12]

[1] Data expressed as the mean ± standard deviation; [2] Median (minimum–maximum); [3] Estimated frequency of volunteers with inadequate intake; [4] based on estimated average requirement values whenever available, and are in the same units as the first column, except stated otherwise; in the case of carotenoids (β-carotene and lycopene), the reference value was taken as the daily intake level considered prudent for maintaining health; [5] EAR is used to assess adequacy of carbohydrate and protein intake, but usual intake expressed as en% are, respectively 45–65 and 5–10 [14]. AMDR: acceptable macronutrient distribution ranges; en%: macronutrient intake as a percentage of energy intake; 24hR-MSM: two 24-h recalls were used, and data were assessed by the Multiple Source Method; BMI: body mass index; EAR: Estimated Average Requirement.

3.3. *Serum Vitamin A and E Were Not Associated with Their Changes in Breast Milk Concentration throughout Lactation*

Serum vitamin A was adequate in all volunteers in early- and mid-lactation (Table 3). In contrast, 68 and 84% of the volunteers were at risk of developing vitamin E deficiency in early- and mid-lactation, respectively. Although serum retinol concentration did not vary throughout lactation, retinol in breast milk showed a significant 13% decrease from early- to mid-lactation (Table 3). In early lactation, retinol concentration in the milk of all volunteers was above the limit considered adequate [1,3] for the formation of infant liver reserves. After 10 weeks of lactation, however, milk retinol concentration became inadequate in 21% of the nursing women [1]. A similar trend was observed with breast milk contents of β-carotene, lutein+zeaxanthin and α-tocopherol, which significantly decreased from early- to mid-lactation, irrespective of the serum concentrations (Table 3).

Table 3. Concentrations of fat-soluble vitamins (μmol/L) in the serum and breast milk of adult Brazilian nursing women (n = 19), in early- (2nd to 4th week) and mid- (12th to 14th week) lactation, and respective cut-off values for inadequacy [1].

Vitamin	Serum				Breast Milk			
	Lactation Period			Undernutrition Cut-Off Value	Lactation Period			Inadequacy Cut-Off Value
	2nd–4th Week	12th–14th Week	p		2nd–4th Week	12th–14th Week	p	
Retinol	1.50 ± 0.30	1.48 ± 0.31	0.913	0.7 [28]	2.3 ± 0.78	2.0 ± 0.72	0.013 *	1.05 [1,28]
β-Carotene	0.61 ± 0.07	0.59 ± 0.05	0.628	—	0.17 ± 0.02	0.14 ± 0.3	0.001 *	—
α-Carotene	0.43 ± 0.09	0.44 ± 0.08	0.720	—	0.04 ± 0.01	0.03 ± 0.01	0.304	—
Lycopene	0.20 ± 0.03	0.18 ± 0.04	0.530	—	0.04 ± 0.01	0.04 ± 0.00	1.000	—
Lutein + zeaxanthin	0.24 ± 0.04	0.23 ± 0.07	0.633	—	0.07 ± 0.02	0.06 ± 0.01	0.026 *	—
α-Tocopherol	11.1 ± 1.11	10.1 ± 1.23	0.089	11.6 [12]	1.29 ± 0.25	1.07 ± 0.13	0.001 *	7.4 [28]
γ-Tocopherol	0.76 ± 0.15	0.75 ± 0.13	0.896	—	0.38 ± 0.04	0.35 ± 0.04	0.436	—

[1] Data expressed as the mean ± standard deviation. * Significant differences between lactation periods, paired t-test.

3.4. *Breast Milk Concentration of Fat-Soluble Vitamins from Early- to Mid-Lactation Is Associated with Dietary Vitamin A, Serum β-Carotene and Tocopherols*

Multiple regression analysis was used to investigate the determinants of vitamin A and E and carotenoid concentration in breast milk (Table 4). Retinol concentration in breast milk was determined by the dietary intake of vitamin A, and this association was stable from early- to mid-lactation (Table 4; models 1 and 4). In contrast, the determinants of milk β-carotene changed from early- to mid-lactation (Table 4; models 2 and 5). Regarding vitamin E, serum concentration was the sole determinant of its contents in breast milk (Table 4; models 3 and 6).

Table 4. Multiple regression models of the concentrations of vitamin A and E (μmol/L) in the milk of Brazilian nursing women (n = 19), to assess its associations with the intake [1] and serum contents of these vitamins.

Model N	Dependent Variable *Breast Milk* [2]	Independent Variables *Serum* [A] and *Diet* [B]	Coefficients		Weight in the Model [3]	Adj. R^2	Error (%) [4]	p [5]
			Value	p				
			Early-Lactation: 2nd–4th Week					
1	Retinol	Vitamin A [B]	5.33×10^{-3}	<0.0001	100%	94.9	9%	<0.0001
2	β-Carotene	β-Carotene [A]	2.25×10^{-1}	0.0045	63%	87.7	14%	<0.0001
		β-Carotene [B]	2.52×10^{-5}	0.0430	37%			
3	α-Tocopherol	α-Tocopherol [A]	1.24	<0.0001	100%	96.2	18%	<0.0001
			Mid-Lactation: 12th–14th Week					
4	Retinol	Vitamin A [B]	4.79×10^{-3}	<0.0001	100%	94.7	14%	<0.0001
5	β-Carotene	β-Carotene [A]	2.34×10^{-1}	<0.0001	100%	78.4	17%	<0.0001
6	α-Tocopherol	α-Tocopherol [A]	1.03	<0.0001	100%	97.9	12%	<0.0001

[1] Data from the average of two 24-h recalls corrected by the Multiple Source Method (Vitamin A, μg RE/day; β-Carotene, μg/day); [2] Concentrations of fat-soluble vitamins in milk; [3] Weight in the model = independent variable coefficient × variable average content in samples; [4] Relative error of estimate = (estimated absolute error × 100%)/average value of the dependent variable; [5] Model significance. Superscript letters indicate whether the vitamins included as independent variables in the model were serum concentration ([A]) or dietary intake ([B]). Variables included in the starting analysis matrices before running the backward stepwise regression analysis (p-to-remove ≥ 0.05): model 1, vitamin A intake (RE), serum retinol and fat intake; model 2, β-carotene intake and serum β-carotene; model 3, vitamin E intake and serum α-tocopherol; model 4, vitamin A intake (RE), serum retinol and fat intake; model 5, β-carotene intake and serum β-carotene; model 6, vitamin E intake and serum α-tocopherol. Adj. R^2: adjusted coefficient of determination for the fitted model.

3.5. *Vitamin A and E and Carotenoids Distributed Differently in Lipoprotein Fractions during Lactation*

There were no significant changes from early- to mid-lactation in the relative distribution of vitamin A and E and carotenoids in serum lipoprotein fractions (Figure 1). Retinol and γ-tocopherol were distributed equally between HDL+serum binding proteins and LDL+VLDL fractions, in both lactation periods. β-Carotene and α-carotene, lycopene and α-tocopherol were enriched in the LDL+VLDL fraction. In contrast, approximately 70% of lutein+zeaxanthin was concentrated in the HDL+binding proteins fraction, in both lactation periods.

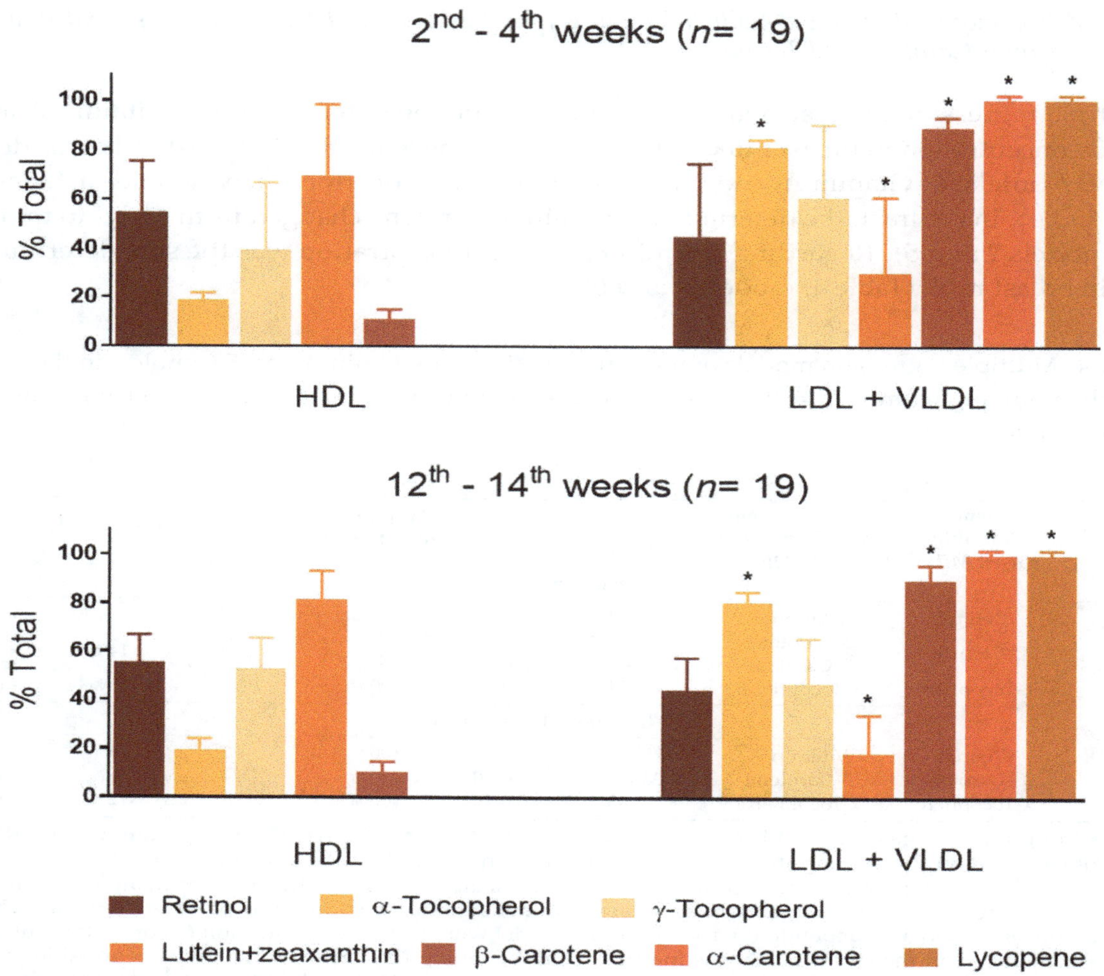

Figure 1. Distribution of fat-soluble vitamins in blood serum lipoprotein fractions in early- and mid-lactation. * Significantly different from the contents (%) in the HDL fraction (paired *t*-test; $p < 0.05$). Error bars represent standard deviations.

4. Discussion

Adequate breast milk contents of vitamins and minerals are crucial for infant development. In the present work, the maternal nutritional status of vitamin A and E was evaluated, and the factors associated with their content in breast milk in adult Brazilian nursing mothers. The most striking result was the fact that despite constant serum levels, the content of vitamin A and E in breast milk decreased throughout lactation, which we hypothesize as a consequence of the sustained inadequate dietary intake from early- to mid-lactation. This sub-adequate intake was insufficient to affect biochemical markers of vitamin status in serum, but negatively affected breast milk, being potentially detrimental to the lactating infant. Therefore, vitamin A and E in breast milk seem to be more sensitive markers of maternal nutrition status than their respective blood concentrations. Since the distribution of vitamin A and E in fasting serum lipoproteins did not change from early- to mid-lactation, this factor is unlikely to be related to the decrease in the transfer of fat-soluble vitamins into milk during lactation.

4.1. *Dietary Intake, Nutritional Status and Milk Transfer of Vitamin A and E, and Carotenoids*

Vitamin A intake was sub-adequate in 74% of the subjects [13] and was insufficient to maintain adequate breast milk levels throughout lactation. Maternal vitamin A requirement increases during lactation to fulfill the increased demand imposed by the mammary gland, and vitamin A in breast milk is essential to build up the infant's liver stores, contributing to the prevention of vitamin A deficiency when lactation ends [4,29]. A high intake of β-carotene could compensate the low intake of retinol, but the former nutrient was in the range considered prudent (3000–6000 μg/day [12]) in only 53% of the volunteers, thus it is likely that the breastfed infants were at risk of vitamin A deficiency [4,30]. Despite that, all subjects showed serum retinol levels above the cutoff value for inadequacy risk (>0.7 μmol/L [1]) throughout lactation [3].

Retinol in breast milk is also seen as a reliable marker of vitamin A nutritional status on a population basis. According to the World Health Organization, when retinol concentration in milk is below 1.1 μmol/L, the infant's body stores may be below the estimated critical amounts to supply for the increased requirements in the second half of childhood [1]. In all subjects in the present study, the breast milk concentration of retinol in early lactation was above this cutoff value. However, in mid-lactation, 21% of the nursing women were below the adequacy cutoff. Possibly, these results indicate that these nursing women presented subclinical vitamin A deficiency, which worsened throughout lactation, and that their lactating newborns were at risk of vitamin A deficiency to build up liver stores [4,29]. However, concentrations of fat-soluble vitamins are usually higher at the beginning of lactation, suffering a progressive fall as lactation progresses [3], but levels should be above the safe cut-off value throughout lactation.

The retinol concentration in breast milk in the two lactation periods evaluated was near the average values previously reported for Brazilian nursing women [5,21,30] and for Korean nursing women (2.0 to 3.0 μmol/L) [31]. As these previous works did not assess dietary intake, further discussion regarding the factors involved in the regulation of the concentration of vitamins in breast milk was not possible. Retinol content in breast milk is associated with maternal dietary fat intake, stressing the importance of dietary lipids to retinol transport and absorption [31]. It is suggested that during lactation, a large proportion of retinol from the maternal diet is transported directly into the mammary gland via blood lipoproteins, bypassing the liver [3]. Breast milk vitamin A might be more strongly affected by dietary fat intake than by serum retinol concentration, especially in groups with a low dietary intake of vitamin A and inadequate nutritional status of this vitamin [31]. Consistently, in the present study, fat intake was correlated with breast milk retinol, both in early ($r = 0.47$; $p = 0.042$) and in mid-lactation ($r = 0.46$; $p = 0.046$) and vitamin A intake was a determinant of breast milk retinol concentration in both lactation periods investigated (Table 4).

The intake of vitamin E was also sub-adequate in all volunteers [12]. Vitamin E intake might have been underestimated in the present study, because its principal dietary source was vegetable oil, and it is inherently difficult to assess cooking oil intake [32]. In Brazil, soybean oil is by far the most consumed oil and the main source of vitamin E in the subjects' diets. In contrast, it should also be considered that the possibility that vitamin E EAR (16 mg/day [12]) is overestimated, which could contribute to the high frequency of inadequacy in the present study [32]. In this sense, the recommended daily intake of vitamin E for Brazilian nursing women [32] is nearly half that recommended in North America by the Institute of Medicine [4,12]. The vitamin E status biomarker (serum α-tocopherol/cholesterol ratio; μmol/mmol) indicates that the prevalence of vitamin E deficiency (<2.25 μmol/mmol) [2,4] increased from 37 to 63% of the volunteers from early- to mid-lactation.

β-Carotene was the major carotenoid present in the serum and breast milk throughout lactation, consistent with maternal usual diets, representing over 50% of total carotenoids in milk [21,33]. Serum and breast milk β-carotene were strongly associated, as expected [34,35] and, in early-lactation, breast milk β-carotene was also associated with maternal intake, highlighting the importance of both dietary intake and blood concentration to β-carotene in breast milk [34,35]. It is noteworthy that the concentration of β-carotene and lutein+zeaxanthin in breast milk was, respectively, approximately 8- and 6-fold higher than observed in a previous study with Brazilian nursing women [21]. Compared to the values of a recent study that addressed the effect of prematurity on the content of carotenoids in the colostrum, the results of the present study were sensibly lower, particularly for lutein+zeaxanthin and lycopene concentrations, which were approximately 10-fold lower [36]. These differences might be related to the stage of lactation and also to potential differences in the habitual diets of the volunteers of both studies. The concentration of α-tocopherol in breast milk was determined by its concentration in the serum. It is important to highlight that the intake of α-tocopherol was entered as an independent variable in the multiple regression analysis matrix. However, the model did not adjust, and significance was reached only after dietary data were excluded from the analysis matrix.

4.2. Vitamin A and E, and Carotenoids Distribution among Serum Lipoprotein Fractions Was Stable from Early- to Mid-Lactation

Highly nonpolar carotenes partition more easily into lipoprotein particles that are richer in neutral lipids (VLDL+LDL), and the more polar xanthophylls partition into HDL particles [37]. Indeed, our results showed that approximately 68% of serum lutein+zeaxanthin was in the HDL fraction in both early- and mid-lactation and serum carotenes were predominant in the serum fraction of LDL+VLDL. An important quality control of the protocol used for the differential precipitation of serum lipoproteins was the analysis of HDL-c in whole serum and in the HDL fraction, after precipitation of LDL+VLDL. There was no significant difference between HDL-c concentration in whole serum and in this lipoprotein fraction, indicating that there was no co-precipitation of HDL with LDL+VLDL. Retinol was evenly distributed between HDL and non-HDL serum fractions and was unchanged from early- to mid-lactation, consistently with previous reports [3]. However, the protocol used herein to precipitate LDL+VLDL does not allow the discrimination between free retinol, transported bound to retinol binding protein (RBP), and the HDL fraction. It is worth investigating in the future whether RBP-mediated retinol transport varies during lactation. γ-Tocopherol was evenly distributed in the serum fractions of HDL and LDL+VLDL. In contrast, α-tocopherol was more concentrated in the LDL+VLDL fraction, possibly because vitamin E is transferred to HDL, and then promptly transfers into all other circulating lipoproteins [5], which possibly favors its uptake by the mammary glands and transfer into breast milk.

In summary, the distribution of fat-soluble vitamins among plasma lipoprotein fractions, HDL and LDL+VLDL, in lactating women was similar to that of non-pregnant non-lactating women [37], despite the high adipose tissue turnover that is common to exclusive lactation. In addition, this distribution pattern was stable from early- to mid-lactation in the present study. From data in Figure 1, we estimated the sample size required to assess potential differences between early- and mid-lactation in the distribution of vitamin A and E, and carotenoids among HDL and LDL+VLDL fractions (Supplementary Table S1). Accordingly, it may be speculated that for the carotenes (α- and β-carotene and lycopene) and for retinol, it is unlikely that variations in their distribution between the lipoprotein fractions would be reasonably detectable—or that if detectable, they would have a biological role. Therefore, in the case of retinol and β-carotene, it is very unlikely that the decrease in the concentrations in breast milk, until mid-lactation, is related to their distribution between HDL and LDL+VLDL serum fractions. However, changes in the distribution of the xantophylls (Lut + Zea) and tocopherols (α and γ) in serum fractions might be detected between early- and mid-lactation with sample sizes of approximately 100 and 500 depending on the nutrient (Supplementary Table S1) and, in the case of α-tocopherol and the xantophylls, this metabolic distribution among serum lipoproteins might have a role in the decreasing transfer to breast milk from early- to mid-lactation, if confirmed in future studies. The major limitation of this work is the limited number of subjects, that limited reaching a significance level in some analyses and the capacity to extrapolate the results found to larger population groups. However, our results indicate new potentially interesting points to be investigated in the future, which might improve nutrition guidance for lactating women, especially if at high risk of sub-adequate intake of vitamin E.

5. Conclusions

Despite constant serum levels, the content of vitamin A and E in breast milk decreased throughout lactation, imposing risks of deficiency to the breastfed infants. Subclinical vitamin A deficiency in the lactating mothers was undetectable by serum retinol concentration in early- or mid-lactation. On the other hand, dietary assessment by the MSM was fairly sensitive to detect vitamin A inadequacy and might be used in the future to identify population groups at risk and guide maternal dietary advice on food choices or eventually supplementation in order to prevent sub-adequate nutritional status in breastfed newborns. A similar trend was observed for vitamin E, because breast the milk concentration of α-tocopherol seemed largely more sensitive than its serum concentration to the sub-adequate intake of the vitamin. Future prospective clinical trials providing nutritional advice to lactating mothers with sub-adequate vitamin A and E intake and the assessment of breast milk levels and infant nutritional status of these vitamins would contribute to widen the impact of this research.

Supplementary Materials:
Figure S1: Representative chromatograms by HPLC-UV-Vis of the analysis of: (A) retinol (325 nm) and tocopherols (292 nm) standards; (B) carotenoid standards (450 nm). Refer to materials and methods for detailed methods description. Table S1: Calculated sample size necessary to disclose differences between early- and mid-lactating women in the distribution of vitamin A and E, and carotenoids in HDL and LDL+VLDL serum fractions.

Author Contributions: Conceptualization, A.G.T. and F.K.; methodology, A.G.T., F.K. and M.R.M.; formal analysis, A.G.T., J.C.N. and M.R.M.; investigation, M.R.M.; resources, A.G.T. and F.K.; data curation, A.G.T. and M.R.M.; writing—original draft preparation, M.R.M.; writing—review and editing, A.G.T. and T.E.-B.; visualization, A.G.T., F.K., J.C.N., M.R.M. and T.E.-B.; supervision, A.G.T., F.K. and J.C.N.; project administration, A.G.T.; funding acquisition, A.G.T and F.K.

Acknowledgments: The authors acknowledge the contribution of the breastfeeding mothers that participated in this study, without any direct compensation. The assistance of the clinical dietitians Danúbia Incuto Silva and Vivianne Magalhães Gomes during sample and data collection is greatly appreciated. The assistance of conticom.com.br designing the graphical abstract is greatly acknowledged.

References

1. World Health Organization (WHO). *Global Prevalence of Vitamin A Deficiency in Populations at Risk 1995–2005*; WHO: Geneva, Switzerland, 2009; pp. 9–18.
2. Ribeiro, K.D.S.; Lima, M.S.R.; Medeiros, J.F.P.; Rebouças, A.S.; Dantas, R.C.S.; Bezerra, D.S.; Osório, M.M.; Dimenstein, R. Association between maternal vitamin E status and alpha-tocopherol levels in the newborn and colostrum. *Matern. Child Nutr.* **2016**, *12*, 801–807. [CrossRef] [PubMed]
3. De Vries, J.Y.; Pundir, S.; Mckenzie, E.; Keijer, J.; Kussmann, M. Maternal circulating vitamin status and colostrum vitamin composition in healthy lactating women—A systematic approach. *Nutrients* **2018**, *28*, 687. [CrossRef] [PubMed]
4. Da Silva, A.G.C.L.; Rebouças, A.S.; Mendonça, B.M.A.; Silva, D.C.N.; Dimenstein, R.; Ribeiro, K.D.S. Relationship between the dietary intake, serum, and breast milk concentrations of vitamin A and vitamin E in a cohort of women over the course of lactation. *Matern. Child Nutr.* **2019**, *22*, e12772. [CrossRef] [PubMed]
5. Grilo, E.C.; Medeiros, W.F.; Silva, A.G.A.; Gurgel, C.S.S.; Ramalho, H.M.M.; Dimenstein, R. Maternal supplementation with a megadose of vitamin A reduces colostrum level of α-tocopherol: A randomized controlled trial. *J. Hum. Nutr. Diet.* **2016**, *29*, 652–661. [CrossRef] [PubMed]
6. World Health Organization (WHO). *Obesity: Preventing and Managing the Global Epidemic*; WHO Technical Report Series 894; WHO: Geneva, Switzerland, 2000; pp. 1–253.
7. Harttig, U.; Haubrock, J.; Knüppel, S.; Boeing, H. The MSM program: Web-based statistics package for estimating usual dietary intake using the Multiple Source Method. *Eur. J. Clin. Nutr.* **2011**, *65*, 87–91. [CrossRef] [PubMed]
8. Sartorelli, D.S.; Barbieri, P.; Perdona, G.C. Fried food intake estimated by the multiple source method is associated with gestational weight gain. *Nutr. Res.* **2014**, *34*, 667–673. [CrossRef] [PubMed]
9. U.S. Department of Agriculture, Agricultural Research Service. USDA National Nutrient Database for Standard Reference, Release 25. Available online: https://www.ars.usda.gov/northeast-area/beltsville-md-bhnrc/beltsville-human-nutrition-research-center/nutrient-data-laboratory/docs/sr25-home-page/ (accessed on 20 July 2016).
10. University of Campinas (UNICAMP)—Core Centre for Research in Food (NEPA). *Brazilian Food Composition Table, Taco*, 4th ed.; NEPA/UNICAMP: Campinas, Brazil, 2011; pp. 1–161.
11. Institute of Medicine. *Dietary Reference Intakes Research Synthesis: Workshop Summary*; National Academy Press: Washington, DC, USA, 2007; pp. 127–150.

12. Institute of Medicine. *Dietary Reference Intakes for Vitamin C, Vitamin E, Selenium and Carotenoids*; National Academy Press: Washington, DC, USA, 2000; pp. 186–283.
13. Institute of Medicine. *Dietary Reference Intakes for Vitamin A, Vitamin K, Arsenic, Boron, Chromium, Copper, Iodine, Iron, Manganese, Molybdenum, Nickel, Silicon, Vanadium, and Zinc*; National Academy Press: Washington, DC, USA, 2001; pp. 82–161.
14. Institute of Medicine. *Dietary Reference Intakes—Energy, Carbohydrate, Fiber, Fat, Fatty Acids, Cholesterol, Protein, and Amino Acids*; The National Academy Press: Washington, DC, USA, 2002; pp. 936–967.
15. Lopes-Virella, M.F.; Stone, P.; Ellis, S.; Colwell, J.A. Cholesterol determination in high-density lipoproteins separated by three different methods. *Clin. Chem.* **1977**, *23*, 882–884. [PubMed]
16. Lucas, A.; Gibbs, J.A.; Lyster, R.L.; Baum, J.D. Creamatocrit: Simple clinical technique for estimating fat concentration and energy value of human milk. *Br. Med. J.* **1978**, *1*, 1018–1020. [CrossRef]
17. Perry, N.A.; Doan, F.J. A picric acid method for the simultaneous determination of lactose and sucrose in dairy products. *J. Dairy Sci.* **1950**, *33*, 176–185. [CrossRef]
18. Costa, T.H.M.; Dorea, J.G. Concentration of fat, protein, lactose and energy in milk of mothers using hormonal contraceptives. *Ann. Trop. Pediatr.* **1992**, *12*, 203–209. [CrossRef]
19. Lowry, O.H.; Rosebrough, N.; Farr, A.L.; Randall, R.J. Protein measurement with the Folin phenol reagent. *J. Biol. Chem.* **1951**, *193*, 265–275. [PubMed]
20. Trugo, N.M.F.; Donangelo, C.M.; Koury, J.C.; Silva, M.I.; Freitas, L.A. Concentration and distribution pattern of selected micronutrients in preterm and term milk from urban Brazilian mothers during early lactation. *Eur. J. Clin. Nutr.* **1988**, *42*, 497–507. [PubMed]
21. Meneses, F.; Trugo, N.M.F. Retinol, β-carotene, and lutein+zeaxanthin in the milk of Brazilian nursing women: Associations with plasma concentrations and influences of maternal characteristics. *Nutr. Res.* **2005**, *25*, 443–451. [CrossRef]
22. Hass, D.; Keller, H.E.; Oberlin, B.; Bonfanti, R.; Schüep, W. Simultaneous determination of retinol, tocopherols, carotenes and lycopene in plasma by means of High-Performance Liquid-Chromatography on reversed phase. *Int. J. Vitam. Nutr. Res.* **1991**, *61*, 232–238.
23. Liu, Y.; Xu, M.J.; Canfield, L.M. Enzymatic hydrolysis, extraction, and quantitation of retinol and major carotenoids in mature human milk. *J. Nutr. Biochem.* **1998**, *9*, 178–183. [CrossRef]
24. Silva, L.O.; Castelo-Branco, V.N.; Carvalho, A.G.A.; Monteiro, M.C.; Perrone, D.; Torres, A.G. Ethanol extraction renders a phenolic compounds-enriched and highly stable jussara fruit (*Euterpe edulis* M.) oil. *Eur. J. Lipid Sci. Technol.* **2017**, *119*, e201700200. [CrossRef]
25. Rodriguez-Amaya, D.B.; Kimura, M. *Harvest Plus Handbook for Carotenoid Analysis*; International Food Policy Research Institute (IFPRI): Washington, DC, USA, 2004; pp. 1–57.
26. World Health Organization (WHO). *Prevention and Control of Iron Deficiency Anaemia in Women and Children*; United Nations Children's Fund (UNICEF): Geneva, Switzerland, 1999; pp. 17–30.
27. Expert Panel on Detection, Evaluation and Treatment of High Blood Cholesterol in Adults. Executive summary of the third report of the National Cholesterol Education Program (NCEP) expert panel on detection, evaluation, and treatment of high blood cholesterol in adults (Adult treatment panel III). *JAMA* **2001**, *285*, 2486–2497. [CrossRef] [PubMed]
28. Joint FAO/WHO Expert Consultation on Human Vitamin and Mineral Requirements (FAO/WHO). *Vitamin and Mineral Requirements in Human Nutrition*, 2nd ed.; WHO: Geneva, Switzerland, 2004; pp. 1–362.
29. Deminice, T.M.M.; Ferraz, I.S.; Monteiro, J.P.; Jordão, A.A.; Ambrósio, L.M.C.S.; Almeida, C.A.N. Vitamin A intake of Brazilian mothers and retinol concentrations in maternal blood, human milk, and the umbilical cord. *Nutr. Res. Pract.* **2018**, *46*, 1555–1569. [CrossRef]
30. Lira, L.Q.; De Souza, A.F.; Amâncio, A.M.; Bezerra, C.G.; Pimentel, J.B.; Moia, M.N.; Dimenstein, R. Retinol and betacarotene status in mother-infant dyads and associations between them. *Ann. Nutr. Metab.* **2018**, *72*, 50–56. [CrossRef]
31. Kim, H.; Jung, B.; Lee, B.; Kim, Y.; Jung, J.A.; Chang, N. Retinol, α-tocopherol, and selected minerals in breast milk of lactating women with full-term infants in South Korea. *Nutr. Res. Pract.* **2017**, *11*, 64–69. [CrossRef]
32. Ministry of Health, Brazil; National Sanitary Surveillance Agency (ANVISA). *Resolution RDC N° 269, Technical Regulation on Recommended Daily Intake (IDR) of Protein, Vitamins and Minerals*; ANVISA: Brasilia, DF, Brazil, 2005; pp. 1–6.

33. Garretto, D.; Kim, Y.-K.; Quadro, L.; Rhodas, R.R.; Pimentel, V.; Crnosija, N.A.; Nie, L.; Bernstein, P.; Tropper, P.; Neal-Perry, G.S. Vitamin A and β-carotene in pregnant and breastfeeding post-bariatric women in an urban population. *J. Perinat. Med.* **2019**, *47*, 183–189. [CrossRef] [PubMed]
34. Xu, X.; Zhao, X.; Berde, Y.; Low, Y.; Kuchan, M. Milk and plasma lutein and zeaxanthin concentrations in Chinese breast-feeding mother-infant dyads with healthy maternal fruit and vegetable intake. *J. Am. Coll. Nutr.* **2019**, *38*, 179–184. [CrossRef] [PubMed]
35. Zielinska, M.; Hamulka, J.; Wesolowska, A. Carotenoid content in breastmilk in the 3rd and 6th month of lactation and its associations with maternal dietary intake and anthropometric characteristics. *Nutrients* **2019**, *11*, 193. [CrossRef] [PubMed]
36. Xavier, A.A.O.; Diaz-Salido, E.; Arenilla-Velez, I.; Aguayo-Maldonado, J.; Garrido-Fernandez, J.; Fontecha, J.; Sanchez-Garcia, A.; Perez-Galvez, A. Carotenoid content in human colostrum is associated to preterm/full-term birth condition. *Nutrients* **2018**, *10*, 1654. [CrossRef] [PubMed]
37. Schweigert, F.J.; Bathe, K.; Chen, F.; Büscher, U.; Dudenhausen, J.W. Effect of the stage of lactation in humans on carotenoid levels in milk, blood plasma and plasma lipoprotein fractions. *Eur. J. Nutr.* **2004**, *43*, 39–44. [CrossRef] [PubMed]

13

Impact of Fenugreek on Milk Production in Rodent Models of Lactation Challenge

Thomas Sevrin [1,2], Marie-Cécile Alexandre-Gouabau [2], Blandine Castellano [2], Audrey Aguesse [2], Khadija Ouguerram [2], Patrick Ngyuen [3], Dominique Darmaun [2,4] and Clair-Yves Boquien [2,*]

1 Laboratoire FRANCE Bébé Nutrition, 53000 Laval, France; thomas.sevrin@etu.univ-nantes.fr
2 Nantes Université, INRA, UMR 1280 PhAN, CRNH-Ouest, IMAD, F-44000 Nantes, France; Marie-Cecile.Alexandre-Gouabau@univ-nantes.fr (M.-C.A.-G.); Blandine.Castellano@univ-nantes.fr (B.C.); Audrey.Aguesse@univ-nantes.fr (A.A.); Khadija.Ouguerram@univ-nantes.fr (K.O.); Dominique.Darmaun@chu-nantes.fr (D.D.)
3 ONIRIS, NP3, CRNH-Ouest, F-44000 Nantes, France; patrick.nguyen@oniris-nantes.fr
4 CHU Nantes, F-44000 Nantes, France
* Correspondence: clair-yves.boquien@univ-nantes.fr

Abstract: Fenugreek, a herbal remedy, has long been used as galactologue to help mothers likely to stop breastfeeding because of perceived insufficient milk production. However, few studies highlight the efficacy of fenugreek in enhancing milk production. The aims of our study were to determine whether fenugreek increased milk yield in rodent models of lactation challenge and if so, to verify the lack of adverse effects on dam and offspring metabolism. Two lactation challenges were tested: increased litter size to 12 pups in dams fed a 20% protein diet and perinatal restriction to an 8% protein diet with eight pups' litter, with or without 1 $g.kg^{-1}.day^{-1}$ dietary supplementation of fenugreek, compared to control dams fed 20% protein diet with eight pups' litters. Milk flow was measured by the deuterium oxide enrichment method, and milk composition was assessed. Lipid and glucose metabolism parameters were assessed in dam and offspring plasmas. Fenugreek increased milk production by 16% in the litter size increase challenge, resulting in an 11% increase in pup growth without deleterious effect on dam-litter metabolism. Fenugreek had no effect in the maternal protein restriction challenge. These results suggest a galactologue effect of fenugreek when mothers have no physiological difficulties in producing milk.

Keywords: fenugreek; milk flow; milk composition; litter size; maternal protein restriction; plasma metabolic parameters

---

1. Introduction

The World Health Organisation recommends exclusive breastfeeding for infants up to six months of age, based on the clear health benefits of breastfeeding on mother-infant dyad [1]. Indeed, there is a consensus regarding the association of breastfeeding with a reduced risk of respiratory and gastro-intestinal infections during the first year of life. Infants, who were breastfed for longer periods, may also have a lower risk of developing obesity and type II diabetes at adulthood [2,3]. For mothers, breastfeeding could limit the risk of developing ovarian cancer and type II diabetes [4,5]. Despite these benefits, breastfeeding prevalence remains relatively low, particularly in several high-income countries in North America and Europe, where only 40% of mothers breastfeed six months after delivery [6]. Exclusive breastfeeding rate is about 60% at four months in Scandinavian countries, 35% in the Netherlands, 16% in the UK [7], and 10% in France [7,8].

Early cessation of breastfeeding clearly is multifactorial [9]. One of the main factors is the maternal perception of insufficient milk secretion to quell infant's hunger or support infant growth and leads to early cessation of breastfeeding in 35% of cases [9–11]. Perception of insufficient milk production is a complex, multifactorial issue that can have biological, social, or psychological determinants, and it often remains unclear whether the low milk secretion is real or only perceived [9]. Indeed, as a result of the lack of an objective marker of insufficient milk production and the importance of maternal psychology in breastfeeding duration, perceived milk insufficiency is probably much more common than true insufficient production [9–11]. True insufficient milk secretion can result from many causes, ranging from inability to lactate due to breast abnormalities or endocrine disorder (5% of women) to difficulties in breastfeeding management, maternal stress and anxiety, or early food diversification in the infant. Although maternal milk production can be often increased through psychological support or maternal breastfeeding education [9,10,12], many healthy mothers are eager to enhance their milk production through various nutritional supplements.

Several drugs and herbal preparations have traditionally been prescribed as galactologues: i.e., substances that promote initiation or increase of lactation [13]. Drugs like domperidone®or metoclopramide®carry the risk of adverse side effects such as arrhythmia or hypothyroidism in mother-children dyad [12]. That is why herbal galactologues like fennel, anise, barley, milk thistle, or garlic are becoming more and more popular for increasing lactation. Among these herbal compounds, fenugreek probably is the most widely consumed [12–14]. Fenugreek has been used since antiquity in traditional Persian, Chinese, and Egyptian medicine for its range of therapeutic effects. It is now increasingly consumed in Western countries for its presumed protective effects against diabetes, atherosclerosis, inflammation, and hypertriglyceridemia, as well as its putative role as a galactologue [12,15] due, in part, to trigonelline, one of its main active ingredients [15]. There is, however, little evidence for its effectiveness on milk yield [13]. Whereas a positive effect of fenugreek on milk production was observed in various mammals, such as rabbit [16], buffalo [17], goat [18], or ewe [19]; the wide range of doses tested (from 180 mg.kg-1.d-1 [17] to 2.1 g.kg-1.d-1 [18]) led to large discrepancies in the reported effect on milk production (ranging from a 10% increase [16] to a 110% [18] increase), which makes it difficult to determine the effective dose of fenugreek. Moreover, other studies failed to demonstrate an effect in rabbits [20] and goats [21]. In these studies, milk production was measured either by the weight–suckle–weight method (in rabbit), or by milking (in larger animals). The latter methods do not, however, directly assess milk production in response to physiological suckling by the pups. Moreover, these studies evaluated the effectiveness of fenugreek to increase milk production with the aim of productivity, under otherwise optimal conditions of lactation, as opposed to mothers challenged by their perception of insufficient milk production. Finally, none of these studies evaluated the metabolic status of mother-infant dyad following fenugreek supplementation. Thus, the true efficacy of fenugreek on milk production in an animal model submitted to a breastfeeding challenge remains to be ascertained.

To that purpose, the current study used the deuterium oxide enrichment method [22], which meets all criteria to adequately assess breast milk supply even in small animals and, in turn, evaluate the putative galactologue effect of substances such as fenugreek. Indeed, it has been shown to be precise and to provide a smoothed value of several days milk production obtained under physiological conditions of lactation [22]. Moreover, in order to simulate conditions where mothers are unable to feed their own pups optimally, two classical models of lactation challenges were used. The first one mimics conditions in which mothers can adapt their milk production but still fail to adequately cover the litters' needs, leading to suboptimal growth of the offspring. This model, obtained by increasing litter size through pup adoption, is known to induce extra-uterine growth restriction (EUGR) in the offspring due to a reduced milk intake in individual pups due to their larger number [23,24]. The second model mimics conditions in which mothers are truly unable to produce sufficient milk due to a perinatal restriction in dietary protein intake when fed a diet containing 8% protein instead of 20% in the standard diet. This model is also notably known to induce EUGR [25] due to a 34% drop in milk production [22].

The specific aims of this study were: (a) to verify the ability of our stable isotope method to detect changes in milk production in two rodent models of lactation challenge; (b) to test the galactologue effect of fenugreek on milk production and composition in these models of lactation challenge; and (c) to explore the effect of fenugreek on maternal metabolism during the lactation period and the short and long-term metabolic outcome in the offspring.

2. Materials and Methods

2.1. Animal Experiment

Housing and Diets

The experimental protocol was approved by the Animal Ethics committee and the French Ministry of Research (protocol APAFIS 2018121018129789). Pregnant Sprague-Dawley rats were purchased from Janvier Labs (Le Genest-Saint-Isle, France) at gestational day one (G1). They were housed individually in cages with wood chips located on ventilated racks kept at a constant temperature of 22 ± 1 °C and at a relative humidity of 50% ± 3%. Cages were placed in a room with a fixed 12 h light–dark cycle (light from 7:00 a.m. to 7:00 p.m.). Pregnant rats had access to water and food ad libitum.

During gestation, dams received a standard normal protein diet based on AIN-93G diet [26] with 20 g protein per 100 g of food (NP diet) or an isoenergetic, low-protein diet with 8 g protein per 100 g of food (LP diet).

During lactation, dams received experimental diets based on NP and LP diets and supplemented with a dry water extract of fenugreek seeds (Plantex, Sainte-Geneviève-des-Bois, France) named NPF and LPF diets, respectively, in the following. Fenugreek, as an oxytocic substance [13], was provided to dams only during the lactation period. The amount of fenugreek in NPF and LPF diets was calculated to reach a consumption of 1 g.kg body weight^{-1}.day^{-1} in rat as an equivalent as the traditionally recommended [12,13] 6 g daily dose in women weighing 60 kg and assuming that metabolic rate per unit of body weight is 10 fold higher in rats than in humans [27]. The four diets (i.e., NP, LP, NPF, and LPF) were manufactured by the "Unité de Préparation des Aliments Expérimentaux" (INRA-UPAE, Jouy-en-Josas, France). The composition and energy of each diet is provided in Supplementary Table S1.

After weaning, offspring were fed ad libitum with a standard growth diet A03 (SAFE, Augy, France).

2.2. Experimental Design

On the first day of gestation (G1), seventy-two female rats (i.e., 4 consecutive series of 18 animals), were randomly assigned to be fed experimental diets during gestation: 52 females received the NP diet and 20 females received the LP diet. Delivery occurred at the 21st day of gestation that was considered as day 0 of lactation (L0). At birth, pups born from protein-restricted dams (LP dams) were discarded and killed to avoid the bias due to intrauterine growth restriction. Only pups born from control dams (NP dams) were randomly adopted by NP or LP dams, taking care to balance pup's birth weights between groups. The litter size was adjusted to either 8 or 12 pups per dam with a female/male ratio of 1/1, as described in Figure 1.

Five groups were defined (47 dams). In the NP:8 group (our reference group, n = 8), dams suckled 8 pups per litter and were fed the NP diet. The NP:12 group (n = 11) corresponded to the first model of lactation challenge by increasing litter size (12 pups per litter) with dams under the NP diet. In the LP:8 group (n = 8), dams suckled 8 pups per litter and were fed the LP diet. The LP:8 group corresponded to the second model of lactation challenge with a known decreased milk flow due to perinatal protein restriction [22,25]. In the two other groups NPF:12 (12 suckled pups per litter, n = 11) and LPF:8 (8 suckled pups per litter, n = 9), dams were respectively fed an NP and LP diet supplemented with fenugreek.

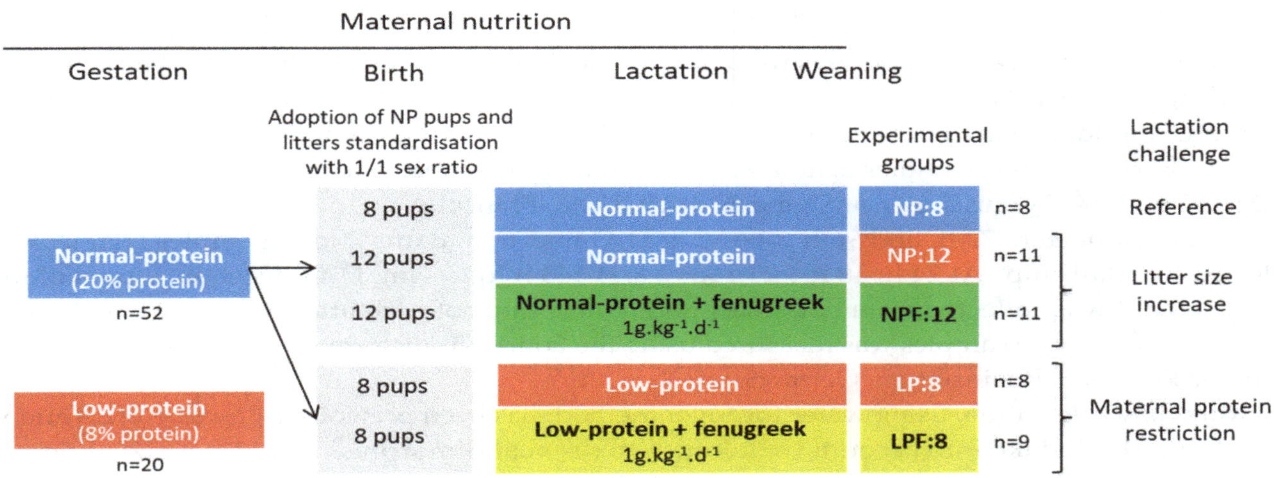

Figure 1. Representation of the 5 experimental groups of dams.

At weaning (L20), 4 pups (2 males and 2 female) per litter were killed and perirenal, subcutaneous and brown adipose tissues were collected and weighed. Two other males and two females per litter were weaned and placed with 3 animals per cage with ad libitum access to food and water until post-natal day 75 (PND75), and then killed. Liver, gastrocnemius muscle, perirenal, subcutaneous, and visceral adipose tissues were removed from PND75 offspring and weighed.

At L21, mothers were fasted for 4h and then sacrificed. Liver, left inguinal mammary gland, perirenal, subcutaneous, and visceral adipose tissues were removed, weighed, sampled, and immediately frozen in liquid nitrogen before storage at −80 °C.

Sacrifice was performed by intracardiac injection of 0.5 mL Exagon®(Richter pharma, Wels, Austria) when animal tissues were collected, whereas supernumerary dams or supernumerary weaned pups were killed by carbon dioxide anaesthesia or by decapitation for pups at birth.

During lactation, dams' weight, food and water consumption, and both male and female litters' weight were recorded every two days from L0 to L11, and every day from L11 to L21. For dams, weight loss (in g) during the lactation period was calculated by subtracting weight at L0 (delivery) from the daily weight. For male and female offspring, pups' mean weight (expressed as g) was obtained by dividing litter weight by the number of pups. Weight gain (in g) was calculated by subtracting birth weight (L0) from the daily weight. Daily growth rate (in g.day^{-1}) was calculated by subtracting weight at day d-1 from the weight at day d. Food and water relative intakes (in g.kg^{-1}.day^{-1}) were obtained by dividing daily intakes by daily weight.

2.3. Biological Samples Collection

Milk samples were collected from lactating dams at L18, as previously described [28]. Briefly, dams were separated from their pups and received an intraperitoneal injection of oxytocin (1 unit of Syntocinon®; Sigma-Tau, Ivry-sur-Seine, France) to stimulate milk ejection. After 20 min, dams were anaesthetized with 4% of isoflurane, and by applying manual pressure to nipples, about 200 to 400 µL of milk were collected before storage at −20 °C.

Blood samples were collected before animal sacrifice by an intra-cardiac puncture in EDTA-tubes (Pfizer-Centravet, Plancoët, France). Otherwise, blood samples were collected on alert dams by a tail snip in EDTA-tubes. Blood samples were centrifuged at 1132 g for 15 min at 4 °C, and plasma was collected in Eppendorf before storage at −20 °C until analysis.

For urine, pups were first separated from the mother for 30 min to avoid urine loss by maternal stimulation. Urine samples were then collected from pups by stimulation of lower bellies with an iced cotton bud and pooled for the male and female litter.

2.4. Milk Flow Measurement by Water Turnover Method

The water turnover method was used as previously described [22]. Briefly, at L8, plasma and urine samples were collected prior to maternal deuterated water (D_2O) injection to determine baseline body D_2O abundance in dams and litter, respectively. At L11, when lactation was well established, following 4% isoflurane anaesthesia, mothers received an intravenous tail injection of 4.95 ± 0.13 g.kg^{-1} D_2O (99.9 mole % D_2-enrichment) (Sigma-Aldrich, Lyon, France).

At 2 h, 24 h, 48 h, 72 h, and 96 h following D_2O injection, dams' blood samples (300 μL) were collected by a tail snip. At 24 h, 48 h, 72 h, 96 h, and 168 h following D_2O-injection, a pool of urine (about 300 μL) was collected from both male and female pups of each litter. The D_2O enrichment of both plasma and urine samples was measured using the Fourier Transform infrared spectrophotometer Alpha II®(Brucker, Rheinstetten, Germany).

Milk flow calculation, using water turnover method, has been previously described [22] and was refined in order to take into account both intra-litter sexual dimorphism and litter size differences between experimental groups. Regarding sexual dimorphism, instead of a bi-compartmental model (dam-litter), a four-compartment model (Figure 2) was used, in which 2 single-compartments corresponded to the turnover of total body water (TBW) of both male (3) and female (4) pups in the same litter, and the other 2 single-compartments corresponded to the turnover of TBW of their own dam (1 and 2, with 1 = 2). Each mother compartment was related by water flow to one pup compartment (male or female). Absolute production rates are represented in Figure 2: R10, R20 (R20 = R10), R30, and R40 are the inputs into the body of dam and its male and female litter, respectively, arising from water drinking and non-dietary water as metabolic water production; R01, R02, R03, and R04 are the outputs of water by transpiration, urine or faeces of dam and its male and female litter, respectively; R31 and R42 are water flows from the dam to male litter and from the dam to female litter, respectively. The model has five unknown parameters: i) K01 and K02 are equal and represent the output flow constants of the dam; ii) K03 and K04 are the output flow constants from male and female litter, respectively and iii) K31 and K42 are the output flow constants from the dam to its male and female litter, respectively.

Using the isotope dilution method, the mass of dam's TBW (TBWd, in g) was calculated by dividing the amount of D_2O injected by the D_2O value extrapolated from the D_2O concentration curve to the intercept with the y-axis at time 0 (Supplementary Table S2). TBWd (in %) was calculated by dividing the mass of TBWd (in g) by dams' mean mass from L11 to L15.

Flow constants of the model (K01, K03, K04, K31, and K42) were then determined using the SAAM II®software. As litter size (8 or 12 pups) presumably impacts D_2O dilution in the litter, we used values of D_2O mass instead of D_2O concentrations for calculations in our model. To this end, D_2O concentration, obtained after baseline concentration deduction, was multiplied by animal mass at each day of sampling, following Equation (1):

$$D_2O\ concentration\ \left(\mu g.g^{-1}\right) * animal\ mass\ (g) = D_2O\ mass\ (\mu g) \tag{1}$$

This calculation implicitly assumes that dams' and pups' TBW (in %) are equivalent, which is probably the case considering that suckled pups have about 75% of TBW [29], which is similar to suckling dams' TBW [22]. Moreover, in order to indicate that compartment (1) and (2) represent the same individual (dam), the same data were incremented for both compartments, and K02 was forced to be equal to K01. Flow constants of the model were obtained directly with SAAM II®from a fit of plasma and urine D_2O mass–time curves. The water flows, from mother to male litter R31 (g.h^{-1}) and from the dam to female litter R42 (g.h^{-1}), were calculated as the product of TBWd (g) and K31 or K42, respectively. These values were then multiplied by 24 to obtain the daily milk production (g.day^{-1}).

In this model, R31 and R42 were associated to milk flows between the dam and its male litter or between the dam and its female litter, respectively, assuming milk was the only external source of water for the pups. Thus, milk flow corresponds to the milk produced by the dam, as determined from the D2O transfer from the dam to litter, after the dam received a D2O injection. As the water content of each individual milk was not accurately measured, milk flow was directly calculated from water flow without correction. We assumed that this does not alter conclusions concerning group comparisons. Total milk production of the dam was calculated by summing R31 and R42 and represented the mean milk production throughout the sampling period (L11 to L18). Milk consumption by male and female litters was obtained by dividing R31 and R42, respectively, by the number of males or females pups (4 in NP:8, LP:8 and LPF:8 groups or 6, in NP:12 and NPF:12 groups).

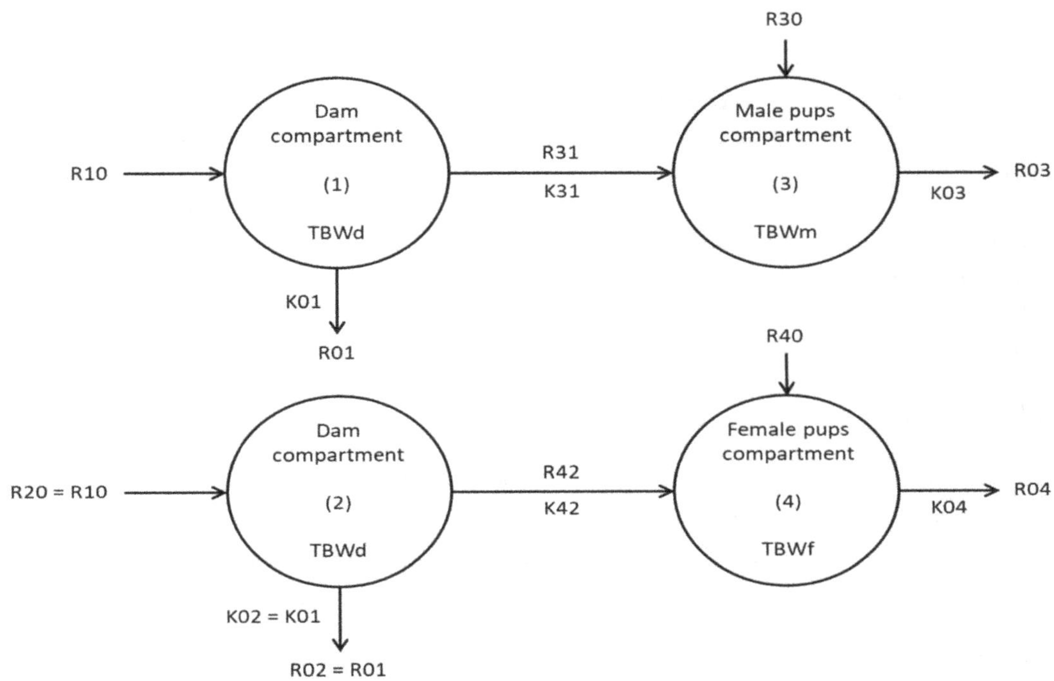

Figure 2. Four-compartment model of water turnover. TBWd, TBWm, TBWf: total body water (expressed in g) of dam, male, and female litter respectively; K01 and K02 (in h^{-1}) are equal and represent the output flow constants from the dam; K03 and k04 (in h^{-1}) are the output flow constants from the male and female litters, respectively; K31 and K42: (in h^{-1}) are the output flow constants from the dam to its male litter and from the dam to its female litter, respectively; R10, R20, R30, and R40 (in $g.h^{-1}$) are input water flows into the body of dam (R10 is equal to R20) and its male and female litter respectively; R01 and R02 (in $g.h^{-1}$) are equal and represent output water flows from the dam; R03 and R04 (in $g.h^{-1}$) are output water flows from male and female litters respectively; R31 and R42 (in $g.h^{-1}$) are water flows from the dam to its male litter and from the dam to its female litter and are associated to milk flow.

2.5. Milk Protein, Lactose, and Fatty Acid Analysis

Milk protein concentration was determined using a colourimetric Pierce BCA Protein Assay Kit (ThermoFisher Scientific, Waltham, MA, USA) with milk diluted at 1/40 in osmosed water and bovine serum albumin (fraction V) as standard. Milk lactose concentration was estimated using an enzymatic Lactose/D-Galactose Assay Kit K-LACGAR®(Megazyme, Bray, Ireland) with milk diluted at 1/20 in osmosed water and α-lactose monohydrate as standard. Milk total lipids were not fractionated. Fatty acids (FAs) were extracted using the modified liquid–liquid extraction method of Bligh-Dyer, as previously described [28]. Briefly, FAs were extracted from 30 μL milk in methanol–chloroform mix (1:1, *v/v*). Heptadecanoic acid was used as the internal standard. Total FAs were transesterified using boron trifluoride in methanol, and fatty acid methyl esters were analysed by gas chromatography using an Agilent Technologies 7890A®instrument. Each FA was expressed as a percentage of the total identified FAs, and only FAs whose percentage was above 0.5% were taken into account. The sum of FAs (in g.L^{-1}) was assumed to represent total milk lipid (free fatty acids, triacylglycerols and phospholipids) content.

The energy content of milk was calculated by multiplying lactose, proteins, and lipid content by their energy content, assuming 4 kcal.g^{-1} for both carbohydrate (lactose) and protein and 9 kcal.g^{-1} for fat. Milk macronutrient production and milk energy production by the dam were then calculated by multiplying total milk production by macronutrient concentrations or energy content of milk respectively.

2.6. *Dams and Offspring Metabolic Markers and Offspring Glucose Tolerance Test*

At PND60, blood samples (300 μL) were collected from 6 h fasted offspring. An oral glucose tolerance test (OGTT) was performed in offspring at PND61 and PND62. Following 6 hours of fasting, all rats received a 2 g/kg BW dose of glucose by gavage. Blood samples (100 μL) were collected to determine plasma insulin concentration before (T0) and after 15 (T15) and 30 min (T30) gavage with glucose. Blood glucose was measured at T0, T15, T30, T45, T60, T90, and T120 after glucose intake, using a Performa Accu-Chek®glucometer (Roche Diabetes Care France, Meylan, France).

Insulin (Rat Insulin ELISA kit®, ALPCO, Salem, USA), glucose (Glucose GOD FS®, DiaSys, Holzheim, Germany), triglycerides (Triglycerides FS®, DiaSys, Holzheim, Germany), and cholesterol (Cholesterol FS®, DiaSys, Holzheim, Germany) were measured in plasma, following manufacturers' instructions. Optical density was read with a microplate reader Varioskan Lux®(ThermoFisher Scientific, Waltham, USA).

2.7. *Trigonelline Quantification in Experimental Diet, Dams' Plasma, and Milk*

Ten μL of the labelled internal standard: trigonelline-D3 (CIL, Sainte Foy la Grande, France) at 50 μM, and 100 μL of acetonitrile were added to 10μL of diet solution (mixed diet in water, 100 g.L^{-1}), dams' plasma or milk. Samples were centrifuged for 10 min at 11,000 g, and the supernatant was injected into the LC–MS/MS using a hydrophilic interaction liquid chromatography system (Acquity H-Class®UPLC^{TM} device, Waters) coupled with a triple quadrupole mass spectrometry detector (Xevo®TQD) with an electrospray interface. Data acquisition and analyses were performed with MassLynx®and TargetLynx®software, both versions 4.1 (Waters). Trigonelline was separated over 6 min on a HILIC column (2.1 × 100 mm; 1.7 μM), (Waters) held at 45 °C with a linear gradient of mobile phase A (10 mM ammonium acetate in water) in mobile phase B (98% acetonitrile in water), each containing 0.1% formic acid, at a flow rate of 400 μL/min. Trigonelline was detected by the Xevo®TQD that allowed the multiple reaction monitoring (MRM) mode to be performed, with the electrospray interface operating in the positive ion mode (capillary voltage, 1.5 kV; desolvation gas (N_2) flow and temperature, 650 L/h and 150 °C; source temperature, 150 °C). Based on specific collision-induced fragmentation of precursor ions, the MRM precursor/fragment pairs were based on the following transitions *m/z*: 138.06→93.98 amu for trigonelline and 141.03→97.00 amu for the internal standard. Chromatographic peak area ratios between trigonelline and its internal standard constituted the detector response. Trigonelline standard solutions (concentrations from 1 nM to 10 μM) were used for calibration.

2.8. *Statistical Analysis*

To maximise the power of analysis, parametric tests were favoured using one-way ANOVA or two-way ANOVA with an experimental group factor and a day or a sex factor. The validity of the parametric tests was checked by assessing normality of residuals with a Shapiro–Wilk test. In the case of absence of residual normality non-parametric, the Kruskal–Wallis test was used instead of one-way ANOVA. Multiple comparison tests used after ANOVA were: Dunnett's post-hoc test to compare several levels to one level of interest (Table 1), Tukey's post-hoc test to compare levels altogether (Table 2) and Sidak's post-hoc test when there were only two levels in a factor (Table 4). After the Kruskal–Wallis test, the non-parametric Dunn's post-hoc test was used. To determine the strength of the link between two variables, Pearson's correlation tests were used, and simple linear regression was performed to determine the relation between two variables. All tests were performed with the GraphPad prism®software, version 6.

3. Results

3.1. Dams and Litter Characteristics in the Reference Group NP:8

For all groups, we took care to balance pups' birth weight, following the adoption of NP pups and litter standardization. Mean pup birth weight was 7.1 ± 0.0 g, with no difference between groups ($p = 0.37$), although males were significantly bigger than females (7.3 ± 0.0 g versus 6.9 ± 0.0 g, $p < 0.001$). NP:8 dams weighed 344.3 ± 8.7 g at delivery. Maternal weight loss during the lactation period and food and water intakes are given in Table 1. Litter growth rate was 22.9 ± 0.7 g·day^{-1}, which represented a pup growth rate of 2.86 ± 0.09 g·day^{-1} and did not differ between genders ($p = 0.23$). In the water turnover models, output flow constants (K3,1 and K4,2), as reported in Supplementary Table S3, were determined with good accuracy due to a forecast standard deviation (FSD) of each group lower than 5%, allowing the milk flows to be determined with confidence. For the NP:8 group, milk flow was 46.0 ± 1.6 g·day^{-1}, which represented a mean milk consumption of 5.74 ± 0.20 g·day^{-1} per pup, with no significant sexual dimorphism ($p = 0.36$).

Table 1. Effect of fenugreek on dams' lactation follow up, pups growth, and milk flow in two models of lactation challenges. Results are expressed as mean ± SEM.

Lactation Challenges	*Control*	*Litter Size Increase*		*Maternal Protein Restriction*	
Experimental Groups	**NP:8**	**NP:12**	**NPF:12**	**LP:8**	**LPF:8**
n	8	11	10	7	9
Dams (L0–L21)					
Weight loss, g	−6.2 ± 2.4	−13.5 ± 4.0	−7.7 ± 2.9	−8.0 ± 3.7 **	−7.9 ± 2.2 $$$
Food intake, g.d^{-1}	43.3 ± 1.5	50.7 ± 1.0 ***	57.4 ± 1.2 $$$ £££	37.2 ± 1.3 **	37.7 ± 0.7 $$
Water intake, g.d^{-1}	49.6 ± 1.5	58.0 ± 1.4 ***	58.5 ± 2.0 $$	30.3 ± 1.5 ***	29.1 ± 1.1 $$$
Pup growth (L11–L18)					
Litter growth rate, g.d^{-1}	22.9 ± 0.7	27.6 ± 0.7 ***	30.1 ± 0.8 $$$ £	10.3 ± 0.6 ***	10.0 ± 0.3 $$$
Pups growth rate, g.d^{-1}	2.86 ± 0.09	2.30 ± 0.06 ***	2.51 ± 0.06 $$ ▪	1.31 ± 0.08 ***	1.25 ± 0.04 $$$
Milk flow (L11–L18)					
Total milk production, g.d^{-1}	46.0 ± 1.6	54.3 ± 2.8 *	63.0 ± 3.1 $$$ £	25.9 ± 1.3 ***	26.6 ± 1.2 $$$
Pups milk consumption, g.d^{-1}	5.74 ± 0.20	4.52 ± 0.23 ***	5.25 ± 0.25 ▪	3.24 ± 0.16 ***	3.32 ± 0.16 $$$

NP:8, 20% protein diet with 8 pups per litter; NP:12, 20% protein diet with 12 pups per litter, NPF:12, 20% protein diet with fenugreek (1 g.kg BW^{-1}.d^{-1}) with 12 pups per litter, LP:8, 8% protein diet with 8 pups per litter and LPF:8, 8% protein diet with fenugreek (1g.kg BW^{-1}·day^{-1}) with 8 pups per litter. Dams and pup growth results for each individual are mean value through the indicated period (L0 to L21 or L11 to L18). The two lactation challenges (NP:12 and LP:8) were compared to NP:8 with one-way ANOVAs followed by Dunnett's post-hoc tests. * $p<0.05$, ** $p<0.01$ and *** $p<0.001$ compared to NP:8 group. Each fenugreek group (NPF:12 and LPF:8) were compared to its lactation challenge control (NP:12 or LP:8) and to NP:8 with one-way ANOVA followed by Dunnett's post-hoc test. $ $p < 0.05$, $$ $p < 0.01$, $$$ $p < 0.001$ compared to NP:8 and ▪ $p < 0.10$, £ $p < 0.05$, ££ $p < 0.01$, £££ $p < 0.001$ compared to challenge model control.

3.2. Lactation Challenges Impact both Physiological Characteristics of Dam and Litter Compared to the Control Group NP:8

As no global sex effect was observed for pups' growth and milk flow variables, results from the female and male offspring were pooled. Except for weight at delivery (similar for all groups, mean of 348.4 ± 5.2 g), every variable characterizing lactating dams, pups' growth and milk flow was significantly affected by both lactation challenges (Table 1).

In the litter size increase challenge, dam's weight loss during the entire lactation period was similar between NP:8 and NP:12 dams. Food and water intakes of lactating dams increased significantly (+17%) in NP:12, compared with the NP:8 group. Similarly, the litter growth rate between L11 and L18 was significantly increased (+21%). The increase of litter size led to extra-uterine growth restriction

(EUGR) in the offspring during the lactation period since pup growth rate was 20% lower in NP:12, compared to the NP:8 litters. The enhancement in milk production with larger litter size remained insufficient to cope with increased demand: although total milk production of NP:12 dams was 18% greater than for NP:8 dams ($p = 0.029$), NP:12 pups' milk consumption was 21% lower than in NP:8 pups ($p < 0.001$).

In the maternal protein restriction challenge, dam's weight loss during the entire lactation period was 4.6-fold greater for LP:8 than for the NP:8 ($p = 0.002$) group. Food and water intakes of lactating dams were significantly decreased for LP:8 dams compared to NP:8 dams (−14% and −40%, respectively). Similarly, litter and pup growth rates were significantly decreased (−53%) in LP:8 pups, confirming EUGR occurred in response to maternal protein restriction. The maternal dietary protein restriction challenge was very effective since both values of total milk production, and milk consumption by pups was much lower for the LP:8 group than for the NP:8 group (−44%).

3.3. Correlation between Milk Flow Variables, Pups' Growth Variables, and Lactating Dams' Intakes Variables

Pearson's correlations were calculated between milk flow variables and lactating dam's intakes or pup's growth variables. Total milk production was strongly correlated with litter growth rate (Figure 3a), dams' food ($r = 0.86$, $p < 0.001$) and water ($r = 0.93$, $p < 0.001$) intakes. Similarly, pups milk consumption was strongly correlated with pup growth rate (Figure 3b).

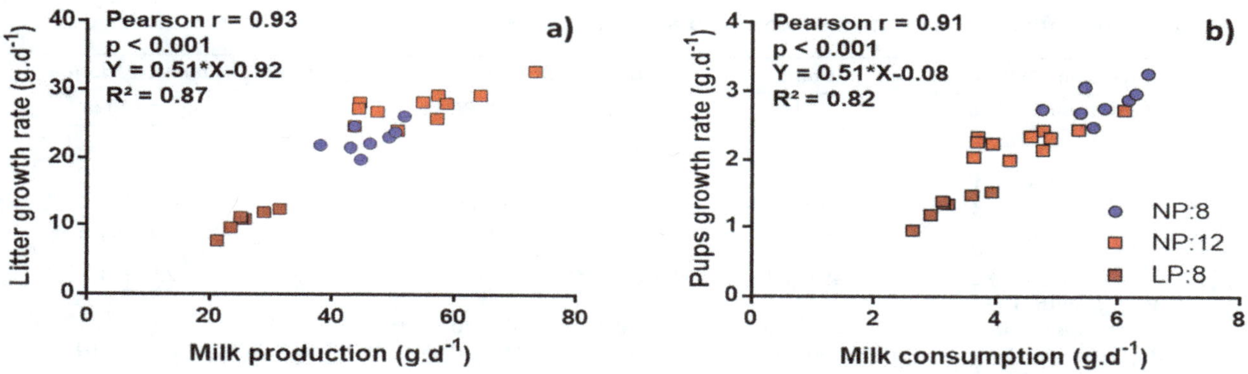

Figure 3. Correlation between pup growth and milk flow variables in three different conditions of lactation physiology (NP:8, NP:12, and LP:8). (**a**) Correlation between total milk production and litter growth rate from L11 to L18. (**b**) Correlation between pup milk consumption and pup growth rate from L11 toL18. NP:8, 20% protein diet with 8 pups per litter; NP:12, 20% protein diet with 12 pups per litter, and LP:8 groups, 8% protein diet with 8 pups per litter.

3.4. Determination of Galactologue Effect of Fenugreek in Two Models of Lactation Challenges

Fenugreek intake was close to 1 g.kg $BW^{-1}.d^{-1}$ for both supplemented groups (i.e., 1.01 ± 0.02 g.kg $BW^{-1}.d^{-1}$ for NPF:12 dams and 0.93 ± 0.02 g.kg $BW^{-1}.day^{-1}$ for LPF:8 dams), but consumption was 7.8% higher in the NPF:12 group than in LPF:8 group ($p = 0.018$). Trigonelline was measured in the diet as a marker of fenugreek content, and was 12.5 μg.kg^{-1} and 14.9 μg.kg^{-1} for the NPF:12 and LPF:8 diet, respectively (SD1), leading to a slightly higher trigonelline intake for NPF:12 (1.99 ± 0.05 mg.kg $BW^{-1}.day^{-1}$) than LPF:8 dams (1.73 ± 0.04 mg.kg $BW^{-1}.day^{-1}$).

In the litter size increase challenge, no significant difference was observed for NPF:12 dams on delivery weight (367.0 ± 11.1 g, $p = 0.28$), weight loss, or water intake during lactation when compared to NP:12 dams (Table 1), although food intake was 13.1% higher in NPF:12 than NP:12 dams $p = 0.001$). However, when intake was reported to dam's body weight, the difference in food intake was no longer significant (153.8 ± 2.1 and 161.0 ± 3.6 g.$kg^{-1}.day^{-1}$, respectively). Moreover, water intake of NPF:12 dams (163.9 ± 3.7 g.$kg^{-1}.day^{-1}$) became significantly lower compared to NP:12

dams (175.8 ± 4.2 g.kg^{-1}.d^{-1}, $p = 0.045$), but was still significantly higher compared to NP:8 dams (146.8 ± 2.2 g.kg^{-1}.day^{-1}, $p = 0.008$).

In this challenge, fenugreek promoted pup growth when comparing NPF:12 and NP:12 groups (Figure 4a). This significant difference was observed from L12 ($p = 0.022$) to L18 ($p = 0.002$). However, NPF:12 pups failed to reach the growth observed in NP:8 pups. The final weight gain of NPF:12 pups was increased by 10.6% compared to NP:12 pups but was 12.2% lower compared to NP:8 pups (Figure 4b).

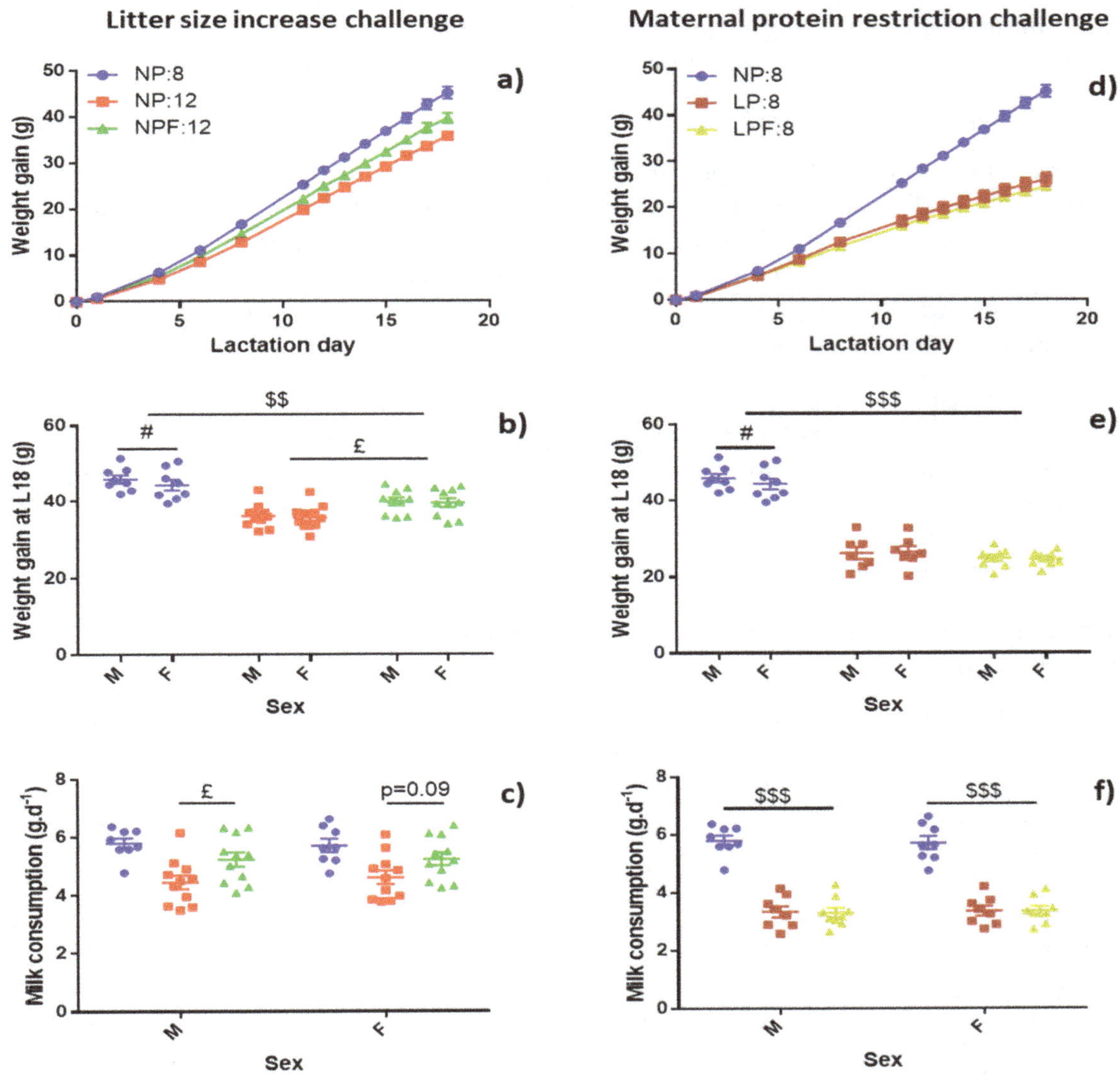

Figure 4. Effect of fenugreek on pup growth and pup milk consumption in 2 models of lactation challenges by litter size increase (**a**,**b**,**c**) or by maternal protein restriction (**d**,**e**,**f**). Weight gain during lactation was represented in graphs (**a**) and (**d**). Values were mean of male and female pups' weight gain. Final weight gain at L18 was represented in graphs (**b**) and (**e**) and pup milk consumption was represented in graphs (**c**) and (**f**) for both males (M) and females (F). Results were analysed with two-way ANOVAs with group and day factors for graphs (**a**) and (**d**) and with group and sex factors for other graphs. Pairwise comparisons were realised with Dunnett's post-hoc test to compare fenugreek supplemented groups to their challenge control and NP:8 and with Sidak's *post-hoc* tests for sex factors. £ $p < 0.05$ represented the significant difference between NPF:12 or LPF:8 and their own lactation challenge model control. $$ $p < 0.01$ and $$$ $p < 0.001$ represented the significant difference with NPF:12 or LPF:8 and NP:8. # $p < 0.05$ represented the significant difference between male and female pups.

Fenugreek promoted milk flow: total milk production was 16.1% higher in NPF:12 dams (63.0 ± 3.1 g.day^{-1}), compared with NP:12 dams ($p = 0.048$) (Table 1). Milk consumption per pup also tended to be higher ($p = 0.059$) with a greater increase for males (+17.7%, $p = 0.028$) than females (+13.8%, $p = 0.088$), although no overall sex effect was observed (Figure 4c).

In the maternal protein restriction challenge, fenugreek had no effect on dam's weight loss during lactation, nor on water and food intakes when comparing with the non-supplemented group LP:8. No significant difference was also observed for pup growth between LPF:8 and LP:8 groups neither for growth rate (Table 1), nor for weight gain during overall lactation or at a specific day (Figure 4d,e). Fenugreek had no effect on milk production (Table 1) and pups milk consumption (Figure 4f).

3.5. Fenugreek Enhances Milk Lactose and Trigonelline Content in the Litter Size Increase Challenge

In the litter size increase challenge, milk composition was similar between the NP:8 and NP:12 groups. Fenugreek had no effect on milk fatty acids (FAs), protein, and energy content, but led to a 27% increase in lactose concentration compared to NP:12 (Table 2). Every macronutrient flow was significantly increased in the NPF:12 group compared to the NP:12 group (+29.6%, +49.1%, and +28.9% for protein, lactose and FAs, respectively), leading to a 30.5% increase in energy flow for the NPF:12 group, while no difference was observed between the NP:12 and NP:8 groups.

The maternal protein restriction challenge had no significant effect on lactose and FAs concentrations and energy of milk but resulted in a significant 16% decrease in protein concentration (LP:8 vs. NP:8). Flow was significantly decreased for every macronutrient and for energy in the LP:8 group compared to NP:8 (−52.8%, −51.1%, −34.0%, and −38.9% for protein, lactose, FAs, and energy, respectively). Fenugreek failed to induce a modification in macronutrient composition or energy (in concentration and in flow) between LPF:8 and LP:8 milk.

Table 2. Effect of fenugreek on energy and macronutrient composition of milk and on energy and macronutrient flows.

Lactation Challenges	**Control**	**Litter Size Increase**		**Maternal Protein Restriction**	
Experimental Groups	**NP:8**	**NP:12**	**NPF:12**	**LP:8**	**LPF:8**
n	**7**	**8**	**9**	**7**	**9**
Macronutrient concentration, g.L^{-1}					
Protein	97.1 ± 4.9	91.7 ± 1.5	98.3 ± 3.3	81.5 ± 2.2 **	77.4 ± 2.1 $$$
Lactose	30.1 ± 1.9	29.4 ± 1.2	37.4 ± 0.9 $$ £££	27.4 ± 1.3	25.3 ± 1.1
Fatty acids	147.1 ± 12.8	129.4 ± 6.6	137.8 ± 7.2	174.3 ± 13.6	176.5 ± 9.2
Energy, kcal.dL^{-1}	183.2 ± 12.0	165.1 ± 5.5	178.3 ± 6.9	200.4 ± 11.7	199.9 ± 8.8
Macronutrient flow, g.day^{-1}					
Protein	4.49 ± 0.32	4.87 ± 0.26	6.31 ± 0.41 $$ £	2.12 ± 0.12 ***	2.06 ± 0.12 $$$
Lactose	1.38 ± 0.09	1.60 ± 0.12	2.38 ± 0.10 $$$ £££	0.71 ± 0.04 ***	0.68 ± 0.06 $$$
Fatty acids	6.79 ± 0.66	6.81 ± 0.31	8.78 ± 0.53 $ £	4.48 ± 0.34 *	4.72 ± 0.42 $
Energy flow, kcal.day^{-1}	84.6 ± 6.6	87.2 ± 4.0	113.8 ± 6.2 $$ ££	51.6 ± 3.0 ***	± 4.4 $$$

Values were mean ± SEM and were analysed by one-way ANOVA followed by a Tukey post-hoc test to compare all groups of each lactation challenge. * $p < 0.05$, ** $p < 0.01$, *** $p < 0.001$ represented significant differences between NP:12 or LP:8 and NP:8. £ $p < 0.05$, ££ $p < 0.01$, £££ $p < 0.001$ represented significant differences between NPF:12 or LPF:8 and their own lactation challenge control.$ $p < 0.05$, $$ $p < 0.01$, $$$ $p < 0.001$ represented significant differences between NPF:12 or LPF:8 and NP:8.

Trigonelline concentration was measured in milk at L18 as a marker of fenugreek content. NPF:12 milk had a trigonelline concentration 17.1-fold higher than NP:12 milk (2575.6 ± 132.9 nM and 150.3 ± 22.9 nM, respectively, $p < 0.001$). Similarly, LPF:8 milk had a significant 5-fold increased trigonelline concentration compared to LP:8 milk (2683.2 ± 141.9 nM and 533.7 ± 118.2 nM respectively, $p < 0.001$).

3.6. *Effect of Fenugreek on Metabolic Status of Dams and Offspring at Short and Long Term for the Litter Size Increase Challenge*

As fenugreek had a positive effect on milk production and quality only in the litter size increase lactation challenge, the metabolic status of dams and offspring was assessed exclusively in the NP:8, NP:12, and NPF:12 groups.

Dams' metabolic parameters were determined in plasma sampled at L12 without a fasting period and at L21 after a 4 h-fasting period (Table 3). Milk cholesterol, triglycerides (TGs), and glucose concentrations rose significantly between L12 (mid lactation) and L21 (end of lactation). A larger rise in cholesterol was observed in the NPF:12 group (+20,7%, $p < 0.001$) compared to the NP:12 group (+5%), but no significant difference was observed between the NPF:12 and NP:12 groups, at both days of lactation. Insulin concentration was significantly lower in the NPF:12 group than in NP:12 group (−42.4%, $p = 0{,}018$) transitory at L12, but no significant difference was observed between the NPF:12 group and NP:8 group.

Table 3. Effect of fenugreek on metabolic parameters in dams' plasma at L12 and L21 in the litter size increase lactation challenges.

Parameter	Groups			Two-Way ANOVA		
	NP:8	NP:12	NPF:12	Global Effects		
n	8	11	11	Inter	Group	Day
Cholesterol, mg.dL^{-1}						
L12	101.3 ± 6.0 ^{a,1}	94.6 ± 3.9 ^{a,1}	92.2 ± 3.8 ^{a,1}	0.050	0.57	0.002
L21	105.8 ± 5.6 ^{a,1}	99.2 ± 4.1 ^{a,1}	111.3 ± 6.9 ^{a,2}			
Triglycerides, mg.dL^{-1}						
L12	54.6 ± 7.0 ^{a,1}	43.5 ± 2.8 ^{a,1}	52.8 ± 5.2 ^{a,1}	0.027	0.062	<0.001
L21	132.0 ± 16.6 ^{a,2}	189.9 ± 25.1 ^{ab,2}	224.3 ± 23.7 ^{b,2}			
Glucose, mg.dL^{-1}						
L12	125.1 ± 6.4 ^{a,1}	120.6 ± 3.7 ^{a,1}	117.4 ± 3.7 ^{a,1}	0.72	0.62	<0.001
L21	148.0 ± 3.1 ^{a,2}	150.7 ± 6.5 ^{a,2}	144.7 ± 6.2 ^{a,2}			
Insulin, ng.mL^{-1}						
L12	0.60 ± 0.09 ^{a,1}	1.65 ± 0.25 ^{b,1}	0.95 ± 0.26 ^{a,1}	0.12	0.004	0.22
L21	0.68 ± 0.06 ^{a,1}	0.98 ± 0.09 ^{a,2}	0.94 ± 0.15 ^{a,1}			

Values were mean ± SE and were analysed with two-way ANOVA with group and day factors and with repeated values for day factor. ANOVA was followed by Tuckey's post-hoc test for comparisons between groups and by Sidak's post-hoc test for comparisons between days. For each biomarker, different letters represented significant differences ($p < 0.05$) between groups at each day and the difference between numbers represented significant difference ($p < 0.05$) between days for each group.

As expected, trigonelline content was largely increased at L12 in NPF:12 dams' plasma compared to NP:12 (3258.7 ± 200.4 nM and 464.3 ± 78.5 nM respectively, $p < 0.001$).

Offspring's metabolism was determined in the short (PND20) and long-term (PND60) when pups reached early adulthood. Selected plasma parameters of lipid and glucose metabolism are presented in Table 4. At PND 20, lactation challenge by litter size increase did not affect cholesterol, TGs, or insulin concentration in offspring's plasma, whereas it tended to increase glucose concentration (+7.5%, $p = 0.052$) in the NP:12 group vs. the NP:8 group. At PND 60, it tended to a decrease TGs concentration (−17.8%, $p = 0.10$) mainly for males (−21.7%, $p = 0.047$). Fenugreek had no effect on glucose, insulin, and TGs concentration although, at PND 20, a significant decrease in plasma cholesterol concentration was observed in the NPF:12 group compared to the NP:12 group (−10.0%, $p = 0.024$), greater for female (−11.8%) than for male (−8.1%). Fenugreek no longer had any effect on cholesterol concentration at PND 60.

Table 4. Effect of fenugreek on offspring's metabolism in the short and long term.

Parameter	Groups			Two-way ANOVA		
	NP:8	NP:12	NPF:12	Global Effects		
		PND 20		Inter	Group	Sex
n for each sex	8	22	11			
Cholesterol, mg.dL^{-1}						
Male	143.2 ± 10.1 ^{a,1}	144.5 ± 3.9 ^{a,1}	132.8 ± 3.0 ^{a,1}	0.225	0.005	0.039
Female	167.5 ± 12.4 ^{a,1}	151.5 ± 4.1 ^{a,b,1}	133.5 ± 6.1 ^{b,1}			
Triglycerides, mg.dL^{-1}						
Male	260.2 ± 39.2 ^{a,1}	272.0 ± 21.1 ^{a,1}	258.8 ± 56.3 ^{a,1}	0.853	0.763	0.969
Female	284.5 ± 46.1 ^{a,1}	267.8 ± 23.3 ^{a,1}	235.0 ± 35.9 ^{a,1}			
Glucose, mg.dL^{-1}						
Male	157.1 ± 7.4 ^{a,1}	164.4 ± 3.8 ^{a,1}	164.5 ± 3.5 ^{a,1}	0.446	0.055	0.655
Female	152.7 ± 3.7 ^{a,1}	168 ± 3.0 ^{a,1}	159.7 ± 3.5 ^{a,1}			
Insulin, ng.mL^{-1}						
Male	0.19 ± 0.04 ^{a,1}	0.35 ± 0.05 ^{a,1}	0.41 ± 0.09 ^{a,1}	0.958	0.037	0.282
Female	0.28 ± 0.04 ^{a,1}	0.41 ± 0.05 ^{a,1}	0.46 ± 0.07 ^{a,1}			
		PND 60				
n for each sex	10	22	16			
Cholesterol, mg.dL^{-1}						
Male	76.8 ± 2.5 ^{a,1}	85.0 ± 2.5 ^{a,1}	81.5 ± 2.1 ^{a,1}	0.433	0.208	0.170
Female	84.8 ± 3.1 ^{a,1}	85.7 ± 2.6 ^{a,1}	82.3 ± 3.0 ^{a,1}			
Triglycerides, mg.dL^{-1}						
Male	135.8 ± 11.7 ^{a,1}	106.4 ± 7.0 ^{b,1}	123.2 ± 12.0 ^{ab,1}	0.390	0.095	<0.001
Female	66.0 ± 3.7 ^{a,2}	59.5 ± 5.2 ^{a,2}	64.1 ± 6.3 ^{a,2}			

Values were mean ± SE and were analysed with two-way ANOVA with group and sex factors followed by Tukey's post-hoc test for comparisons between groups and by Sidak's *post-hoc* test for comparisons between sexes. For each biomarker, different letters represented significant ($p < 0.05$) differences between groups for each sex and different numbers represented significant differences ($p < 0.05$) between sexes for each group.

Long-term glucose metabolism was assessed in offspring by OGTT only for NP:12 and NPF:12 groups (Figure 5). Before oral glucose gavage (T0), no significant difference was observed between NPF:12 and NP:12 groups for plasma glucose and insulin concentrations, but females had significantly lower concentrations than males (−25.0%, $p = 0.014$), greater in the NPF:12 group (−37.1%, $p = 0.064$) than in the NP:12 group (−17.4%, $p = 0.33$). After oral glucose gavage, no difference was observed in glycaemia neither between sexes nor between groups (Figure 5a,b). Fenugreek decreased the insulin area under curve (AUC) in NPF:12 compared to the NP:12 group (−38.4%, $p = 0.004$) (Figure 5d) and this difference was greater for females (−60%, $p = 0.044$) than for males (−29.7%, $p = 0.094$). Insulin peak was delayed in the NPF:12 (30 min) group compared to the NP:12 group (15 min) (Figure 5c).

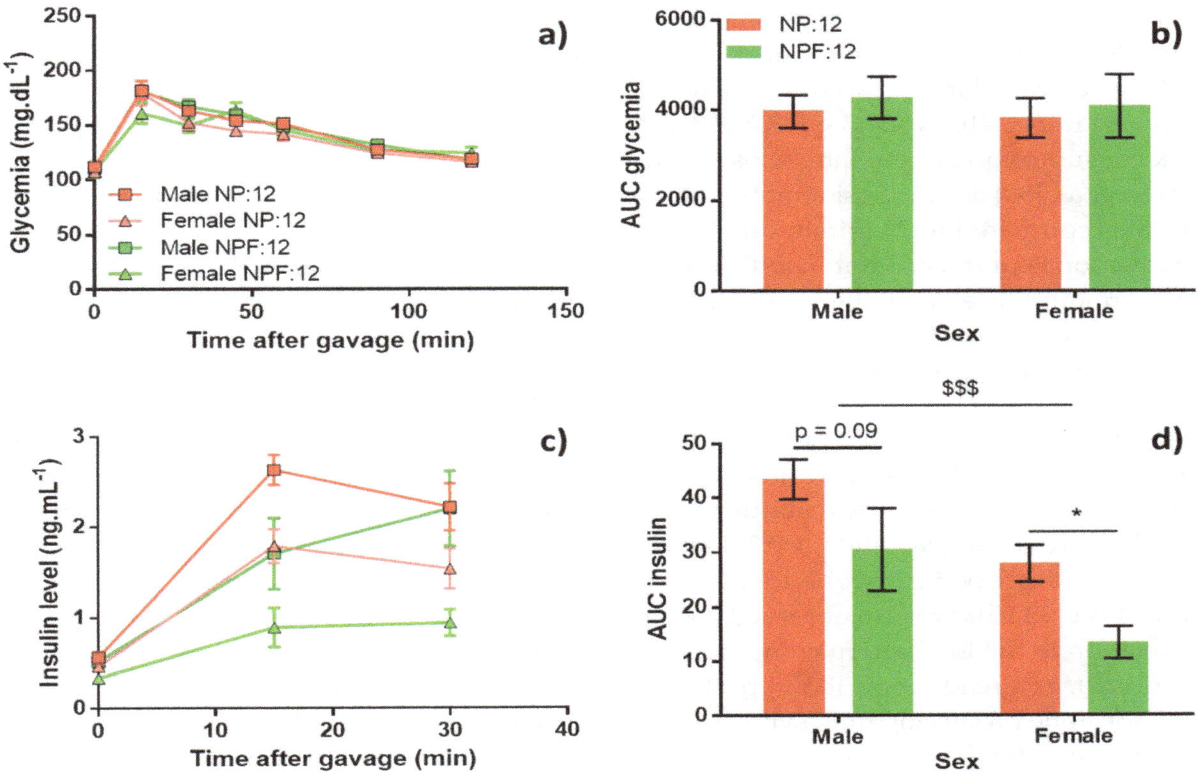

Figure 5. Effect of fenugreek on long-term glucose metabolism assessed by oral glucose tolerance test for NP:12 and NPF:12 groups. At PND 60, after 6 h fasting, 2 g.kg^{-1} of glucose was injected to rats by gavage. (**a**) Time course of glycaemia after glucose gavage; (**b**) area under curve (AUC) of glycaemia; (**c**) time course of insulin concentration after glucose gavage; (**d**) AUC of insulin concentration. For NP:12, $n = 12$ per sex and for NPF:12, $n = 8$ per sex. Values were mean ± SEM and were analysed with two-way ANOVA with group and sex factors followed by Sidak's post-hoc test. $$$ $p < 0.001$ represents significant difference between sexes and * $p < 0.05$ represents significant difference between groups.

4. Discussion

To the best of our knowledge, this study is the first to explore the effect of fenugreek on milk production in a rat model. The effect on milk production, measured using stable isotope labelled water, was assessed in two separate models of lactation challenge: (a) litter size increase from 8 to 12 pups, and (b) maternal, perinatal dietary protein restriction (from 20% to 8%). We found that when dams were under appropriate physiological conditions for lactation and confronted with a litter size increase, fenugreek produced an increase in milk flow. In contrast, when dams were placed under inappropriate physiological conditions of lactation following dietary protein restriction, fenugreek was ineffective.

4.1. Effect of Lactation Challenges on Pup Growth and Milk Production

First, we verified that litter size increase and maternal, perinatal protein restriction both led to a decrease in milk consumption by the pups, resulting in Extra-Uterine Growth restriction (EUGR), confirming that dams had difficulties producing milk sufficiently to meet the demand.

When litter size was increased from 8 to 12 pups, dams adjusted their milk production, suggesting dams' adaptations to the increased demand from pups. Indeed, the litter size increase led to a 21% increase in litter growth rate, along with an 18% increase in milk flow. These results are in accordance with those from Morag et al. [23] and Kumaresan et al. [30] who reported a 43% and 22% increase of milk yield, measured by weight-suckle weight method, for a litter size increase from 9 or 8 pups to 12 pups, respectively. However, this rise of milk production was not sufficient to compensate the litter size increase, resulting in EUGR with a 26% lower overall pup weight gain, presumably due to a 21% decrease in milk consumption per pup. Kumaresan et al. [30] found similar results, with a 20% decrease in milk availability per pup at L14 when litter size was increased from 8 to 12 pups, and an 11% decreased in pup weight at L18 (31.1 g for 8 pups to 27.6 g for 12 pups) compared to the 18% decrease in our study (52.3 g for NP:8 and 42.9 g for NP:12 at L18). Our values of pup growth and milk consumption are probably closer to physiological values than those of Morag et al. [23] and Kumaresan et al. [30] as we considerably reduced the stress of dam/pup separation (from 8 h to 10 h in these studies compared to 30 min in ours). These conditions in which the dams' capacity to increase milk production is preserved but insufficiently to produce optimal pup growth, as observed in a litter of 12 or more pups, are likely the most suitable to test the effect of a galactologue compound [23,30].

In the other lactation challenge (maternal dietary protein restriction), we confirmed that 8% perinatal protein restriction led to an EUGR due to an impaired ability of dams to produce milk. This challenge led to a 44% reduced milk flow, confirming data from our earlier studies [22], and resulted in impaired pup growth with a 42% decrease in pup weight gain at L18 (as already observed by Bautista et al. [25] and Martin-Agnoux et al. [31]). The impaired ability of mothers to produce milk suggests the dams' physiological status was impaired due to undernutrition during gestation and lactation. Indeed, during lactation, LP:8 dams exhibited a 4.5-fold greater weight loss than NP:8 dams, which is a well-described consequence of nitrogen store depletion on milk-protein synthesis in states of malnutrition [32,33]. We also observed a significant 36% reduction in mammary gland weight at the end of lactation in the LP:8 group compared to the NP:8 group (5.73 ± 0.67 g for NP:8 vs. 3.67 ± 0.75g for LP:8 dams), as already reported in protein-restricted dams [32]. Finally, secretion of prolactin, the principal hormone promoting milk synthesis, has been shown to decrease by 70% in the serum of dams fed a low protein diet [32]. Altogether, these physiological changes contribute to a decrease in dams' capacity to produce sufficient milk to meet the offspring requirement.

4.2. Correlation between Milk Flow, Pups' Growth, and Lactating Dams' Intakes of Food and Water

Secondly, we confirmed that the use of the water turnover method, with D_2O values as mass, reliably measures milk flow. When considering the three lactation models altogether, the changes in total milk production were strongly correlated with litter growth rate ($r = 0.93$), and changes in milk production and milk consumption accounted for at 87% and 82% of the change in growth rate in the two models tested (Figure 3). As litter or pup growth rate and milk production or consumption are expressed in the same unit (g.day^{-1}), the slopes of 0.51 with intercept close to 0 in both regression lines suggest that the consumption of 1g of milk produced a weight gain of 0.51 g per day between L11 and L18. These results are also supported by the strong correlations between milk production and the dams food and water intake ($r = 0.86$ and $r = 0.91$, respectively), representing the increasing needs of the lactating mother for milk production with large litters [33]. Altogether these results suggest that the water turnover method, with values of D_2O mass, accurately measures milk production regardless of the dam conditions.

4.3. Galactologue Effect of Fenugreek in Two Models of Lactation Challenge

In the litter size increase challenge, dietary supplementation of fenugreek at a dose of 1 g.kg^{-1}.d^{-1} increased milk flow by 16% and increased pup growth rate and final weight gain, by 9% and 11%, respectively. The galactologue effect of fenugreek is consistent with the rise in milk production observed in other mammals (+13% at a fenugreek dose of 2 g.kg^{-1}.day^{-1}in goat [18] and +18% at a fenugreek dose of 270 mg.kg^{-1}.d^{-1} in buffalo [17]). Other authors found a stronger effect of fenugreek with a 42% greater pup growth at the end of lactation in rabbit (fenugreek dose of 0.5 g.kg^{-1}.day^{-1}) [16] and a 110% increase in milk yield in ewe (fenugreek dose of 1.2 g.kg^{-1}.day^{-1}) [19]. The stronger galactologue effects in the rabbit could be explained by the fact that they only nurse their litter once a day [24], suggesting that pups have important growth with only a small milk intake. Otherwise, in ewes, fenugreek supplementation is associated with greater crud protein and energy content in the ration compared to the control group, which could also affect milk production.

In contrast, in the maternal protein restriction challenge, fenugreek failed to affect pup growth or milk production. Undernutrition likely produced profound alterations in global metabolism and mammary gland development and function that could not be reversed by a galactologue.

The mechanisms underlying the impact of fenugreek in the litter size challenge raise many questions. The reported increase in plasma prolactin and growth hormone may play an important role [17,18]. Fenugreek might also act by allowing dams to maintain their weight during lactation. Indeed, a significant correlation was found between dam mass and pup growth in rats [24]. Yet, NPF:12 dams' weight at L11 was significantly higher than NP:12 dams ($p = 0.021$) although no significant difference was observed at L0. Increased food intake in the fenugreek-supplemented group likely played a minor role in maintaining dam weight since the increased energy intake barely compensated for the increasing energy output that accounted for increased milk production. Thus, fenugreek probably promotes energy storage, which in turn could positively affect the mother's lactation performance [24]. Finally, the effect of fenugreek may be mediated by trigonelline [15]. Indeed, a 7-fold rise in dam plasma trigonelline was observed following fenugreek supplementation at 1 g.kg^{-1}.day^{-1}. Trigonelline is a precursor of niacin or nicotinic acid (B3 vitamin) involved in the formation of nicotinamide adenine dinucleotide (NAD^+) [34]. This coenzyme factor may play a key role in various metabolic pathways such as i) ATP formation, via its reduction in NADH in glycolysis, beta-oxidation, and citric acid cycle [35], ii) cell survival, as NAD^+ is the sole precursor of PARP, a DNA repair enzyme, and iii) transcriptional regulation as it is a main cofactor of sirtuins [36]. Thus, in the mammary gland, an increase in trigonelline could increase NAD^+ content, and thus, enhance lactation by promoting energy supply for milk synthesis, as well as mammary cell longevity and function.

4.4. *Effect of Fenugreek on Milk Composition*

A separate collection of milk secreted at the beginning and at the end of each suckling is not feasible. Milk composition was assessed at L18, which corresponds to the end of the lactation period in the rat. As rat milk composition changes during lactation [37], macronutrient composition reported at L18 may not reflect day to day variations in milk composition during the entire period during which the milk production was determined (L11–L18). As observed by earlier studies [38], the increase in litter size did not alter milk macronutrient concentration. Fenugreek increased milk lactose by 27%, whereas lipids and proteins remained unchanged. Discrepant results of fenugreek supplementation on milk macronutrient content have been reported in the literature in several animal models (rabbit, buffalo, goat, and ewe) [16–19]. However, lactose was the most affected by fenugreek, especially in our model, and its concentration is increased in most cases [16,17]. The key osmotic regulatory role of lactose on milk secretion could explain the positive effect of fenugreek on total milk production through an increase in water flow from the mammary epithelial cells into the mammary secretory vesicles and subsequently into the alveolar lumen [39].

Increasing litter size did not increase macronutrient and energy flow although milk flow was significantly increased, suggesting that the increase in milk production was offset by a dilution of macronutrients, likely due to the osmotic role of lactose. Indeed, NP:12 milk had the lower mean value of protein, fat, and energy, leading to even lower intakes for the pups. In contrast, macronutrient and energy flows were all increased when dams were supplemented with fenugreek suggesting that, with the increase in total milk production, the activity of the synthesis pathways of the three milk macronutrients was enhanced to maintain baseline concentrations. Further molecular investigations would be needed at the mammary gland level to confirm this hypothesis. In terms of pups' intake, the increase in macronutrient and energy flow led to a similar intake of the three macronutrients by the NPF:12 pups and NP:8 pups (Figure S2). As lactose concentration was increased in NPF:12 milk, the mean lactose intake by NPF:12 pups was slightly, but not significantly larger than the lactose intake in NP:8 pups. Larger lactose intake, however, did not allow NPF:12 pups to achieve the same growth rate as NP:8 pups. This suggests that lactose is not the major nutrient that promotes pup growth. Moreover, as the three macronutrients were consumed in similar amounts in both groups despite different growth trajectories, this suggests that micronutrients and/or other bioactive compounds of milk likely impact pup growth. In the maternal protein restriction model, fenugreek had no effect on milk composition. Once again, important modifications of milk composition due to maternal undernutrition [28] cannot be overcome by fenugreek.

4.5. Effect of Fenugreek on Dams Metabolism during Lactation and on Short- and Long-Term Offspring Metabolism

At mid-lactation, fenugreek did not modify dams' plasma cholesterol, triglycerides, and glucose concentrations as previously found in ewe [19] or in goat [21], suggesting that fenugreek did not alter maternal blood metabolic biomarkers during lactation. However, plasma insulin concentration was significantly increased in the NP:12 group and returned near to the baseline level in the NPF:12 group. Among metabolic adaptations reported during lactation, mammary gland displays enhanced insulin sensitivity while other tissues developed insulin resistance, leading to a redirection of energy substrates toward the mammary gland [40]. These changes result in a decrease in plasma insulin concentration, which is inversely related to milk production [41] and is consistent with the increased milk production and lower insulin concentration observed in NPF:12 dams at L12.

Contrary to the overall lactation period, the suckling phase leads to a rise in plasma insulin concentration [41,42]. Yet, plasma was sampled just after dam/pup separation, and pups were allowed to suckle until separation. The greater number of pups in NP:12 litters compared to NP:8 litters probably led to greater suckling, explaining the greater dams' insulin level observed. All these results in insulin must be relativized, knowing that at L12, dams' plasma was sampled without a fasting period.

At the end of the lactation period, both cholesterol and triglycerides were greatly increased in NPF:12 than in NP:12 dams' plasma compared to mid-lactation, which could be explained by the higher milk production of NPF:12 dams. Indeed, during lactation, the mammary gland becomes the main site of lipogenesis with a rate 5-fold higher than in liver [33], which in contrast, increases its hepatic cholesterol synthetic activity [43] and in detriment of adipose tissue, which exhibits an increased lipolytic activity [33]. These changes are associated with a large rise in triglyceride and cholesterol uptake from circulating chylomicrons in the mammary gland thanks to the increased activity of prolactin-mediated lipoprotein lipase (LPL) [44]. At the end of lactation, the prolactin-mediated LPL activity in the mammary gland drops rapidly [43], although lipolytic activity in adipose tissues and cholesterol synthesis in liver persist for a while. This leads to higher plasma triglyceride [43] and cholesterol concentration, which could presumably be further increased when milk production is enhanced. This would be consistent with the differences observed in NP:12 and NPF:12 plasma and with the larger rise in plasma triglyceride concentration in NP:12 dams compared to NP:8 dams.

Finally, the current study was the first to demonstrate the absence of adverse effects of dams' fenugreek supplementation on offspring metabolism. In the short-term, only cholesterol plasma concentration was decreased by fenugreek supplementation. Fenugreek is known to have a hypocholesterolemic effect that has been attributed to the large amount of fibre in fenugreek seed [45], or to steroid saponin such as diosgenin [15]. The effect of fenugreek on plasma cholesterol concentration of the offspring in the short-term may be mediated by the consumption of these components in milk. Indeed, milk trigonelline concentration increased 17-fold upon maternal supplementation, implying many components of fenugreek appear in mothers' milk. Alternatively, as pups begin to eat dams' pellet food at the end of lactation, the hypocholesterolemic effect of fenugreek might be directly mediated by solid food consumption. When fenugreek consumption stopped at L20, cholesterol concentration became indistinguishable from those of control offspring at PND 60, suggesting only a short-term hypocholesterolemic effect of fenugreek.

In the long run, no difference was observed between NPF:12 and NP:12 offspring in glucose concentration after glucose gavage, although NPF:12 offspring had lower concentrations of insulin with a delayed peak. Although a delayed peak of insulin is generally associated with insulin resistance [46], it is often related to an increased glucose concentration and area-under-curve, which is not the case in our study. Conversely, the decrease in insulin area under curve could reflect greater insulin sensitivity, and fenugreek is known to have antidiabetic properties [15], notably via the action of trigonelline [47]. The increased consumption of milk trigonelline by pups during lactation may help them to develop higher insulin sensitivity in the short-term and thus favour long-term glucose metabolism. However, despite the apparent absence of metabolic alterations, fenugreek should not be consumed by women with asthma, digestive disorders, hypertension, heart cardiovascular disease, or hypothyroidism because of its possible side effects [15,48].

5. Conclusions

The current study confirms the galactologue effect of fenugreek in another mammal model, suggesting that this dietary supplement may be helpful in humans. We tested the capacity of dams' fenugreek to increase milk production and subsequent pup growth in two models of the lactation challenges. The galactologue effect of fenugreek was confirmed, but only in the challenge by litter size increase when dams had no physiological impairment in their ability to produce milk. In contrast, the lack of effect of fenugreek under maternal dietary protein restriction suggests that fenugreek cannot overcome the lactation impairment due to undernutrition. Thus, fenugreek supplementation might enhance milk production in the case of insufficient maternal milk production, due to maternal stress, difficulties in breastfeeding management, first parity, or when mothers are breastfeeding twins, but fenugreek is unlikely to be effective in situations that affect lactation physiology, such as undernutrition deficiency, mammary hypoplasia, and hormonal deregulation. Finally, we observed no adverse metabolic effect neither on the dam at mid- and end-lactation nor on offspring, with preliminary evidence that fenugreek might even enhance insulin sensitivity in the long run. The 16% increase in milk production, thanks to fenugreek, is of significance and clearly warrants the design of clinical trials in breastfeeding women

Author Contributions: Conceptualization, T.S., M.-C.A.-G., D.D. and C.-Y.B.; data curation, T.S. and C.-Y.B.; formal analysis, T.S.; funding acquisition, M.-C.A.-G., D.D. and C.-Y.B.; investigation, T.S. and B.C.; methodology, A.A. and K.O.; project administration, C.-Y.B.; resources, A.A. and P.N.; software, K.O.; supervision, M.-C.A.-G. and C.-Y.B.; writing—original draft, T.S.; writing—review and editing, T.S., M.-C.A.-G., D.D. and C.-Y.B.

Acknowledgments: The authors want to thank specifically thank Alexis Gandon (PhAN, Nantes, France), Sandrine Suzanne and Amandine Lefebvre (UTE, Nantes, France) for their precious help during all the animal experiments. We thank Isabelle Grit (PhAN, Nantes, France) for help with every metabolic analysis. Finally, we thank the Mass Spectrometry Core Facility of CNRH-O (Centre de Recherche en Nutrition Humaine Ouest) and Biogenouest, particularly the Corsaire network of analytical platforms, for their support of this project.

References

1. WHO. *Indicators for Assessing Infant and Young Child Feeding Practices: Part 1: Definitions: Conclusions of a Consensus Meeting Held 6–8 November 2007 in Washington, DC, USA*; WHO: Geneva, Switzerland, 2008.
2. Rito, A.I.; Buoncristiano, M.; Spinelli, A.; Salanave, B.; Kunešová, M.; Hejgaard, T.; García Solano, M.; Fijałkowska, A.; Sturua, L.; Hyska, J.; et al. Association between Characteristics at Birth, Breastfeeding and Obesity in 22 Countries: The WHO European Childhood Obesity Surveillance Initiative—COSI 2015/2017. *Obes. Facts* **2019**, *12*, 226–243. [CrossRef]
3. Eidelman, A.I.; Schanler, R.J. Breastfeeding and the Use of Human Milk. *Pediatrics* **2012**, *129*, e827–e841. [CrossRef]

4. Danforth, K.N.; Tworoger, S.S.; Hecht, J.L.; Rosner, B.A.; Colditz, G.A.; Hankinson, S.E. Breastfeeding and risk of ovarian cancer in two prospective cohorts. *Cancer Causes Control* **2007**, *18*, 517–523. [CrossRef] [PubMed]
5. Gunderson, E.P.; Lewis, C.E.; Lin, Y.; Sorel, M.; Gross, M.; Sidney, S.; Jacobs, D.R., Jr.; Shikany, J.M.; Quesenberry, C.P., Jr. Lactation Duration and Progression to Diabetes in Women across the Childbearing Years: The 30-Year CARDIA Study. *JAMA Intern. Med.* **2018**, *178*, 328–337. [CrossRef] [PubMed]
6. Victora, C.G.; Bahl, R.; Barros, A.J.; Franca, G.V.; Horton, S.; Krasevec, J.; Murch, S.; Sankar, M.J.; Walker, N.; Rollins, N.C.; et al. Breastfeeding in the 21st century: Epidemiology, mechanisms, and lifelong effect. *Lancet* **2016**, *387*, 475–490. [CrossRef]
7. Bonet, M.; Marchand, L.; Kaminski, M.; Fohran, A.; Betoko, A.; Charles, M.A.; Blondel, B. Breastfeeding duration, social and occupational characteristics of mothers in the French 'EDEN mother-child' cohort. *Matern. Child Health J.* **2013**, *17*, 714–722. [CrossRef] [PubMed]
8. Salanave, B.d.L.C.; Boudet-Berquier, J.; Castetbon, K. Durée de l'allaitement maternel en France (Épifane 2012–2013). *Bull. Epidémiol. Hebd.* **2014**, *27*, 450–457. [CrossRef]
9. Thulier, D.; Mercer, J. Variables associated with breastfeeding duration. *J. Obstet. Gynecol. Neonatal Nurs.* **2009**, *38*, 259–268. [CrossRef]
10. Gatti, L. Maternal perceptions of insufficient milk supply in breastfeeding. *J. Nurs. Scholarsh.* **2008**, *40*, 355–363. [CrossRef]
11. Murase, M.; Wagner, E.A.; Chantry, C.J.; Dewey, K.G.; Nommsen-Rivers, L.A. The Relation between Breast Milk Sodium to Potassium Ratio and Maternal Report of a Milk Supply Concern. *J. Pediatr.* **2017**, *181*, 294–297. [CrossRef]
12. Javan, R.; Javadi, B.; Feyzabadi, Z. Breastfeeding: A Review of Its Physiology and Galactogogue Plants in View of Traditional Persian Medicine. *Breastfeed. Med.* **2017**, *12*, 401–409. [CrossRef] [PubMed]
13. Forinash, A.B.; Yancey, A.M.; Barnes, K.N.; Myles, T.D. The use of galactogogues in the breastfeeding mother. *Ann. Pharmacother.* **2012**, *46*, 1392–1404. [CrossRef] [PubMed]
14. Abascal, K.; Yarnell, E. Botanical Galactagogues. *Altern. Complement. Ther.* **2008**, *14*, 288–294. [CrossRef]
15. Bahmani, M.; Shirzad, H.; Mirhosseini, M.; Mesripour, A.; Rafieian-Kopaei, M. A Review on Ethnobotanical and Therapeutic Uses of Fenugreek (*Trigonella foenum-graceum* L.). *J. Evid. Based Complement. Altern. Med.* **2016**, *21*, 53–62. [CrossRef] [PubMed]
16. Abdel-Rahman, H.; Fathalla, S.I.; Ezzat Assayed, M.; Ramadan Masoad, S.; Abdelaleem Nafeaa, A. Physiological Studies on the Effect of Fenugreek on Productive Performance of White New-Zealand Rabbit Does. *Food Nutr. Sci.* **2016**, *7*, 1276–1289. [CrossRef]
17. Mahgoub, A.A.S.; Sallam, M.T. Effect of Extract Crushed Fenugreek Seeds as Feed Additive on some Blood Parameters, Milk Yield and Its Composition of Lactating Egyptian Buffaloes. *J. Anim. Poult. Sci.* **2016**, *7*, 269–273. [CrossRef]
18. Alamer, M.A.; Basiouni, G.F. Feeding effect of Fenugreek seed (*Trigonella foenum-graecum* L.) on lactation performance, some plasma constituent and growth hormone level in goats. *Pak. J. Biol. Sci.* **2005**, *8*, 1553–1556.
19. Al-Sherwany, D.A.O. Feeding effects of fenugreek seeds on intake, milk yield, chemical composition of milk and some biochemical parameters in Hamdani ewes. *Al-Anbar J. Vet. Sci.* **2015**, *8*, 49–54.
20. Eiben, C.; Rashwan, A.; Kustos, K.; Gódor-Surmann, K.; Szendrő, Z. Effect of Anise and Fenugreek supplementation on performance of rabbit does. In Proceedings of the 8th World Rabbit Congress, Puebla, Mexico, 7–10 September 2004.
21. Al-Shaikh, M.A.; Al-Mufarrej, S.I.; Mogawer, H.H. Effect of Fenugreek Seeds (*Trigonella foenumgraecum* L.) on Lactational Performance of Dairy Goat. *J. Appl. Anim. Res.* **1999**, *16*, 177–183. [CrossRef]
22. Sevrin, T.; Alexandre-Gouabau, M.C.; Darmaun, D.; Palvadeau, A.; Andre, A.; Nguyen, P.; Ouguerram, K.; Boquien, C.Y. Use of water turnover method to measure mother's milk flow in a rat model: Application to dams receiving a low protein diet during gestation and lactation. *PLoS ONE* **2017**, *12*, e0180550. [CrossRef]
23. Morag, M.; Popliker, F.; Yagil, R. Effect of litter size on milk yield in the rat. *Lab. Anim.* **1975**, *9*, 43–47. [CrossRef] [PubMed]
24. Rodel, H.G.; Prager, G.; Stefanski, V.; von Holst, D.; Hudson, R. Separating maternal and litter-size effects on early postnatal growth in two species of altricial small mammals. *Physiol. Behav.* **2008**, *93*, 826–834. [CrossRef] [PubMed]

25. Bautista, C.J.; Boeck, L.; Larrea, F.; Nathanielsz, P.W.; Zambrano, E. Effects of a maternal low protein isocaloric diet on milk leptin and progeny serum leptin concentration and appetitive behavior in the first 21 days of neonatal life in the rat. *Pediatr. Res.* **2008**, *63*, 358–363. [CrossRef] [PubMed]
26. Reeves, P.G.; Nielsen, F.H.; Fahey, G.C., Jr. AIN-93 purified diets for laboratory rodents: Final report of the American Institute of Nutrition ad hoc writing committee on the reformulation of the AIN-76A rodent diet. *J. Nutr.* **1993**, *123*, 1939–1951. [CrossRef] [PubMed]
27. Osowska, S.; Duchemann, T.; Walrand, S.; Paillard, A.; Boirie, Y.; Cynober, L.; Moinard, C. Citrulline modulates muscle protein metabolism in old malnourished rats. *Am. J. Physiol. Endocrinol. Metab.* **2006**, *291*, E582–E586. [CrossRef] [PubMed]
28. Martin Agnoux, A.; Antignac, J.P.; Boquien, C.Y.; David, A.; Desnots, E.; Ferchaud-Roucher, V.; Darmaun, D.; Parnet, P.; Alexandre-Gouabau, M.C. Perinatal protein restriction affects milk free amino acid and fatty acid profile in lactating rats: Potential role on pup growth and metabolic status. *J. Nutr. Biochem.* **2015**, *26*, 784–795. [CrossRef]
29. Von Dreele, M.M. Age-related changes in body fluid volumes in young spontaneously hypertensive rats. *Am. J. Physiol. Ren. Physiol.* **1988**, *255*, F953–F956. [CrossRef]
30. Kumaresan, P.; Anderson, R.R.; Turner, C.W. Effect of litter size upon milk yield and litter weight gains in rats. *Rev. Tuberc. Pneumol.* **1966**, *30*, 41–45. [CrossRef]
31. Martin Agnoux, A.; Alexandre-Gouabau, M.C.; Le Drean, G.; Antignac, J.P.; Parnet, P. Relative contribution of foetal and post-natal nutritional periods on feeding regulation in adult rats. *Acta Physiol.* **2014**, *210*, 188–201. [CrossRef]
32. Moretto, V.L.; Ballen, M.O.; Gonçalves, T.S.S.; Kawashita, N.H.; Stoppiglia, L.F.; Veloso, R.V.; Latorraca, M.Q.; Martins, M.S.F.; Gomes-da-Silva, M.H.G. Low-Protein Diet during Lactation and Maternal Metabolism in Rats. *ISRN Obstet. Gynecol.* **2011**, *2011*, 876502. [CrossRef]
33. Williamson, D.H. Integration of metabolism in tissues of the lactating rat. *FEBS Lett.* **1980**, *117*, K93–K105. [CrossRef]
34. Mehrafarin, A.; Qaderi, A.; Rezazadeh, S.; Naghdi Badi, H.; Noormohammadi, G.; Zand, E. Bioengineering of important secondary metabolites and metabolic pathways in fenugreek (*Trigonella foenum-graecum* L.). *J. Med. Plants* **2010**, *3*, 1–18.
35. Stein, L.R.; Imai, S.-i. The dynamic regulation of NAD metabolism in mitochondria. *Trends Endocrinol. Metab.* **2012**, *23*, 420–428. [CrossRef] [PubMed]
36. Braidy, N.; Poljak, A.; Grant, R.; Jayasena, T.; Mansour, H.; Chan-Ling, T.; Guillemin, G.; Smythe, G.; Sachdev, P. Mapping NAD+ metabolism in the brain of ageing Wistar rats: Potential targets for influencing brain senescence. *Biogerontology* **2013**, *15*, 177–198. [CrossRef] [PubMed]
37. Nicholas, K.R.; Hartmann, P.E. Milk secretion in the rat: Progressive changes in milk composition during lactation and weaning and the effect of diet. *Comp. Biochem. Physiol. Part A Physiol.* **1991**, *98*, 535–542. [CrossRef]
38. Fiorotto, M.L.; Burrin, D.G.; Perez, M.; Reeds, P.J. Intake and use of milk nutrients by rat pups suckled in small, medium, or large litters. *Am. J. Physiol.* **1991**, *260*, R1104–R1113. [CrossRef]
39. Bleck, G.T.; White, B.R.; Miller, D.J.; Wheeler, M.B. Production of bovine α-lactalbumin in the milk of transgenic pigs1. *J. Anim. Sci.* **1998**, *76*, 3072–3078. [CrossRef]
40. Jones, R.G.; Ilic, V.; Williamson, D.H. Physiological significance of altered insulin metabolism in the conscious rat during lactation. *Biochem. J.* **1984**, *220*, 455–460. [CrossRef]
41. Widström, A.M.; Winberg, J.; Werner, S.; Hamberger, B.; Eneroth, P.; Uvnäs-Moberg, K. Suckling in lactating women stimulates the secretion of insulin and prolactin without concomitant effects on gastrin, growth hormone, calcitonin, vasopressin or catecholamines. *Early Hum. Dev.* **1984**, *10*, 115–122. [CrossRef]
42. Eriksson, M.; Lindén, A.; Uvnäs-Moberg, K. Suckling increases insulin and glucagon levels in peripheral venous blood of lactating dogs. *Acta Physiol. Scand.* **1987**, *131*, 391–396. [CrossRef]
43. Smith, J.L.; Lear, S.R.; Forte, T.M.; Ko, W.; Massimi, M.; Erickson, S.K. Effect of pregnancy and lactation on lipoprotein and cholesterol metabolism in the rat. *J. Lipid Res.* **1998**, *39*, 2237–2249.
44. Scow, R.O.; Chernick, S.S.; Fleck, T.R. Lipoprotein lipase and uptake of triacylglycerol, cholesterol and phosphatidylcholine from chylomicrons by mammary and adipose tissue of lactating rats in vivo. *Biochim. Biophys. Acta (BBA) Lipids Lipid Metab.* **1977**, *487*, 297–306. [CrossRef]

45. Wani, S.A.; Kumar, P. Fenugreek: A review on its nutraceutical properties and utilization in various food products. *J. Saudi Soc. Agric. Sci.* **2018**, *17*, 97–106. [CrossRef]
46. Hayashi, T.; Boyko, E.J.; Sato, K.K.; McNeely, M.J.; Leonetti, D.L.; Kahn, S.E.; Fujimoto, W.Y. Patterns of Insulin Concentration During the OGTT Predict the Risk of Type 2 Diabetes in Japanese Americans. *Diabetes Care* **2013**, *36*, 1229–1235. [CrossRef] [PubMed]
47. Zhou, J.; Zhou, S.; Zeng, S. Experimental diabetes treated with trigonelline: Effect on β cell and pancreatic oxidative parameters. *Fundam. Clin. Pharmacol.* **2013**, *27*, 279–287. [CrossRef] [PubMed]
48. Panda, S.; Tahiliani, P.; Kar, A. Inhibition of triiodothyronine production by fenugreek seed extract in mice and rats. *Pharmacol. Res.* **1999**, *40*, 405–409. [CrossRef]

14

Maternal Nutrition and Body Composition During Breastfeeding: Association with Human Milk Composition

Agnieszka Bzikowska-Jura [1], Aneta Czerwonogrodzka-Senczyna [1], Gabriela Olędzka [2,*], Dorota Szostak-Węgierek [1], Halina Weker [1] and Aleksandra Wesołowska [3]

1 Department of Clinical Dietetics, Faculty of Health Science, Medical University of Warsaw, E Ciolka Str. 27, 01-445 Warsaw, Poland; agnieszka.bzikowska@wum.edu.pl (A.B.-J.); aneta.senczyna@wum.edu.pl (A.C.-S.); dorota.szostak-wegierek@wum.edu.pl (D.S.-W.); halina.weker@wum.edu.pl (H.W.)

2 Department of Medical Biology, Faculty of Health Science, Medical University of Warsaw, Nowogrodzka Str. 73, 02-018 Warsaw, Poland

3 Laboratory of Human Milk and Lactation Research at Regional Human Milk Bank in Holy Family Hospital, Faculty of Health Science, Department of Neonatology, Medical University of Warsaw, Zwirki i Wigury Str. 63A, 02-091 Warsaw, Poland; aleksandra.wesolowska@wum.edu.pl

* Correspondence: gabriela.oledzka@wum.edu.pl

Abstract: The composition of human milk is dynamic and can vary according to many maternal factors, such as diet and nutritional status. This study investigated the association of maternal nutrition and body composition with human milk composition. All measurements and analyses were done at three time points: during the first (n = 40), third (n = 22), and sixth (n = 15) month of lactation. Human milk was analyzed using the Miris human milk analyzer (HMA), body composition was measured with bioelectrical bioimpedance (BIA) using a Maltron BioScan 920-II, and the assessment of women's nutrition was based on a three-day dietary record. The correlation coefficient (Pearson's r) did not show a significant statistical relationship between human milk composition and nutrients in women's diet at three time points. For women in the third month postpartum, we observed moderate to strong significant correlations (r ranged from 0.47 to 0.64) between total protein content in milk and the majority of body composition measures as follows: positive correlations: % fat mass ($r = 0.60$; $p = 0.003$), fat-free mass expressed in kg ($r = 0.63$; $p = 0.001$), and muscle mass ($r = 0.47$; $p = 0.027$); and negative correlation: % total body water ($r = -0.60$; $p = 0.003$). The variance in milk fat content was related to the body mass index (BMI), with a significant positive correlation in the first month postpartum ($r = 0.33$; $p = 0.048$). These findings suggest that it is not diet, but rather the maternal body composition that may be associated with the nutritional value of human milk.

Keywords: breastfeeding; human milk composition; body composition; maternal diet

---

1. Introduction

Human milk is the best source of nutrition for infants, as it contains essential nutrients in the right balance, and other bioactive factors (e.g., hormones, antibodies, bioactive molecules, stem cells) [1,2]. It is well documented that exclusive breastfeeding for the first six months of life is associated with a decreased incidence of infections and chronic diseases [3,4]. Exclusive breastfeeding has also been shown to trigger a protective effect against later obesity [5,6] and type 2 diabetes in the offspring [7,8]. Nevertheless, this protective effect is controversial, and it may differ in accordance with maternal phenotypes [9,10].

Compared to infant formulas, which have standardized compositions, human milk composition changes dynamically, as it is produced by women with significantly varying genotypes and phenotypes [11].

Table 1 summarizes the milk energy and macronutrient concentration from past studies on different human populations.

The composition of human milk is influenced by many maternal, infant, and physiological factors (Figure 1) [11]. Some of these factors are better investigated than others, involving 24 h variations (peak fat content occurs at midmorning) [12], lactational stage (colostrum is reported to be higher in protein but lower in lactose and fat in comparison to mature milk) [13], and time point in breastfeeding session (hindmilk is higher in fat than foremilk; lactose shows an inverse correlation with the stage of breastfeeding) [14,15]. The influence of other factors, including those contained in this study (maternal nutrition and body composition) do not have well-defined effects.

Previous studies assessing the relationship between maternal factors and human milk composition had some limitations, such as no specific time for the expression of milk samples (time of day, hind- or foremilk), and no information about exclusive breastfeeding or analysis of milk composition, excluding nonprotein nitrogen sources, which lead to inflated protein concentrations. Additionally, most of the existing studies were conducted in the 1980s and 1990s [16–18] and for milk composition analysis, they used separate analytical instruments for protein, fat, and lactose, which may have been flawed and was time-consuming. All of these limitations influence a true-value assessment of these associations.

We investigated the impact of maternal diet and body composition on human milk composition, analyzing women's diets and body composition and the nutritional value of human milk.

Table 1. Variations in mature human milk composition in different sample populations.

Population	Characteristics of Participants	Analytical Technique	Energy [1]	Fat [2]	Lactose [2]	Protein [2]	Reference
			Mean ± SD				
Korea	2632 healthy lactating mothers of full-term infants (32.0 ± 3.3 years)	Infrared spectrophotometry (MilkoScan FT2)	61.1 ± 12.1	3.0 ± 1.4	7.1 ± 0.4	1.4 ± 0.3	Chang, 2015 [13]
China	436 urban Chinese lactating mothers	Infrared spectrophotometry	61.3	3.4	7.1	0.9	Yang, 2014 [19]
Tibet	82 breastfeeding Tibetans living at high and low altitudes in rural villages	Micro Rose–Gottlieb	81.4 ± 17.4	5.3 ± 2.0	7.4 ± 0.5	1.3 ± 0.4	Quinn, 2016 [20]
Philippines	102 Filipino breastfeeding mothers (24.6–25.4 years)	Micro Rose–Gottlieb	68.6 ± 15.0	3.8 ± 1.5	7.3 ± 0.6	1.3 ± 0.5	Quinn, 2012 [21]
Brazil	34 donors of the Human Milk Bank	Infrared spectrophotometry (MilkoScan Minor)	56.7 ± 11.7	3.1± 1.18	6.1 ± 0.6	1.22 ± 0.5	Abranches, 2014 [22]
United States (DARLING study)	58 healthy lactating mothers planning to continue nursing for a minimum of 12 months	Lowry assay (protein), Folch extraction (fat), colorimetric (lactose)	69.7 ± 6.7	3.6 ± 0.7	7.4 ± 0.15	1.2 ± 0.15	Nommsen, 1991 [18]
Australia	23 lactating mothers of healthy term infants (33.0 ± 3 years)	Mid-infrared spectrophotometry (MIRIS)	82.4	5.9	6.3	1.0	Khan, 2013 [23]

[1] Energy is presented as kilocalories (kcal) per 100 mL. [2] Macronutrients are presented as grams per 100 mL. SD, standard deviation.

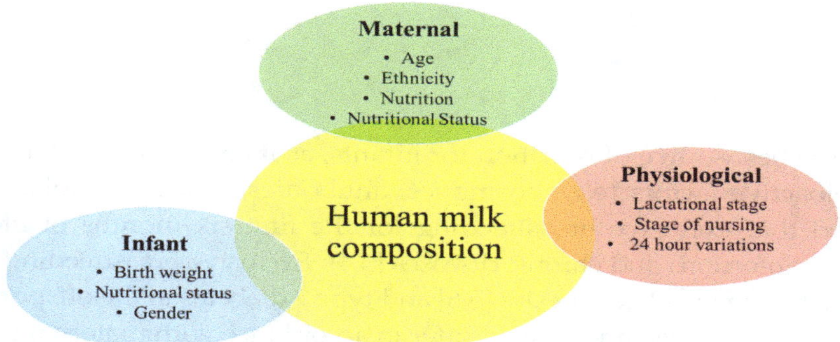

Figure 1. Maternal, infant, and physiological factors that may influence human milk composition.

2. Materials and Methods

2.1. Study Participants

A convenience sample of breastfeeding women (n = 40) was recruited from the community, primarily from the Holy Family Hospital in Warsaw. Participants were enrolled during their first month of lactation. The inclusion criteria were as follows: age $\geq$ 18 years, full-term delivery (gestational age $\geq$ 37 weeks), exclusively breastfeeding, and no contraindications to body composition analysis (metal implants, pacemaker, defibrillator, stents, large implants, implanted devices that emit an electronic signal). Exclusion criteria included the following: preexisting chronic or gestational disease, smoking during pregnancy, multiple pregnancy, low birth weight of the newborn, and low milk supply. All mothers provided written informed consent to participate in the study. The study was approved by the Ethics Committee of the Medical University of Warsaw (KB/172/115).

2.2. Study Session Design

All measurements and analyses were made at three time points: during the first, third, and sixth months of lactation. Participants visited the Holy Family Hospital in Warsaw. At each study session, the mother was weighed, a body composition analysis was performed, and a 24 h milk collection was taken. Twenty-two women provided milk samples at two time points, and 15 women at three time points. A 3-day dietary record was self-reported by each mother and checked by a qualified dietitian.

2.3. Anthropometric Measurements

Body weight and height were measured using a Seca 799 measurement station and column scales ($\pm$0.1 kg/cm; Seca, Chino, CA, USA). The body mass index (BMI) was calculated as the ratio between the body weight and the height squared (kg/m^2). Interpretation of these data followed the classification proposed by the World Health Organization (WHO): below 18.5 kg/m^2, underweight; 18.5–24.9 kg/m^2, normal weight; 25.0–29.9 kg/m^2, pre-obese; $\geq$30 kg/m^2, obese [24].

2.4. Body Composition Analysis with Bioelectrical Impedance (BIA)

Whole-body impedance (wrist to ankle) of the women was measured using the Maltron BioScan 920-II multifrequency bioelectrical impedance analyzer (Maltron Bioscan, Rayleigh, UK) according to the manufacturer's instructions [25]. Total body electrical impedance alternated with four frequencies: 5, 50, 100, and 200 kHz. The subjects were measured in a supine position, on a nonconductive surface, after taking a rest for about 10 min. Before the electrodes were placed, the sites were cleaned using isopropyl alcohol to limit possible errors and to ensure adherence. The whole-body impedance vector components resistance (R) and reactance (Xc) were measured at the same time. On this basis, body fat, lean mass, other components, and REE (resting energy expenditure) were calculated. Before taking the BIA measurement, the women were instructed with the following guidelines (according to Heyward and Stolarczyk [26]): no heavy exercise 12 h before the test, no large meals or caffeinated products 4 h before the test, consumption of liquids limited to 1% of body weight or two 8 oz. glasses of water 2 h before the test.

2.5. Twenty-Four-Hour Human Milk Collection

Human milk samples were collected by participants at home after they were given detailed instructions on taking, storing, and transporting samples to the Holy Family Hospital in Warsaw. Prefeed and postfeed samples were collected from all participants from all time periods (6:00–12:00, 12:00–18:00, 18:00–24:00, 24:00–6:00) to minimize possible circadian influences on the milk composition. A total of 5–10 mL of prefeed and postfeed milk samples were obtained from the breast(s) the infant fed from, by breast pump, or manually. Samples were stored at -20 °C for later analysis.

2.6. Human Milk Composition

Human milk was analyzed using the Miris human milk analyzer (HMA) (Miris, Uppsala, Sweden) with a validated protocol. The HMA is calibrated with human milk standards, and it can measure total and true proteins, fat, lactose, and total solids simultaneously. In addition, the macronutrient content of the milk was used to calculate digestible energy. The concentrations of all macronutrients were reported in grams per 100 mL and energy (kilocalories) was calculated at 4 kcal/g for protein, 9 kcal/g for fat, and 4 kcal/g for carbohydrates. Total protein refers to total nitrogen × 6.25, and true protein is total protein minus 24% for nonprotein nitrogen. Total protein as reported by the Miris analyzer was converted to bioavailable protein (true protein) for the data analysis using the following equation: total protein (grams) × 0.825 [26,27]. The HMA is based on semisolid mid-infrared (MIR) transmission spectroscopy, which is the certified method for milk analysis in the dairy industry according to ISO 9622:1999 by the Association of Official Analytical Chemists (AOAC) and the International Dairy Federation (IDF) [28]. Before analysis, each sample ($n = 77$) was warmed to 40 °C and homogenized for 1.5 s/1 mL of probe using a sonicator (milk homogenizer, Miris, Uppsala, Sweden). From each pool, three samples (~12 mL in total) were taken to analyze the nutritional value, and for the result, we used the average of three measurements.

2.7. Nutritional Value of Daily Food Consumption

The assessment of women's nutrition was based on a 3-day dietary record. Sizes of declared food portions were verified using the "Album of Photographs of Food Products and Dishes" from the National Food and Nutrition Institute [29]. Collected data were used to estimate daily food consumption. Energy and nutritional value of daily food consumption (content of macronutrients, cholesterol, fatty acids, dietary fiber, minerals, and vitamins) were calculated using Dieta 5.0 nutritional software (National Food and Nutrition Institute, Warsaw, Poland).

2.8. Statistical Analysis

Statistical analyses were performed using Statistica 12PL, Tulusa, USA and IBM Statistics 21, New York, NY, USA. A p-value below 0.05 was adopted as statistically significant. Variable distributions were evaluated with Shapiro–Wilk test, and descriptive statistics (means and standard deviations as well as medians and interquartile ranges) were calculated. The mothers' anthropometric data and body composition, and the nutritional value of their diet in the first and sixth months of lactation were compared using a paired 2-sample Student's t-test (normal distribution of differences between all pairs), or a Wilcoxon signed-rank test for paired samples (nonnormally distributed differences between all pairs). A trend analysis of milk composition at three time points was performed with the Jonckheere–Terpstra test, and its effect size was estimated with Kendall's tau-b correlation coefficient. Correlations between milk composition and the mothers' body composition and diet were estimated with Pearson's r correlation coefficient.

3. Results

3.1. Subjects and Human Milk Composition

All participants had a university education and a high socioeconomic status. The subjects' anthropometric data and body composition measures are shown in Table 2. The mean maternal age was 31.1 ± 4.4 years. At the first month postpartum, none of the participants were classified as being underweight (BMI < 18.5 kg/m^2). Most of them ($n = 32$, 80%) had normal body mass, and 20% ($n = 8$) were overweight. We did not observe any statistically significant differences between maternal body composition at the first and third months postpartum. However, there were statistically significant differences between weight and BMI values in the first and sixth months of lactation. The Wilcoxon signed-rank test was 2.59, $p = 0.009$ for weight and 2.67, $p = 0.008$ for BMI.

Table 2. Subjects' anthropometric data and body composition measures.

Characteristic	Month of Lactation 1 (n = 40)	3 (n = 22)	6 (n = 15)	Difference between First and Sixth Month of Lactation (p-Value)
Weight (kg)	64.5 ± 12.2 62.3 (54.8–70.9)	65.1 ± 13.2 62.4 (54.7–70.5)	61.4 ± 10.0 59.5 (54.6–67.0)	0.009 [2,*]
Height (cm)	166.6 ± 6.6 166.5 (162.0–172.5)	166.6 ± 6.6 166.5 (162.0–172.5)	166.6 ± 6.6 166.5 (162.0–172.5)	–
Body mass index (kg/m^2)	23.0 ± 3.6 22.7 (20.4–24.8)	23.3 ± 4.0 23.0 (19.9–25.9)	21.8 ± 2.8 21.5 (19.8–23.7)	0.008 [2,*]
Fat mass (kg)	19.8 ± 10.3 17.9 (11.3–23.0)	19.8 ± 9.5 19.3 (12.6–23.3)	16.9 ± 6.6 17.7 (9.8–21.3)	0.064 [2]
Fat mass (%)	28.2 ± 8.5 28.5 (20.6–33.0)	28.9 ± 8.6 30.2 (21.3–34.6)	26.4 ± 7.1 26.7 (19.2–32.4)	0.174 [1]
Fat-free mass (kg)	45.4 ± 3.9 45.7 (43.0–48.4)	45.3 ± 4.6 45.1 (40.9–49.2)	45.0 ± 4.4 43.5 (40.9–49.4)	0.701 [1]
Total body water (L)	32.4 ± 3.8 31.2 (29.4–35.2)	32.2 ± 4.1 31.0 (28.5–34.7)	31.5 ± 3.7 30.6 (28.5–34.1)	0.695 [2]
Total body water (%)	51.2 ± 5.1 50.3 (46.9–55.3)	50.3 ± 4.9 49.8 (46.5–52.2)	51.2 ± 4.1 50.9 (46.9–54.8)	0.236 [1]
Protein (kg)	9.0 ± 1.4 9.0 (8.5–9.9)	9.3 ± 1.3 9.2 (8.4–10.6)	9.6 ± 1.0 9.4 (8.7–10.6)	0.638 [2]
Muscles (kg)	19.9 ± 1.9 19.8 (18.8–21.4)	19.8 ± 2.0 19.7 (18.3–21.7)	19.3 ± 1.7 18.9 (18.3–21.5)	0.084 [2]

Data are mean ± standard deviation (SD), median, and ranges. [1] Paired two-sample Student's t-test; [2] Wilcoxon signed rank test for paired samples. * $p < 0.05$.

Table 3 provides the average results of the nutritional value of human milk (energy, macronutrients, and dry matter) and changes in the concentrations of the components at three time points. We observed a statistically significant downward trend for total protein (tau-b = −0.31; $p = 0.001$) and true protein (tau-b = −0.30; $p = 0.001$) concentration in human milk. We also noted a decreasing energy value, but the trend was not statistically significant (tau-b = −0.18; $p = 0.052$).

Table 3. Composition of human milk.

	Month of Lactation 1 (n = 40)	3 (n = 22)	6 (n = 15)	Linear Trend (p-Value)	Effect Size (Kendall's Tau-b)
Energy (kcal/100 mL)	65.9 ± 9.9 65.5 (62.0–72.5)	61.8 ± 14.4 61.3 (49.0–71.7)	61.2 ± 14.2 60.0 (47.0–73.7)	0.052	−0.18
Fat (g/100 mL)	3.5 ± 1.0 3.5 (3.1–4.3)	3.2 ± 1.5 3.1 (1.8–4.1)	3.2 ± 1.4 3.1 (1.8–4.5)	0.120	−0.14
Total protein (g/100 mL)	1.2 ± 0.2 1.1 (1.1–1.2)	1.1 ± 0.1 1.0 (1.0–1.1)	1.0 ± 0.3 1.0 (0.9–1.1)	0.001	−0.31
True protein (g/100 mL)	0.9 ± 0.2 0.9 (0.8–1.0)	0.8 ± 0.1 0.8 (0.7–0.9)	0.8 ± 0.2 0.7 (0.7–0.9)	0.001	−0.30
Carbohydrates (g/100 mL)	7.0 ± 0.3 7.0 (6.8–7.2)	7.0 ± 0.4 7.1 (6.9–7.2)	7.1 ± 0.4 7.1 (6.9–7.4)	0.236	0.11
Dry matter (g/100 mL)	11.7 ± 1.3 11.8 (11.2–12.7)	11.4 ± 1.7 11.3 (9.9–12.6)	11.4 ± 1.8 11.0 (9.7–12.9)	0.298	−0.09

3.2. Nutritional Value of Daily Food Consumption

Table 4 presents the results of energy and nutrient intake in relation to Polish nutritional standards [29]. The risk of deficient energy intake was observed in 100% of the women at three time points. There were no significant differences between the intake of macronutrients (protein, fat, and carbohydrates), minerals, and vitamins at each stage of the study. Among all of the women (100%), at every time point we observed an insufficient intake of vitamin D. The majority of women (60%, $n = 24$) at the first month postpartum did not reach the estimated average requirement (EAR) value for calcium.

Table 4. Energy and nutrient intake in relation to Polish nutritional standards 2012 [29].

	Month of Lactation			Difference between First and Sixth Month of Lactation (p-Value)	Nutritional Standards EAR/RDA/AI
	1 ($n = 40$)	3 ($n = 22$)	6 ($n = 15$)		
Energy (kcal)	1822.7 ± 445.7 1798.4 (1504.4–2070.8)	1825.3 ± 462.0 1773.4 (1508.3–2052.2)	1614.6 ± 435.0 1487.3 (1343.3–1957.7)	0.295 *	2555
Protein (g)	77.7 ± 21.4 76.5 (61.0–91.4)	74.9 ± 19.2 74.9 (64.9–86.6)	66.2 ± 19.9 60.2 (53.3–91.0)	0.187 *	1.17 g/kg weight
Protein (% kcal)	17.3 ± 3.3 17.8 (14.6–19.5)	16.7 ± 2.7 16.3 (14.3–18.8)	16.6 ± 3.0 16.4 (14.7–19.2)	0.567 *	15
Fat (g)	63.4 ± 20.0 62.7 (49.3–74.7)	66.3 ± 23.5 62.0 (50.1–72.1)	55.8 ± 22.8 50.8 (40.2–66.6)	0.805 *	90
SFA	23.6 ± 10.1 20.5 (17.9–28.0)	22.8 ± 12.2 21.0 (18.1–25.8)	20.6 ± 7.4 19.2 (15.4–22.5)	0.846 *	–
MUFA	24.04 ± 8.8 23.8 (16.2–27.8)	24.7 ± 8.6 22.9 (20.5–25.9)	21.4 ± 11.1 18.1 (14.2–25.0)	0.989 *	–
PUFA	10.8 ± 4.4 10.3 (7.1–12.7)	13.8 ± 10.4 11.6 (7.2–15.2)	9.3 ± 9.0 6.7 (4.7–8.1)	0.173 **	–
Fat (% kcal)	30.8 ± 5.8 30.2 (26.4–34.4)	31.9 ± 5.3 30.3 (27.93–36.4)	30.4 ± 7.7 30.0 (23.8–35.9)	0.585 *	30
Cholesterol (mg)	265.7 ± 112.4 253.6 (211.5–339.7)	247.7 ± 135.8 219.0 (165.8–362.3)	255.1 ± 139.6 226.4 (139.2–339.3)	0.879 *	–
Carbohydrates (g)	255.3 ± 65.8 253.5 (204.0–297.0)	253.1 ± 62.4 234.0 (208.8–295.2)	229.7 ± 66.3 247.1 (176.2–290.2)	0.217 *	>175
Carbohydrates (% kcal)	51.9 ± 6.6 51.4 (48.1–56.3)	51.4 ± 5.3 50.7 (48.0–56.2)	53.0 ± 9.2 51.6 (46.3–57.6)	0.863 *	45–65
Sucrose (g)	50.4 ± 30.2 42.6 (28.5–69.1)	46.4 ± 32.7 36.1 (25.5–55.0)	48.7 ± 30.4 44.6 (28.0–58.5)	0.687 *	–
Dietary fiber (g)	21.8 ± 7.2 20.7 (172–25.6)	22.7 ± 9.3 21.6 (16.2–29.2)	19.3 ± 7.6 19.0 (14.5–23.7)	0.251 *	–
Sodium (mg)	2612.4 ± 881.6 2588.0 (2036.7–3179.6)	2359.4 ± 804.3 2280.3 (2064.2–2918.6)	2314.2 ± 745.3 2139.1 (1757.5–2663.9)	0.955 *	1500
Potassium (mg)	3132.6 ± 881.6 2923.7 (2512.5–3576.2)	3009.9 ± 745.5 2894.8 (2655.8–3497.3)	2953.8 ± 846.8 2770.0 (25340.0–3532.4)	0.392 *	4000
Calcium (mg)	745.9 ± 347.3 710.0 (548.2–927.3)	613.3 ± 256.1 598.9 (421.9–774.0)	659.0 ± 302.0 566.1 (459.0–897.2)	0.812 *	800.0
Phosphorus (mg)	1326.7 ± 350.2 1255.5 (1046.9–1555.3)	1320.6 ± 314.1 1347.0 (1204.9–1473.0)	1146.5 ± 383.8 1005.3 (824.6–1441.6)	0.234 *	580
Magnesium (mg)	322.1 ± 87.7 305.8 (263.2–363.8)	351.7 ± 129.2 344.5 (258.9–407.2)	315.5 ± 133.8 283.2 (226.1–406.8)	0.820 *	265.0
Iron (mg)	12.8 ± 9.4 11.0 (9.3–13.3)	12.2 ± 3.7 11.6 (9.6–15.1)	12.6 ± 8.7 10.6 (7.9–13.3)	0.955 **	7.0
Zinc (mg)	10.5 ± 3.9 9.8 (8.9–11.0)	10.2 ± 2.2 9.9 (9.5–11.2)	8.6 ± 2.6 7.8 (6.5–10.9)	0.132 *	10.4
Iodine (μg)	106.0 ± 35.6 102.8 (86.2–128.4)	90.8 ± 37.6 87.2 (64.9–111.2)	88.7 ± 35.2 84.6 (58.6–110.5)	0.656 *	210.0
Vitamin A (μg)	1216.1 ± 680.4 1023.9 (838.3–1297.5)	1390.0 ± 1392.0 960.9 (628.6–1701.0)	1049.3 ± 435.4 893.9 (692.4–1539.9)	0.496 **	900
Vitamin D (μg)	3.23 ± 2.6 2.3 (1.5–3.7)	3.2 ± 2.7 1.9 (1.3–5.0)	2.7 ± 2.3 1.6 (1.2–4.6)	0.874 *	15.0

Table 4. *Cont.*

	Month of Lactation			Difference between First and Sixth Month of Lactation (p-Value)	Nutritional Standards EAR/RDA/AI
	1 (n = 40)	3 (n = 22)	6 (n = 15)		
Vitamin E (mg)	10.4 ± 4.6 9.4 (6.8–13.6)	11.9 ± 7.9 9.3 (7.2–16.0)	10.4 ± 6.8 7.9 (6.5–14.8)	0.873 *	11.0
Vitamin B_1 (mg)	1.2 ± 0.4 1.2 (1.0–1.4)	1.4 ± 0.5 1.2 (1.0–1.7)	1.2 ± 0.5 1.1 (0.9–1.5)	0.825 *	1.3
Vitamin B_2 (mg)	1.8 ± 0.6 1.6 (1.3–2.1)	1.6 ± 0.5 1.6 (1.2–1.9)	1.7 ± 0.6 1.5 (1.2–2.1)	0.920 *	1.3
Vitamin PP (mg)	16.2 ± 6.2 14.9 (11.0–18.5)	16.8 ± 6.0 17.8 (11.9–20.3)	16.6 ± 8.8 13.0 (11.0–20.3)	0.936 *	13.0
Vitamin B_6 (mg)	1.9 ± 0.7 1.8 (1.4–2.2)	1.9 ± 0.6 1.9 (1.4–2.2)	4.8 ± 8.3 1.9 (1.3–2.6)	1.00 **	1.7
Vitamin C (mg)	127.8 ± 109.1 92.3 (57.6–139.9)	135.6 ± 83.9 113.8 (79.1–160.7)	163.0 ± 81.2 139.8 (120.7–253.7)	0.730 *	100
Vitamin B_{12} (μg)	3.75 ± 1.7 3.4 (2.3–4.8)	4.04 ± 3.1 3.0 (1.9–4.9)	3.2 ± 1.8 2.9 (1.9–4.1)	0.900 *	2.4
Folic acid (μg)	324.6 ± 141.2 (239.2–379.3)	310.0 ± 109.9 288.4 (239.5–388.6)	436.5 ± 213.7 364.6 (284.6–672.8)	0.099 *	450.0

Data are mean ± standard deviation (SD), median, and ranges. * Paired two-sample Student's t-test; ** Wilcoxon signed rank test for paired samples. SFA, saturated fatty acids; MUFA, monounsaturated fatty acids; PUFA, polyunsaturated fatty acids; EAR, estimated average requirement; RDA, recommended daily allowance; AI, adequate intake.

3.3. Association between Maternal Diet and Milk Composition

Table 5 presents correlation coefficient (Pearson's r) between human milk composition and nutrients in the mother's diet at three time points (first, third, and sixth month of lactation). We did not observe any statistically significant correlation between these factors ($p > 0.05$). The estimated energy value and the macronutrient content in lactating women's average daily food consumption recorded for three days did not allow for the prediction of the variance in their milk composition.

Table 5. Correlations between human milk composition and nutrients in mothers' diet.

Energy and Nutrients in Mothers' Diet	Month of Lactation	Composition of Human Milk					
		Energy [1]	Total Protein [2]	True Protein [2]	Fat [2]	Carbohydrates [2]	Dry Matter [2]
Energy (kcal)	1 3 6	0.06 0.12 −0.15	0.08 −0.05 −0.12	0.13 0.02 −0.05	0.08 0.11 −0.09	−0.14 0.08 −0.22	0.02 0.11 −0.11
Protein (g)	1 3 6	0.08 0.10 0.01	0.02 −0.19 −0.7	0.02 −0.12 −0.05	0.08 −0.13 0.05	−0.05 −0.20 −0.24	0.06 0.05 0.03
Fat (g)	1 3 6	0.09 0.09 −0.01	0.01 0.07 −0.12	0.04 0.10 −0.03	0.08 0.06 0.03	−0.02 0.15 −0.10	0.11 0.10 0.05
Carbohydrates (g)	1 3 6	0.01 0.15 −0.27	0.13 −0.06 −0.08	0.20 0.04 −0.03	0.05 0.14 −0.21	−0.22 0.06 −0.26	−0.09 0.13 −0.25
Percent of energy from protein	1 3 6	0.02 −0.01 0.25	−0.06 −0.18 0.13	−0.13 −0.16 0.05	−0.01 0.05 0.24	0.12 −0.42 −0.01	0.06 −0.06 0.25
Percent of energy from fat	1 3 6	0.13 0.01 0.23	−0.07 0.16 −0.08	−0.09 0.14 −0.04	0.09 −0.02 0.22	0.21 0.22 0.13	0.24 0.05 0.27
Percent of energy from carbohydrates	1 3 6	−0.13 −0.01 −0.27	0.09 −0.06 0.03	0.15 −0.06 0.02	−0.08 −0.01 −0.26	−0.24 0.01 −0.10	−0.24 −0.02 −0.30

Table 5. *Cont.*

Energy and Nutrients in Mothers' Diet	Month of Lactation	Composition of Human Milk					
		Energy [1]	Total Protein [2]	True Protein [2]	Fat [2]	Carbohydrates [2]	Dry Matter [2]
Sodium (mg)	1	0.01	0.20	0.25	−0.03	−0.01	0.08
	3	−0.22	0.02	0.05	−0.22	−0.18	−0.24
	6	−0.17	0.33	0.40	−0.18	0.01	−0.19
Potassium (mg)	1	0.09	−0.02	0.04	0.11	−0.04	−0.05
	3	0.21	−0.01	0.20	0.22	−0.07	0.18
	6	−0.37	−0.03	0.04	−0.34	−0.48	−0.35
Calcium (mg)	1	0.32	0.08	0.08	0.30	0.21	0.29
	3	0.21	−0.20	−0.23	0.19	0.26	0.23
	6	0.11	−0.12	−0.18	0.20	−0.24	0.13
Phosphorus (mg)	1	0.12	−0.03	−0.03	0.13	−0.01	0.09
	3	0.19	0.02	0.08	0.19	−0.06	0.17
	6	−0.04	−0.05	−0.02	0.02	−0.40	−0.02
Magnesium (mg)	1	0.04	−0.04	−0.02	0.03	−0.02	−0.11
	3	0.27	0.26	0.37	0.27	0.00	0.27
	6	−0.34	0.01	0.06	−0.37	−0.32	−0.33
Iron (mg)	1	−0.04	−0.06	−0.01	−0.02	−0.11	−0.13
	3	0.26	0.24	0.43	0.26	−0.01	0.24
	6	0.01	0.10	0.17	−0.04	0.08	0.03
Zinc (mg)	1	−0.06	−0.06	−0.02	−0.05	−0.10	−0.06
	3	0.26	0.24	0.43	0.26	−0.01	0.24
	6	−0.01	0.13	0.20	0.02	−0.24	0.02
Iodine (μg)	1	0.10	0.20	0.18	0.08	0.01	−0.03
	3	0.10	−0.28	−0.24	0.14	−0.21	0.04
	6	−0.12	0.10	0.14	−0.12	−0.18	−0.20
Vitamin A (μg)	1	−0.17	−0.01	0.05	−0.23	−0.07	−0.21
	3	−0.21	−0.10	0.12	−0.20	−0.22	−0.26
	6	−0.14	−0.16	−0.25	−0.13	−0.14	−0.17
Vitamin D (μg)	1	−0.09	−0.09	−0.08	−0.15	−0.09	−0.14
	3	0.23	0.16	0.18	0.28	−0.41	0.16
	6	0.33	0.06	0.08	0.35	0.03	0.33
Vitamin E (mg)	1	0.20	0.02	0.10	0.22	0.06	0.09
	3	0.19	0.06	0.27	0.20	−0.02	0.17
	6	−0.30	−0.02	0.13	−0.34	−0.36	−0.29
Vitamin B_1 (mg)	1	−0.21	−0.14	−0.09	−0.19	−0.22	−0.36
	3	0.12	0.19	0.30	0.14	−0.21	0.08
	6	−0.08	−0.07	−0.01	−0.07	0.07	−0.01
Vitamin B_2 (mg)	1	0.15	−0.02	−0.02	0.18	0.08	0.09
	3	0.08	−0.18	0.02	0.10	−0.10	0.05
	6	0.17	−0.01	−0.02	0.21	−0.04	0.20
Vitamin PP (mg)	1	−0.20	−0.18	−0.15	−0.18	−0.30	−0.24
	3	0.14	−0.02	0.10	0.18	−0.25	0.09
	6	−0.27	0.02	0.05	−0.30	−0.08	−0.19
Vitamin B_6 (mg)	1	−0.08	−0.10	−0.05	−0.07	−0.14	−0.24
	3	0.10	0.02	0.21	0.13	−0.26	0.04
	6	−0.06	−0.00	−0.07	−0.09	0.16	−0.07
Vitamin C (mg)	1	−0.01	0.03	0.09	0.02	−0.02	−0.39
	3	0.08	0.02	0.27	0.11	−0.22	0.03
	6	−0.19	−0.36	−0.23	−0.11	−0.18	−0.25
Vitamin B_{12} (μg)	1	0.21	0.08	0.03	0.15	0.06	0.02
	3	0.10	−0.01	0.16	0.13	−0.29	0.02
	6	0.14	−0.09	−0.08	0.18	−0.29	0.15
Folic acid (μg)	1	0.11	−0.02	0.04	0.16	−0.05	−0.06
	3	0.19	0.02	0.30	0.21	−0.24	0.12
	6	−0.36	−0.07	−0.12	−0.40	0.02	−0.41

[1] Energy is presented as kilocalories (kcal) per 100 mL. [2] Macronutrients and dry matter are presented as grams per 100 mL. Data are presented as Pearson's r coefficients.

3.4. Association between Maternal Body Composition and Milk Composition

Table 6 presents the correlation coefficient (Pearson's r) between human milk composition and lactating mothers' body composition at three time points (first, third, and sixth month of lactation).

For women in the third month postpartum, we observed moderate to strong significant correlations (r ranged from 0.45 to 0.52) between the true protein content in their milk and the majority of body composition measures. In the third month of lactation, the total protein in milk correlated positively with the mothers' weight ($r = 0.63$; $p = 0.002$), BMI ($r = 0.59$; $p = 0.004$), % fat mass ($r = 0.60$; $p = 0.003$), fat-free mass expressed in kg ($r = 0.63$; $p = 0.001$), and muscle mass ($r = 0.47$; $p = 0.027$) and negatively with percentage of total body water ($r = -0.60$; $p = 0.003$).

The variance in milk fat content was related to the lactating women's weight, with a significant positive correlation in the sixth month postpartum ($r = 0.49$; $p = 0.039$), with BMI, and a significant positive correlation in the first month postpartum ($r = 0.33$; $p = 0.048$).

Similar to the protein concentration, the energy value of human milk was highly correlated with the maternal body composition. In the third month postpartum, we found positive correlations with weight ($r = 0.43$; $p = 0.048$), BMI ($r = 0.39$; $p = 0.049$), and muscle mass ($r = 0.44$; $p = 0.041$). There was a negative correlation with % total body water ($r = -0.60$; $p = 0.032$) in the third month of lactation.

We did not observe significant correlations between the carbohydrate content in human milk and measures of the body composition of lactating women, except for a positive correlation with the percentage of intracellular water and a negative correlation with the percentage of extracellular water in the third month postpartum.

Table 6. Correlations between human milk composition and mother's body composition.

Mothers' Body Composition	Month of Lactation	Composition of Human Milk					
		Energy [1]	Total Protein [2]	True Protein [2]	Fat [2]	Carbohydrates [2]	Dry Matter [2]
Weight (kg)	1	0.32 *	0.21	0.18	0.30	0.21	0.52 *
	3	0.43 *	0.63 *	0.51 *	0.37	0.30	0.49 *
	6	0.41	−0.14	−0.21	0.49 *	0.30	0.42
Body mass index (kg/m^2)	1	0.33 *	0.27	0.24	0.33 *	0.20	0.48 *
	3	0.39 *	0.59 *	0.45 *	0.35	0.24	0.45 *
	6	0.44	0.01	−0.05	0.52	0.34	0.45
Fat mass (kg)	1	0.17	0.19	0.14	0.15	0.14	0.33 *
	3	0.42	0.64 *	0.51 *	0.36	0.29	0.48 *
	6	0.43	−0.10	−0.12	0.51	0.24	0.43
Fat mass (%)	1	0.32 *	0.26	0.23	0.29	0.17	0.46 *
	3	0.39	0.60 *	0.47 *	0.33	0.32	0.46 *
	6	0.42	0.01	−0.01	0.48	0.22	0.41
Fat free mass (kg)	1	0.24	0.10	0.06	0.22	0.25	0.52 *
	3	0.37	0.50 *	0.42	0.32	0.29	0.43 *
	6	0.15	−0.34	−0.38	0.22	0.06	0.17
Total body water (L)	1	0.27	0.19	0.15	0.27	0.10	0.49 *
	3	0.35	0.54 *	0.42	0.30	0.27	0.41
	6	0.25	−0.33	−0.38	0.31	0.13	0.26
Total body water (%)	1	−0.27	−0.20	−0.20	−0.23	−0.22	−0.41 *
	3	−0.46 *	−0.60 *	−0.52 *	−0.40	−0.35	−0.52 *
	6	−0.38	−0.06	−0.06	−0.44	−0.17	−0.37
Protein (kg)	1	−0.09	−0.10	−0.07	−0.14	0.12	−0.01
	3	0.16	0.05	0.11	0.14	0.14	0.15
	6	−0.22	−0.21	−0.19	−0.19	−0.21	−0.19
Muscles (kg)	1	0.26	0.10	0.04	0.22	0.28	0.53 *
	3	0.44 *	0.47 *	0.40	0.39	0.37	0.50 *
	6	0.03	−0.10	−0.12	0.08	0.10	0.13

[1] Energy is presented as kilocalories (kcal) per 100 mL. [2] Macronutrients and dry matter are presented as grams per 100 mL. Data are presented as Pearson's r coefficients. * $p < 0.05$.

4. Discussion

In our study, we found that protein (total and true) and carbohydrate concentrations in human milk were significantly different, depending on the period of lactation. From the first to the sixth month of lactation, total and true protein concentrations significantly decreased. We did not find any relationships between the nutritional value of maternal daily food consumption and milk composition. Maternal BMI and adiposity were positively associated with the protein content of milk.

The total milk protein content in our study was high compared to mature milk from Chinese (0.9 g/100 mL [19]), Brazilian (1.1 g/100 mL [22]), and Australian mothers (1.0 g/100 mL [23]). The analysis of carbohydrates by HMA MIRIS in human milk is affected by the presence of lactose and nonlactose carbohydrates, primarily human milk oligosaccharides (HMOs) [27]. Some of the divergence between the findings for lactose concentrations may be related to the inclusion of HMOs in the mid-infrared (mid-IR) transmission spectroscopy measurements [28]. Since the reference laboratory analysis for lactose concentration, high-pressure liquid chromatography (HPLC), does not measure HMOs, it is probable that lactose levels measured by mid-infrared transmission spectroscopy were a result of absorbing terminal or core lactose moieties of HMOs [30]. The measured concentration of carbohydrates in our study (7.0–7.1 g/100 mL) was consistent with the normal range in human milk [31]; however, it has been reported that lactose concentration can vary from 6.3 to 8.1 g/100 mL [32]. The reasons for this variability may relate to the time point in the breastfeeding session (pre- or postfeeding), the time of feeding, feeding frequency, or the milk analysis method [33]. Fat is known to be the most variable macronutrient in human milk. In the first month postpartum, the median fat concentration in milk was 3.5 g/100 mL. Our finding was consistent with those in Japan (3.6 g/100 mL) [19], China (3.4 g/100 mL) [34], and the United States (3.6 g/100 mL) [35].

It is reported that sampling protocols are of prime importance when investigating the association between human milk composition and maternal factors. The direct relationship between the dietary intake of single nutrients and their presence within human milk is hard to study for many reasons. These include difficulties in collecting nutrition data and the availability of reliable human milk samples. In the present study, the procedure of milk collection (using a 24-h period) was performed to minimize errors. We also confirmed a systemic change between fore- and hindmilk samples for concentrations of energy and macronutrients. Additionally, all of the milk samples were from mothers practicing exclusive breastfeeding.

We found no evidence for associations between the maternal intake of any dietary nutrients and the milk composition in this sample. This is consistent with past studies, which showed that milk nutrient composition appears to be mainly independent of the nutritional value of maternal daily food consumption [36]. This absence of an effect of maternal diet is evident in both observational and experimental studies, in which nutritional supplements were shown to result in minimal or trifling changes to milk macronutrient content [21,35]. Some compensatory physiological mechanisms might be responsible for the comparatively stable milk macronutrient composition related to the nutritional variations of maternal diet [33]. Tigas et al. [37] reported that increased glucose demands during lactation are met by increased glucose production as a result of increased glycogenolysis, but not gluconeogenesis, or by an increased use of free fatty acids. These results are consistent with the hypothesis that human milk composition might be buffered against variations in the maternal dietary intake of each component [15]. For instance, Rakicioğlu et al. [38] found that short-term fasting or dieting by lactating women has not been associated with milk composition, despite the fact that the nutritional status of lactating women was affected by Ramadan fasting, when all macronutrient intake decreased.

The concentration of lactose in human milk is known to be the least variable of the macronutrients [32]. No significant relationships were found between milk lactose and a maternal diet high in fat and low in carbohydrates, compared with a diet low in fat and high in carbohydrates [39]. Additionally, there were no significant differences between milk lactose and a high-protein diet [40], or between vegetarian and non-vegetarian diets [41]. Considering the total protein concentration, studies from Europe and the

United States did not report any relationship between milk total protein and maternal intake of animal and vegetable protein [42]. The variation of total fat concentration in human milk also appears to be independent of maternal diet [30]. Nevertheless, the specific fatty acids that form the total lipid fraction are sensitive to maternal nutrition. These fatty acids are either taken up from the maternal plasma, or synthetized endogenously by the mammary glands. Both of these sources are influenced by maternal diet composition [37,43–45].

While there is a lack of a relationship between milk composition and maternal nutrition, we observed that concentrations of several nutrients in milk were correlated with maternal body composition, depending on the postpartum period.

Previous studies based on maternal BMI reported a positive relationship with fat concentration in human milk [13,19,45], which is consistent with our results. We found that in the first month postpartum, maternal BMI was correlated with milk fat content (0.33; $p = 0.048$). Chang et al. [13] reported that the mother's current BMI was positively correlated with lipid levels at 1–2 weeks (0.151; $p < 0.05$), 2–3 months (0.151; $p < 0.05$), and 7–8 months (0.153; $p < 0.05$). Contrary to these findings, Bachour et al. [46] suggested that there were no associations between maternal body mass index and fat concentration in human milk. Interestingly, Quinn et al. [21] observed that women in Cebu with lower BMI tended to produce milk with higher fat contents than women with higher BMI. The significant inverse association between milk fat and BMI suggests that the sample BMI was indexing lean mass. In our study, we found no evidence for an association between maternal body composition and fat concentration in milk at any time point. Although past research has at times reported a relationship between maternal fat mass and milk fat content, these associations were often limited to overweight or obese women [47,48]. It has been also suggested that increasing maternal adiposity may be related to impaired milk sugar synthesis, and that the lipid increase reflects this decrease in lactose [49].

A few studies investigating the associations between human milk protein concentration and maternal nutritional status are contradictory, with some reporting a positive relationship between protein and maternal adiposity as assessed by BMI [13,18,45,50] and one a negative association between total protein content and maternal BMI [21]. However, it must be stressed that BMI is not a direct measure of adiposity, so that the strength of the relationship between protein concentration and BMI may not reflect the true value of these associations. Kugananthan et al. [51] and Quinn et al. [52] observed that a higher maternal fat mass percentage, but not BMI, was associated with higher protein concentrations in milk. Using advanced techniques to evaluate maternal body composition, we found that maternal body composition was highly correlated with total protein concentration in milk. We reported a positive correlation with maternal weight ($p = 0.002$), BMI ($p = 0.004$), % fat mass ($p = 0.003$), and muscles ($p = 0.027$), and a negative correlation with % total body water ($p = 0.003$) in the third month of lactation. A decreased total body water content is characteristic for women with more adipose tissue, explaining that negative correlation. It is also reported that several serum amino acid concentrations, in particular branched-chain amino acids (BCAAs), are increased in mothers with more adipose tissue [53], leading to more amino acids transferred to the breast and milk [54]. This may explain the positive relationship between maternal adiposity and milk protein concentration [18].

The concentration of carbohydrates in human milk is the least variable of the macronutrients. Considering that a stable concentration of lactose is important for maintaining a constant osmotic pressure in milk [55], maternal nutritional status is not expected to have a meaningful impact on total carbohydrate concentrations in milk. In our study, the measured concentrations of carbohydrates were not related to maternal BMI and body composition at any time point. This is in line with a previous study carried out by Kugananthan et al. [51], which showed that that the lactose concentration in human milk (measured by enzymatic spectrophotometric method) was not related to maternal adiposity profiles (BMI, $p = 0.66$; % fat mass, $p = 0.48$). By contrast, Chang et al. [13] reported that maternal BMI was negatively correlated with lactose concentrations at 4–5 months (0.148; $p < 0.05$) and 6–7 months (0.242; $p < 0.01$) postpartum.

The strengths of this study are the use of advanced techniques to assess maternal body composition and the milk collection protocol, which allowed possible errors in human milk composition to be minimized. The limitations of this study are convenience sampling, the modest number of participants, mainly at six months postpartum, resulting from discontinuation of breastfeeding, and the constraints associated with multiple measurement time points. BIA analysis incorporates various assumptions, and it may also result in less precise estimates, mainly in situations in which the water–electrolyte balance is altered. If used to monitor individuals over time, it can indicate the direction, but not the magnitude of changes in lean mass. Further, our population was Caucasian, with university educations and a high socioeconomic status. All indicated limitations decreased the representativity of the study, and caution should be used when extrapolating the results.

Considering that human milk provides not only energy and nutrients, but also bioactive factors that are crucial for infant growth and development, human milk composition research should continue in order to identify factors that may be associated with changes in its composition. All of these efforts may contribute to accomplishing optimum growth, development, and health in infants.

Author Contributions: Conceptualization, A.B.-J., A.C.-S., G.O., D.S.-W., H.W., and A.W.; Data curation, A.B.-J.; Formal analysis, A.B.-J. and A.W.; Funding acquisition, A.C.-S. and A.W.; Investigation, A.B.-J.; Methodology, A.B.-J., D.S.-W., and A.W.; Project administration, A.B.-J., A.C.-S., and A.W.; Resources, D.S.-W. and A.W.; Supervision, A.C.-S., G.O., D.S.-W., and A.W.; Writing—original draft, A.B.-J.; Writing—review and editing, A.B.-J., A.C.-S., G.O., D.S.-W., H.W., and A.W.

Acknowledgments: All authors read and approved the final manuscript. This study was supported by a Polish Society of Clinical Child Nutrition research grant obtained in 2015 for the project entitled "Association between human milk composition and the nutritional status and body composition of lactating women". Many thanks are extended to all of the mothers from the Holy Hospital in Warsaw who participated in this study.

References

1. Lonnerdal, B. Breast milk: A truly functional food. *Nutrition* **2000**, *16*, 509–511. [CrossRef]
2. Hassiotou, F.; Filgueira, L.; Trengove, N.; Lai, C.T.; Hartmann, P.E. Breastmilk contains primitive stem cells from lactating breast with multi-lineage differentiation potential. *FASEB J.* **2012**, *26*, 913.
3. Eidelman, A.I.; Schanler, R.J.; Johnston, M.; Landers, S.; Noble, L.; Szucs, K.; Viehmann, L. Breastfeeding and the use of human milk. *Paediatrics* **2012**, *129*, 827–841.
4. Kramer, M.S.; Kakuma, R. Optimal duration of exclusive breastfeeding. *Cochrane Database Syst. Rev.* **2012**, *15*, 8. [CrossRef]
5. Owen, C.G.; Martin, R.M.; Whincup, P.H.; Smith, G.D.; Cook, D.G. Effect of infant feeding on the risk of obesity across the life course: A quantitative review of published evidence. *Paediatrics* **2005**, *115*, 1367–1377. [CrossRef] [PubMed]
6. Victora, C.G.; Bahl, R.; Barros, A.J.; Franca, G.V.; Horton, S.; Krasevec, J.; Murch, S.; Sankar, M.J.; Walker, N.; Rollins, N.C. Breastfeeding in the 21st century: Epidemiology, mechanisms, and lifelong effect. *Lancet* **2016**, *387*, 475–490. [CrossRef]
7. Owen, C.G.; Martin, R.M.; Whincup, P.H.; Smith, G.D.; Cook, D.G. Does breastfeeding influence risk of type 2 diabetes in later life? A quantitative analysis of published evidence. *Am. J. Clin. Nutr.* **2006**, *84*, 1043–1054. [CrossRef] [PubMed]
8. Horta, B.L.; Loret de Mola, C.; Victora, C.G. Long-term consequences of breastfeeding on cholesterol, obesity, systolic blood pressure and type 2 diabetes: A systematic review and meta-analysis. *Acta Paediatr.* **2015**, *104*, 30–37. [CrossRef] [PubMed]
9. Buyken, A.E.; Karaolis-Danckert, N.; Remer, T.; Bolzenius, K.; Landsberg, B.; Kroke, A. Effects of breastfeeding on trajectories of body fat and BMI throughout childhood. *Obesity* **2008**, *16*, 389–395. [CrossRef] [PubMed]

10. Beyerlein, A.; von Kries, R. Breastfeeding and body composition in children: Will there ever be conclusive empirical evidence for a protective effect against overweight? *Am. J. Clin. Nutr.* **2011**, *94*, 1772–1775. [CrossRef] [PubMed]
11. Andreas, N.J.; Kampmann, B.; Mehring Le Doare, K. Human breast milk: A review on its composition and bioactivity. *Early Hum. Dev.* **2015**, *91*, 629–635. [CrossRef] [PubMed]
12. Kent, J.C.; Mitoulas, L.R.; Cregan, M.D.; Ramsay, D.T.; Doherty, D.A.; Hartmann, P.E. Volume and frequency of breastfeedings and fat content of breast milk throughout the day. *Paediatrics* **2006**, *117*, 387–395. [CrossRef] [PubMed]
13. Chang, N.; Jung, J.A.; Kim, H.; Jo, A.; Kang, S.; Lee, S.W.; Yi, H.; Kim, J.; Yim, J.G.; Jung, B.M. Macronutrient composition of human milk from Korean mothers of full term infants born at 37–42 gestational weeks. *Nutr. Res. Pract.* **2015**, *9*, 433–438. [CrossRef] [PubMed]
14. Charpak, N.; Ruiz, J.G. Breast milk composition in a cohort of pre-term infants' mothers followed in an ambulatory programme in Colombia. *Acta Paediatr.* **2007**, *96*, 1755–1759. [CrossRef] [PubMed]
15. Mitoulas, L.R.; Kent, J.C.; Cox, D.B.; Owens, R.A.; Sherriff, J.L.; Hartmann, P.E. Variation in fat, lactose and protein in human milk over 24 h and throughout the first year of lactation. *Br. J. Nutr.* **2002**, *88*, 29–37. [CrossRef] [PubMed]
16. Lee, J.S. Changes in specific gravity, total solid and protein contents of human milk during the course of lactation in Korean women. *Korean J. Nutr.* **1988**, *21*, 129–133.
17. Lee, S.G.; Chung, T.H. Lipid content of breast milk in Korean women. *J. Korean Pediatr. Soc.* **1985**, *28*, 977–988.
18. Nommsen, L.A.; Lovelady, C.A.; Heinig, M.J.; Lönnerdal, B.; Dewey, K.G. Determinants of energy, protein, lipid, and lactose concentrations in human milk during the first 12 mo of lactation: The DARLING Study. *Am. J. Clin. Nutr.* **1991**, *53*, 457–465. [CrossRef] [PubMed]
19. Yang, T.; Zhang, Y.; Ning, Y.; You, L.; Ma, D.; Zheng, Y.; Yang, X.; Li, W.; Wang, J.; Wang, P. Breast milk macronutrient composition and the associated factors in urban Chinese mothers. *Chin. Med. J.* **2014**, *127*, 1721–1725. [PubMed]
20. Quinn, E.A.; Diki Bista, K.; Childs, G. Milk at Altitude: Human Milk Macronutrient Composition in a High-Altitude Adapted Population of Tibetans. *Am. J. Phys. Anthropol.* **2016**, *159*, 233–243. [CrossRef] [PubMed]
21. Quinn, E.A.; Largado, F.; Power, M.; Kuzawa, C.W. Predictors of breast milk macronutrient composition in Filipino mothers. *Am. J. Hum. Biol.* **2012**, *24*, 533–540. [CrossRef] [PubMed]
22. Abranches, A.D.; Soares, F.V.; Junior, S.C.; Moreira, M.E. Freezing and thawing effects on fat, protein, and lactose levels of human natural milk administered by gavage and continuous infusion. *J. Pediatr.* **2014**, *90*, 384–388. [CrossRef] [PubMed]
23. Khan, S.; Prime, D.K.; Hepworth, A.R.; Tat Lai, Ch.; Trengove, N.J.; Hartmann, P.E. Investigation of short-term variations in term breast milk composition during repeated breast expression sessions. *J. Hum. Lact.* **2013**, *29*, 196–204. [CrossRef] [PubMed]
24. Euro Who. Available online: http://www.euro.who.int/en/health-topics/disease-prevention/nutrition/a-healthy-lifestyle/body-mass-index-bmi (accessed on 16 August 2018).
25. Maltron International. Maltron Bioscan 920-2 Operating and Service Manual. 1999, pp. 8–30. Available online: http://www.bmgrp.at/fileadmin/user_upload/images/downloads/BioScan_920-II_new.pdf (accessed on 12 July 2018).
26. Heyward, V.H.; Stolarczyk, L.M. *Applied Body Composition Assessment*; Human Kinetics Publishers: Champaign, IL, USA, 1996; pp. 1–215.
27. Groh-Wargo, S.; Valentic, J.; Khaira, S.; Super, D.M.; Collin, M. Human Milk Analysis Using Mid-Infrared Spectroscopy. *Nutr. Clin. Pract.* **2016**, *31*, 266–272. [CrossRef] [PubMed]
28. Smilowitz, J.T.; Gho, D.S.; Mirmiran, M.; German, J.B.; Underwood, M.A. Rapid Measurement of Human Milk Macronutrients in the Neonatal Intensive Care Unit: Accuracy and Precision of Fourier Transform Mid-Infrared Spectroscopy. *J. Hum. Lact.* **2014**, *30*, 180–189. [CrossRef] [PubMed]
29. Szponar, L.; Wolnicka, K.; Rychlik, E. *Album of Photographs of Food Products and Dishes*; National Food and Nutrition Institute: Warsaw, Poland, 2011.
30. Casadio, Y.S.; Williams, T.M.; Lai, Ch.T.; Olsson, S.E.; Hepworth, A.R.; Ed, G.D.; Hartmann, P.E. Evaluation of a Mid-Infrared Analyzer for the Determination of the Macronutrient Composition of Human Milk. *J. Hum. Lact.* **2010**, *26*, 376–383. [CrossRef] [PubMed]

31. Ballard, O.; Morrow, A.L. Human milk compostion: Nutrients and bioactive factors. *Pediatr. Clin. N. Am.* **2013**, *60*, 49–74. [CrossRef] [PubMed]
32. Miller, E.M.; Aiello, M.O.; Fujita, M.; Hinde, K.; Milligan, L.; Quinn, E.A. Field and laboratory methods in human milk research. *Am. J. Hum. Biol.* **2013**, *25*, 1–11. [CrossRef] [PubMed]
33. Keikha, M.; Bahreynian, M.; Saleki, M.; Kelishadi, R. Macro- and micronutrients of human milk composition: Are they related to maternal diet? A comprehensive systematic review. *Breastfeed. Med.* **2017**, *12*, 517–527. [CrossRef] [PubMed]
34. Fomon, S.J. Requirements and recommended dietary intakes of protein during infancy. *Pediatr. Res.* **1991**, *30*, 391–395. [CrossRef] [PubMed]
35. Prentice, A.M.; Prentice, A; Lamb, W.H.; Lunn, P.G.; Austin, S. Metabolic consequences of fasting during Ramadan in pregnant and lactating women. *Hum. Nutr. Clin. Nutr.* **1983**, *37*, 283–294. [PubMed]
36. Bravi, F.; Wiens, F.; Decarli, A.; Dal Pont, A.; Agostoni, C.; Ferraroni, M. Impact of maternal nutrition on breast-milk composition: A systematic review. *Am. J. Clin. Nutr.* **2016**, *104*, 646–662. [CrossRef] [PubMed]
37. Tigas, S.; Sunehag, A.; Haymond, M.W. Metabolic adaptation to feeding and fasting during lactation in humans. *J. Clin. Endocrinol. Metab.* **2002**, *87*, 302–307. [CrossRef] [PubMed]
38. Rakicioğlu, N.; Samur, G.; Topcu, A.; Topcu, A.A. The effect of Ramadan on maternal nutrition and composition of breast milk. *Pediatr. Int.* **2006**, *48*, 278–283. [CrossRef] [PubMed]
39. Mohammad, M.A.; Sunehag, A.L.; Haymond, M.W. Effect of dietary macronutrient composition under moderate hypocaloric intake on maternal adaptation during lactation. *Am. J. Clin. Nutr.* **2009**, *89*, 1821–1827. [CrossRef] [PubMed]
40. Forsum, E.; Lonnerdal, B. Effect of protein intake on protein and nitrogen composition of breast milk. *Am. J. Clin. Nutr.* **1980**, *33*, 1809–1813. [CrossRef] [PubMed]
41. Finley, D.A.; Lonnerdal, B.; Dewey, K.G.; Grivetti, L.E. Inorganic constituents of breast milk from vegetarian and nonvegetarian women: Relationships with each other and with organic constituents. *J. Nutr.* **1985**, *115*, 772–781. [CrossRef] [PubMed]
42. Boniglia, C.; Carratu, B.; Chiarotti, F.; Giammarioli, S.; Sanzini, E. Influence of maternal protein intake on nitrogen fractions of human milk. Int. *J. Vitam. Nutr. Res.* **2003**, *73*, 447–452. [CrossRef] [PubMed]
43. Innis, S.M. Human milk and formula fatty acids. *J. Pediatr.* **1992**, *120*, 56–61. [CrossRef]
44. Innis, S.M. Impact of maternal diet on human milk composition and neurological development of infants. *Am. J. Clin. Nutr.* **2014**, *99*, 734–741. [CrossRef] [PubMed]
45. Prentice, A.M.; Goldberg, G.R.; Prentice, A. Body mass index and lactation performance. *Eur. J. Clin. Nutr.* **1994**, *48*, 78–86.
46. Bachour, P.; Yafawi, R.; Jaber, F.; Choueiri, E.; Abdel-Razzak, Z. Effects of smoking, mother's age, body mass index and parity number on lipid, protein and secretory Immunoglobulin A concentrations of human milk. *Breastfeed. Med.* **2012**, *7*, 179–188. [CrossRef] [PubMed]
47. Barbosa, L.; Butte, N.F.; Villalpando, S.; Wong, W.W.; Smith, E.O. Maternal energy balance and lactation performance of Mesoamerindians as a function of body mass index. *Am. J. Clin. Nutr.* **1997**, *66*, 575–583. [CrossRef] [PubMed]
48. Villalpando, S.; del Prado, M. Interrelation among dietary energy and fat intakes, maternal body fatness, and milk total lipid in humans. *J. Mammary Gland Biol. Neoplasia* **1999**, *4*, 285–295. [CrossRef] [PubMed]
49. Rolls, B.A.; Gurr, M.I.; van Duijvenvoorde, P.M.; Rolls, B.J.; Rowe, E.A. Lactation in lean and obese rats: Effect of cafeteria feeding and of dietary obesity on milk composition. *Physiol. Behav.* **1986**, *38*, 185–190. [CrossRef]
50. Grote, V.; Verduci, E.; Scaglioni, S.; Vecchi, F.; Contarini, G.; Giovannini, M.; Koletzko, B.; Agostoni, C. Breast milk composition and infant nutrient intakes during the first 12 months of life. *Eur. J. Clin. Nutr.* **2016**, *70*, 250–256. [CrossRef] [PubMed]
51. Kugananthan, S.; Gridneva, Z.; Lai, Ch.T.; Hepworth, A.R.; Mark, P.J.; Kakulas, F.; Geddes, D.T. Associations between Maternal Body Composition and Appetite Hormones and Macronutrients in Human Milk. *Nutrients* **2017**, *9*, 252. [CrossRef] [PubMed]
52. Quinn, E.A.; Largado, F.; Borja, J.B.; Kuzawa, C.W. Maternal characteristics associated with milk leptin content in a sample of filipino women and associations with infant weight for age. *J. Hum. Lact.* **2015**, *31*, 273–281. [CrossRef] [PubMed]

53. Xie, G.; Ma, X.; Zhao, A.; Wang, C.; Zhang, Y.; Nieman, D.; Nicholson, J.K.; Jia, W.; Bao, Y.; Jia, W. The metabolite profiles of the obese population are gender-dependent. *J. Proteome Res.* **2014**, *13*, 4062–4073. [CrossRef] [PubMed]
54. De Luca, A.; Hankard, R.; Alexandre-Gouabau, M.C.; Ferchaud-Roucher, V.; Darmaun, D.; Boquien, C.Y. Higher concentrations of branched-chain amino acids in breast milk of obese mothers. *Nutrition* **2016**, *32*, 1295–1298. [CrossRef] [PubMed]
55. Martin, C.R.; Ling, P.R.; Blackburn, G.L. Review of infant feeding: Key features of breast milk and infant formula. *Nutrients* **2016**, *8*, 279. [CrossRef] [PubMed]

15

The Effect of High-Dose Postpartum Maternal Vitamin D Supplementation Alone Compared with Maternal Plus Infant Vitamin D Supplementation in Breastfeeding Infants in a High-Risk Population

Adekunle Dawodu [1,*], Khalil M. Salameh [2], Najah S. Al-Janahi [3], Abdulbari Bener [4] and Naser Elkum [5]

1. Department of Pediatrics, College of Medicine, University of Cincinnati, Cincinnati, OH 45267, USA
2. Division of Pediatrics, Al-Wakra Hospital, Hamad Medical Corporation, Doha, Qatar
3. Department of Obstetrics and Gynecology, Women's Hospital, Hamad Medical Corporation, Doha, Qatar
4. Department of Biostatistics and Medical Informatics, Cerrahpasa Faculty of Medicine, Istanbul University Cerrahpasa and Istanbul Medipol University, 34098 Cerrahpasa-Istanbul, Turkey
5. Sidra Medicine, Doha, Qatar

* Correspondence: adekunle_dawodu@yahoo.com or dawodua@ucmail.uc.edu

Abstract: In view of continuing reports of high prevalence of severe vitamin D deficiency and low rate of infant vitamin D supplementation, an alternative strategy for prevention of vitamin D deficiency in infants warrants further study. The aim of this randomized controlled trial among 95 exclusively breastfeeding mother–infant pairs with high prevalence of vitamin D deficiency was to compare the effect of six-month post-partum vitamin D_3 maternal supplementation of 6000 IU/day alone with maternal supplementation of 600 IU/day plus infant supplementation of 400 IU/day on the vitamin D status of breastfeeding infants in Doha, Qatar. Serum calcium, parathyroid hormone, maternal urine calcium/creatinine ratio and breast milk vitamin D content were measured. At baseline, the mean serum 25-hydroxyvitamin D (25(OH)D) of mothers on 6000 IU and 600 IU (35.1 vs. 35.7 nmol/L) and in their infants (31.9 vs. 29.6) respectively were low but similar. At the end of the six month supplementation, mothers on 6000 IU achieved higher serum 25(OH)D mean ± SD of 98 ± 35 nmol/L than 52 ± 20 nmol/L in mothers on 600 IU ($p < 0.0001$). Of mothers on 6000 IU, 96% achieved adequate serum 25(OH)D (≥50 nmol/L) compared with 52%in mothers on 600 IU ($p < 0.0001$). Infants of mothers on 600 IU and also supplemented with 400 IU vitamin D_3 had slightly higher serum 25(OH)D than infants of mothers on 6000 IU alone (109 vs. 92 nmol/L, $p = 0.03$); however, similar percentage of infants in both groups achieved adequate serum 25(OH)D ≥50 nmol/L (91% vs. 89%, $p = 0.75$). Mothers on 6000 IU vitamin D_3/day also had higher human milk vitamin D content. Safety measurements, including serum calcium and urine calcium/creatinine ratios in the mother and serum calcium levels in the infants were similar in both groups. Maternal 6000 IU/day vitamin D_3 supplementation alone safely optimizes maternal vitamin D status, improves milk vitamin D to maintain adequate infant serum 25(OH)D. It thus provides an alternative option to prevent the burden of vitamin D deficiency in exclusively breastfeeding infants in high-risk populations and warrants further study of the effective dose.

Keywords: vitamin D deficiency; supplementation; breastfeeding; mothers; infants

---

1. Introduction

Chronic vitamin D deficiency resulting in rickets remains a serious childhood public health problem worldwide, particularly in breastfeeding infants who lack sun exposure and vitamin D supplementation in Asia, parts of Africa and the Middle East, including Qatar, and among the immigrant population from the above countries to Europe, Australia and New Zealand [1,2]. Although vitamin D is effective in preventing vitamin D deficiency, recent reports confirmed that nutritional rickets due to vitamin D deficiency is common and the prevalence is significantly higher in Middle Eastern countries [3], some parts of Asia [4] and among children of immigrant and minority populations than the Western population in prospective and cross-section studies [5]. Of 540 Qatari children of less than five years of age attending a primary health care clinic, 24% were found to have nutritional rickets [3]. A national survey of vitamin D deficiency in Mongolian children <5 years found that 42% of the children had serum 25-hydroxyvitamin D [25(OH)D] < 23 nmol/L and 50% of those with serum 25(OH)D < 23 nmol/L had clinical rickets [4]. Despite reports of high prevalence of nutritional rickets, especially in high risk populations worldwide [1–5], and the different recommendations from professional bodies and expert advisory groups on preventive measures [1,6], the prevalence of vitamin D deficiency associated with increased risk of rickets continues to be a significant public health problem, especially in breastfed infants [2,7–9] due to low vitamin D intake from the breast milk, low vitamin D supplementation and lack of sunlight exposure. The prevalence and magnitude of vitamin D deficiency depends on the definition used in the reported studies. The Institute of Medicine defines vitamin D deficiency as serum 25(OH)D < 30 nmol/L [9] while the Endocrine Society defines serum 25(OH)D < 50 nmol/L as vitamin D deficiency [10]. Some studies report the prevalence of 25(OH)D < 25 nmol/L as cutoff for vitamin D deficiency in unsupplemented breastfed infants with 43% in New Delhi, India [11], and 58% in a cohort of Arab breastfed infants in Doha, Qatar [12]. Furthermore, the prevalence of serum 25(OH)D < 30 nmol/L associated with increased risk of nutritional rickets [1] range from 13% in Cincinnati, Ohio [13], and 22% in Mexico City [13]. In a review of global vitamin D status based on articles published in PubMed/Medline, the prevalence of vitamin D deficiency as defined in the present study (serum 25(OH)D < 50 nmol/L) [10] in infants range from 24%, 40%, 46% to as high as 93%, 96% and 99% in Argentina, Australia, Black American (US), in Iran, Kuwait and India respectively [14].

Besides rickets, vitamin D deficiency or suboptimal vitamin D intake in infancy has also been shown to be associated with increased risk of lower respiratory tract infections in infancy and childhood [15,16] and vitamin D deficiency should, therefore, be regarded as a significant public health problem in children and prevention, particularly in the breastfed infants, requires heightened attention. The natural sources of vitamin D after birth in breastfeeding infants are previous transplacental transfer, human milk and sunlight exposure. The infant vitamin D stores at birth are dependent on maternal vitamin D status during pregnancy [17]. There are many documented reports of high prevalence of vitamin D deficiency during pregnancy worldwide associated with lack of sunlight exposure and inadequate vitamin D corrective supplements [8] that will predispose their infants to low vitamin D stores at birth [17]. The few studies that have also reported vitamin D status of breastfeeding mothers, indicate high prevalence of vitamin D deficiency (serum 25(OH)D < 50 nmol/L) ranging from 15% in Cincinnati [13], 51% in Shanghai [13], and 62% in Mexico City [13] which would theoretically be associated with low milk vitamin D intake for the nursing infant.

Since human milk contains low vitamin D (20–70 IU/L), it would be insufficient to meet the recommended daily intake of 400 IU of vitamin D for infants [6,9] when infant sun exposure is limited and the mothers are vitamin D deficient. Therefore, the current recommendation from professional body in the U.S. [6], and experts' opinion [1,9,10] is that all infants receive direct oral supplementation of 400 IU vitamin D/day to maintain adequate vitamin D status to prevent vitamin D deficiency. Compliance with vitamin D supplementation in breastfeeding infants has been reported to be very low and recent studies from the US found vitamin D supplementation rate of 5%–19% in fully breastfed infants during the first six months of life [18,19]. In addition, vitamin D supplementation of breastfeeding infants does not address the concomitant high prevalence of vitamin D deficiency in their mothers. Therefore, ensuring maternal vitamin D sufficiency has been suggested as part of the strategy to prevent vitamin D deficiency in breastfed infants and their mothers [8,20]. This led to a pilot study of high-dose maternal vitamin D supplementation alone to prevent vitamin D deficiency in breastfeeding mother and her nursing infant.

Because of increasing reports of rickets [21] and the high prevalence of vitamin D deficiency in breastfeeding infants [6,8,21] and the new data in adults on the safety of up to 10,000 IU/day of vitamin D supplementation [22], a larger study from Charleston, South Carolina in the US, compared the effect of daily high-dose maternal vitamin D supplementation alone of 6400 IU with maternal supplementation of 400 IU/day and direct infant supplementation of 300 IU/day for six months on vitamin D status of breastfeeding infants [23]. The authors found significantly increased maternal serum 25(OH)D and breast milk vitamin D content in the maternal high-dose group [23]. The mean serum 25(OH)D in the nursing infants following high-dose maternal supplementation alone were similar to those in infants following maternal plus infant supplementation. There were no safety concerns related to vitamin D supplementation in mothers and infants as measured by serum calcium levels and urine calcium–creatinine ratio [23]. In a more recent large National Institute of Health-funded randomized controlled trial the same group from Charleston, South Carolina, compared the effectiveness of maternal vitamin D_3 supplementation of 6400 IU/day alone with maternal plus infant supplementation with 400 IU/day in 334 exclusively breastfeeding mother–infant pairs. The authors confirmed that maternal supplementation alone with 6400 IU/day significantly increased maternal vitamin D status to meet the requirement of the nursing infant without safety issues [24]. The vitamin D content of the breast milk was not measured in this later study to assesses the contribution of milk vitamin D. In view of the reported high prevalence of vitamin D deficiency in Arab mother–infant breastfeeding dyads [8], reported low rate of infant vitamin D supplementation, and the possible effect of baseline vitamin D status on the response to supplementation dose [25,26], the present randomized controlled trial was conducted to compare the effect of high-dose maternal vitamin D supplementation alone with combined maternal and direct infant vitamin D supplementation on vitamin D status of breastfeeding infant in this high-risk population. To our knowledge, this was the first study to further examine and compare with previous landmark US studies the effect of daily maternal vitamin D supplementation alone on maternal and breast milk vitamin D status as part of a strategy to reduce the burden of vitamin D deficiency in breastfeeding mother–infant pairs in a population with endemic vitamin D deficiency.

1.1. *Primary Aim*

The effect of 6000 IU/day maternal vitamin D_3 supplementation alone was compared with maternal supplementation of 600 IU/day plus direct infant supplementation of 400 IU/day vitamin D_3 on the serum 25(OH)D levels of breastfeeding mothers and their infants including the percentage of mothers and infants that achieved a priori criteria of adequate serum 25(OH)D levels of $\geq$50 nmol/L [9].

1.2. *Secondary Aim*

The effect of maternal high-dose (6000 IU/day) vitamin D_3 and 600 IU/day maternal vitamin D_3 supplementation on human milk vitamin D content was also evaluated.

The hypothesis was that 6000 IU/day maternal vitamin D_3 supplementation alone would optimize vitamin D status of exclusively breastfeeding mother and maintain vitamin D status of the nursing infant at equivalent level to that of an infant on direct oral vitamin D_3 supplementation of 400 IU/day plus maternal 600 IU/day vitamin D_3 supplementation.

2. Materials and Methods

2.1. *Trial Design, Setting and Participants*

This was a randomized, controlled, double-blind trial of the effect of 6000 IU/day maternal vitamin D_3 supplementation alone versus maternal vitamin D_3 supplementation of 600 IU/day plus direct infant vitamin D_3 supplementation of 400 IU/day on the vitamin D status of breastfeeding infants in a sunny environment of Doha, Qatar. Arab breastfeeding mothers in Doha and Al-Wakra, Qatar, who delivered at term (37–42 weeks) at Al-Wakra Hospital, Hamad Medical Corporation (HMC) and planned to fully breastfeed their babies for the first 4–6 months postpartum were eligible for the study and were enrolled within four weeks of delivery and followed up for six months (during the period of August 2013–May 2016).

The study was approved by Hamad Medical Corporation and Weill Cornell Medical College Qatar Joint Institutional Review Board (JIRB No. 13-00036), and Cincinnati Children's Hospital Medical Center Institutional Review Board (IRB) (study No. 2013–4909). Subjects were included in the study if they met the following criteria: (1) Arab women who delivered at term and presented for routine follow-up within 4 weeks after delivery, (2) were self-reported to be in good health, (3) agreed to blood and milk collection at enrollment and follow up to blood draw from the infant for study investigations, (4) planned to fully breastfeed for at least 4–6 months and (5) would be available for follow up visits. Exclusion criteria were mothers with pre-existing calcium disorders, active thyroid disease, Type 1 diabetes or liver diseases, which are likely to affect vitamin D status of the mothers and those of the infants. Mothers of infants with major or multiple congenital anomalies were also excluded.

2.2. *Initial Visit and Baseline Data*

Each mother completed questionnaires on socio-demographic and health status. These included maternal age, nationality, and educational level and occupation of herself and the father of the infant. Pregnancy and delivery information, and infant dietary and neonatal history including growth parameters were recorded. Maternal and infant sunlight exposure behaviors was based on usual outdoor clothing and included body surface area (BSA) exposed to sunlight, duration of sun exposure outdoor (h/week) and sun index score (%BSA x h/week of sun exposure), which correlate with serum vitamin D status in adults and infants [18,27]. The season in which the blood samples were drawn were defined as "hot season" (April–September) and "cool season" (October–March). Baseline biochemical parameters including serum vitamin D status and calcium homeostasis were assessed as a function of season and sunlight exposure characteristics at first visit. The data provided information with which to compare the results derived from different supplementation groups and at other different time points.

Maternal weight and height were recorded to determine the body mass index (BMI), (weight (kg)/height (meter squared)). BMI was not included as criterion for exclusion because of the high prevalence of overweight and obesity in the Arab population. It was taken into account in the analysis as possible confounding variable.

2.3. *Interventions*

Vitamin D Supplementation, Randomization, Blinding

The mother's vitamin D tablets of 6000 IU or 600 IU were of similar color and taste and were manufactured and supplied by Tischon Corp (Salisbury, Maryland) as in our previous randomized controlled trial (RCT) [25] and each mother received a 100-day supply for three months visit and was repeated at the fourth visit. Biotics Research Corporation (Rosenberg, Texas, USA) manufactured and supplied infant vitamin D_3 drops and the placebo administered daily to each infant. The medication met FDA guidelines and has been used in breastfeeding infants in the USA [24]. The vitamin D drops contained 0 IU (placebo) and 400 IU that were similar in taste, appearance and smell. Mothers were instructed to administer one drop daily to their nursing infants. The investigators, patients, and health care providers were blinded to treatment.

The onsite physician-investigators, assisted by research nurse coordinators, enrolled eligible patients after obtaining informed consent. The consented mother–infant pairs were randomly assigned to compare two treatment regimens of vitamin D_3 supplementations: (a) high-dose maternal supplementation with 6000 IU/day of vitamin D_3 and the infant received placebo and (b) maternal supplementation with 600 IU/day of vitamin D_3 plus the infant receiving 400 IU/day of vitamin D_3 orally. The literature suggests that 1000 IU vitamin D supplementation would increase milk vitamin D by 80 IU/L [23,28]; therefore, high-dose 6000 IU vitamin D_3 maternal supplementation was chosen to improve maternal vitamin D status and increase milk vitamin D to a level that could meet the current need of the nursing infant. The current recommended lactating mother vitamin D intake of 600 IU and 400 IU infant intake [9] were chosen as control. The sampling procedure was designed by a statistician to achieve a seasonally balanced study population so that equal number of each group were enrolled during each of the two major seasons. A random assignment conducted as a stratified block design was computer generated to ensure equal number of mothers were randomly assigned to each of the two treatment groups monthly. Mothers on 6000 IU/day were provided with infant vitamin D drops with 0 IU vitamin D_3, and mothers on 600 IU/day were provided with infant vitamin D drops with 400 IU vitamin D_3. A secretary not involved in the project kept a list of randomization code.

2.4. Follow Up of Subjects

Research nurses assisted in the screening, enrollment, data collection and the follow up of mothers and the infants. The research coordinators completed the questionnaires and schedule appointments for blood draw for vitamin D and calcium homeostatic parameters, anthropometric measurement, pill count, as well as urine and breast milk collection. A computer generated calendar served as a reminder to contact the patients prior to their appointment. Each month, the study data manager and the research nurses generated electronic report on patient recruitment and retention, and every effort was made to reschedule patient for missed appointment.

2.5. Measurement of Outcome Variables

Maternal serum 25(OH)D, parathyroid hormone (PTH) and calcium were monitored at visit 1(enrollment) within 4 weeks postpartum, visit 4 (4 months postpartum after 3 months of vitamin D supplementation), and visit seven (seven months postpartum after six months of vitamin D supplementation). Infant serum 25(OH)D, PTH, and Ca, were also monitored at visits 1, 4 and 7. Serum calcium and maternal urine Ca/Cr ratio detects any possible episodes of hypercalcemia and hypercalciuria. The PTH versus vitamin D status relationship was included to compare response to vitamin D supplementation. Maternal urine pregnancy tests were performed monthly. If the mother was found to be pregnant, she would be informed and exit the study because of the uncertainty of the effect of giving high-dose maternal medication to the mother during the first trimester of pregnancy.

2.6. Laboratory Methods

Maternal and infant serum 25(OH)D and intact PTH. Total serum 25(OH)D levels were measured in HMC chemical laboratory by direct competitive chemiluminescence immunoassay on DiaSorin liaison platform (DiaSorin Liaison, Saluggia, VC, Italy). Serum intact PTH levels were measured also by chemiluminescence immunoassay (Unicel DxL 600, Beckman Coulter, Inc, CA, USA) as previously reported [12]. Vitamin D deficiency was defined a priori as serum 25(OH)D levels < 50 nmol/L [10] and vitamin D adequacy as serum 25(OH)D 50 nmol/L or greater [9] for this study.

Maternal and infant calcium measurement. The serum concentrations of calcium and urinary calcium and creatinine were measured in HMC Clinical Laboratory using standard analytic methods.

Breast milk vitamin D content. A 25 ml aliquot of full breast milk expression was collected at visits 1, 4 and 7 and frozen. The milk vitamin D content was measured by the use of LC-MS/MS Mass spectrometry techniques. Solvents were removed under a vacuum and samples were purified with the use of 2 chemically different HPLC systems. The final quantitation of the vitamin D and 25(OH)D was achieved by LC_MS/MS. The day-to-day inter-assay and intra-assay CVs for quantification were $\leq$ 12% [29]. The milk vitamin D contents were converted to antirachitic activity (ARA) using accepted conversion methods [29,30].

2.7. *Safety Outcome*

Each mother was monitored monthly for hypercalciuria. Vitamin D metabolites, serum calcium and urinary calcium/creatinine (Ca/Cr) ratio were monitored closely, and the results checked to detect any values in cautionary or higher than the predetermined parameters. Vitamin D_3 supplementation was stopped if maternal serum calcium was >2.75 mmol/L and urine Ca/Cr ratio > 1 mmol/mmol [31]. Serum 25(OH)D > 95 ng/ml was defined as upper limit of serum 25(OH)D [10]. In recent studies with high-dose vitamin D supplementation of lactating women there were no evidence of toxicity as shown by either hypercalcemia or hypercalciuria [23,24]. Nonetheless, to ensure safety, Data Safety Monitoring Board (including chemical pathologist, endocrinologist, and a pediatrician) monitored reports of adverse events and compliance.

2.8. *Sample Size Calculation*

The primary outcome was infant serum 25(OH)D concentration at the seventh month postpartum and the secondary outcome was percentage of infants that achieved adequate vitamin D status defined a priori as serum 25(OH)D 50 nmol/L or greater. Based upon the data from published study [23], we calculated a percentage of infants in each group with serum 25(OH)D levels of at least 50 nmol/L (20 ng/ml) as successful outcome. Using these percentages as probability of a successful outcome, we estimated that the sample size of 160 mother–infant pairs will provide 90% power to show statistical non-inferiority (defined as <5% difference in success rate) in infants whose mothers alone were supplemented with vitamin D compared with infants whose mothers were supplemented with 600 IU and the infants also received oral supplementation and allowing for unexpected attrition rate which resulted in a total of 190 mother–infant pairs with 95 mother–infant pairs per group. This sample size also allowed us to compare maternal serum and milk vitamin D levels in between the groups over time using appropriate statistical analysis including linear mixed model.

2.9. *Statistical Analysis*

All patient demographic and outcome data were entered into a Red Cap database. The primary variables collected were maternal and infant serum 25(OH)D concentrations at visits 1, 4 and 7. Univariate statistics were generated to examine their distribution as well as missing values and potential outliers. We investigated the distribution of measured variables across groups to observe if there were any differential distribution problems. Kolmogorov Smirnov test, histogram, Q-Q plot, and box plot were used to control for normality. If variables were not normally distributed, they were presented as medians and differences examined by non-parametric tests. Student-t test was used to ascertain the significance of differences between mean values of two continuous variables and confirmed by non-parametric Mann–Whitney test. Spearman's rank correlation coefficient was used to evaluate the strength of concordance between variables. A series of simple linear regressions were conducted to examine the contribution of each of the potential confounder or covariate variables on the outcome. Variables found to be significant in this analysis were included in the final model. The model was a general linear mixed model that incorporates the repeated nature of the data as well as potential confounder variables. Specifically, we used PROC and GENMOD with an identity link function and generalized estimating equation approach to model the relationship between vitamin D and the dose group while accounting for the potential confounding variables. We compared as secondary outcome the percentage of breastfeeding infants in the two groups that achieved serum 25(OH)D levels 50 nmol/L or greater at each time point in the study using Chi-squared test.

As secondary aim, analysis of variance was conducted to test the difference in terms of milk vitamin D content between the two maternal supplementation dose groups at the different time points. This was followed up with pairwise tests of the groups using Tukey's post hoc tests to adjust for the potential multiple testing and control for other factors that may be associated with changes in vitamin

D levels. Statistical analyses were performed using SAS 9.3 (SAS Institute Inc., Carry, NC, USA). The level $p < 0.05$ was considered as the cut-off value for significance.

3. Results

Of the 420 mothers that were assessed for eligibility, 190 consented to participate and were randomized with IRB acceptance to two treatment groups: maternal 6000 IU/day group plus infant placebo (0 IU/day vitamin D) versus maternal 600 IU/day group plus direct infant supplementation with 400 IU/day vitamin D_3. Sixty-two (32%) of the mothers did not continue participation after randomization without any specific explanation but their baseline data were included in the analysis. One hundred twenty-eight mothers (67%) continued active participation through visit 4 while 104 (55%) completed the study to visit 7 for analysis (Figure 1).

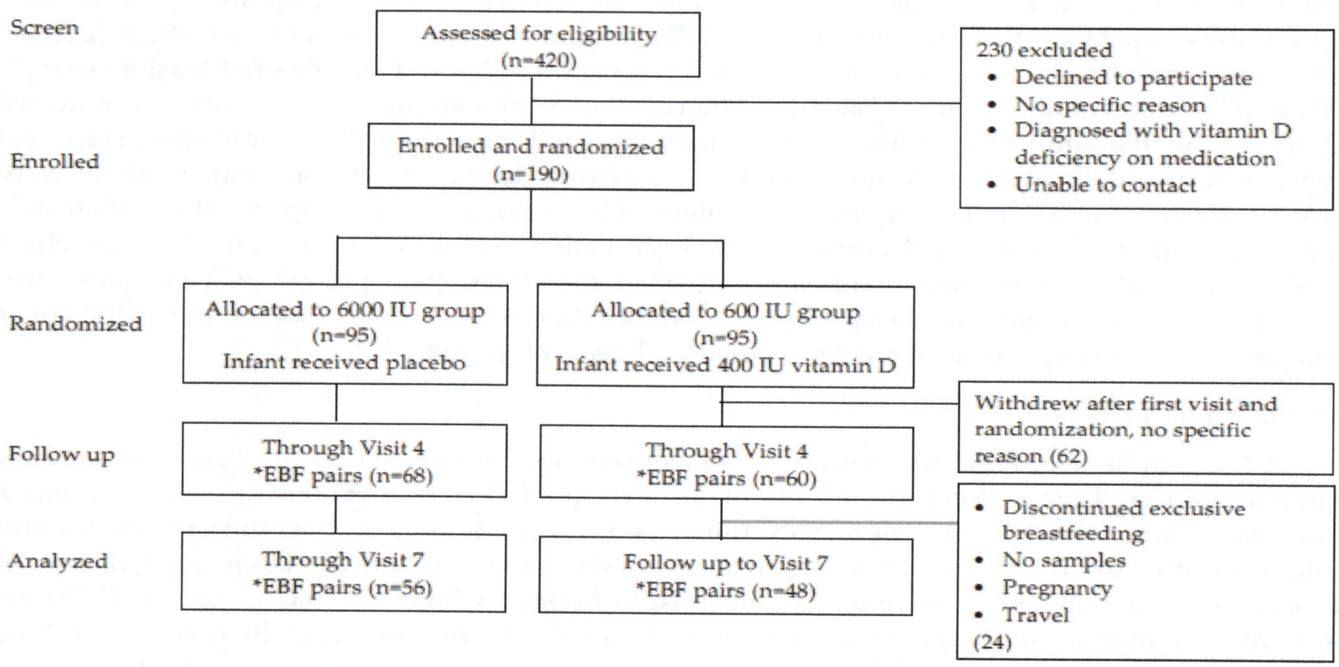

Figure 1. Flow chart of the participants throughout the study. *EBF—Exclusive Breastfeeding.

The mean age of the mothers was 29.6 years, weight was 76 kg, and BMI 29.3. There were no significant differences in all the baseline characteristics including vitamin D status of the mothers and infants between the two groups and breast milk vitamin D content (Tables 1 and 2). Of the mothers and infants with available data, 83% of the mothers were vitamin D deficient (serum 25(OH)D < 50 nmol/L) and 21% had serum 25(OH)D < 25 nmol/L, which is below serum 25(OH)D considered to be associated with osteomalacia [9]. Similarly, 82% of the infants were vitamin D deficient and 47% had serum 25(OH)D < 25 nmol/L, values which are associated with rickets [9]. The mean percentage of maternal body surface area (BSA) exposure outdoors of 13% with 0.32 hr/wk of sun exposure and mean sun index score of 6.6 were low. Although the infants BSA exposure outdoors (26%) was higher than in the mothers, the duration of sun exposure, 0.13 hr/wk, was lower. All the results indicated low maternal and infant sunlight exposure. On univariate analysis, maternal 25(OH)D correlated with BSA (rs = 0.2, $p = 0.005$) and infant 25(OH)D correlated with maternal BSA (rs = 0.19, $p = 0.009$) (Spearman's correlation).

Table 1. Baseline (Visit 1) characteristics and vitamin D status of exclusively breastfeeding mothers by maternal supplementation group.

Variables	N++	6000 IU Group (n = 95) Mean ± SD	N++	600 IU Group (n = 95) Mean ± SD	p-value
Age (years)	95	29.7 ± 5.0	95	29.5 ± 4.6	0.87
Weight (Kg)	95	77.4 ± 16.4	95	75.4 ± 16.4	0.40
Body Mass Index	95	29.4 ± 5.6	95	29.1 ± 6.0	0.33
Education	95		95		
• None/elementary		4		3	0.76
• High school		17		14	
• College/University		74		78	
Subjective health score	95	7.6		7.6	0.95
Season at enrollment (hot) %	95	50.5	95	51.6	0.88
Sun exposure behavior	95		95		
• % BSA exposure outdoors		11.7 ± 7.2		13.6 ± 12.1	0.19
• Sun exposure (h/week)		0.27 ± 0.88		0.38 ± 1.55	0.56
• Sun index score (% BSA x sun exposure h/week)		4.5 ± 15.9		8.7 ± 34.9	0.29
Serum Ca (mmol/L)	95	2.36 ± 0.08	94	2.34 ± 0.07	0.11
Urine CA/Cr ratio (mmol/mmol)	90	0.17 ± 0.15	90	0.14 ± 0.12	0.24
Serum 25(OH)D (nmol/L)	94	35.1 ± 16.3	94	35.7 ± 13.6	0.76
Serum PTH (pg/ml)	94	46.4 ± 25.7	93	50.4 ± 25.2	0.29
Breast milk vitamin D (IU/L)	92	25.5 ± 72.0	90	17.4 ± 42.4	0.36

++ N = number of observations. No significant differences between the two groups. PTH = parathyroid hormone.

Table 2. Baseline (visit 1) characteristics and vitamin D status of exclusively breastfeeding infants by maternal supplementation group.

Variables	N++	6000 IU Group (n = 95) Mean ± SD	N++	600 IU Group (n = 95) Mean ± SD	p-value
Weight (g)	95	3404 ± 509	95	3338 ± 448	0.34
Length (cm)	95	50.8 ± 2.9	95	50.8 ± 2.1	0.86
Head circumference (cm)	95	34.8 ± 2.2	95	34.7 ± 1.4	0.58
Sun exposure behavior					
• % BSA exposure outdoors	95	25.6 ± 13.2	95	26.3 ± 16.8	0.75
• Sun exposure (h/week)	95	0.15 ± 0.5	95	0.11 ± 0.39	0.55
• Sun index score (% BSA x sun exposure h/week)	95	5.1 ± 18.1	95	3.95 ± 14.7	0.63
Serum Ca (mmol/L)	95	2.70 ± 0.08	94	2.69 ± 0.09	0.79
Serum 25(OH)D (nmol/L)	93	31.9 ± 21.7	94	29.6 ± 16.1	0.41
Serum PTH (pg/ml)	91	30.4 ± 21.4	91	31.1 ± 21.8	0.84

++ N = number of observations. No significant differences were observed between the two groups.

3.1. Follow Up

3.1.1. Primary Outcome

The primary outcomes of the study were the serum 25(OH)D concentrations in both the mothers and the infants. Following intervention, maternal and infant serum 25(OH)D increased in both groups from baseline. The mean 25(OH)D concentrations were higher at visit 4 (88 nmol/L vs. 51 nmol/L, $p < 0.0001$) and at visit 7 (98 nmol/L vs. 51 nmol/L, $p < 0.0001$) in mothers on 6000 IU/day than those on 600 IU/day (Table 3). There was a higher serum 25(OH)D level in infants on direct vitamin D supplementation of 400 IU/day plus maternal supplementation of 600 IU/day than in infants of mothers on 6000 IU/day alone without infant supplementation ($p < 0.001$) at visit 4. At visit 7, serum 25(OH)D was slightly higher in infants on direct 400 IU/day vitamin D plus maternal 600 IU/day vitamin D supplementation compared with infants whose mothers alone were supplemented with 6000 IU/day vitamin D_3 ($p < 0.03$) (Table 3).

Table 3. Comparison of serum 25(OH)D concentrations in exclusively breastfeeding mothers and infants by group and visit.

Variables	Visit	N++	6000 IU Group (n = 95) Mean ± SD	N++	600 IU Group (n = 95) Mean ± SD	p-value
Maternal Serum 25(OH)D nmol/L	1	94	35.1 ± 16.3	94	35.7 ± 13.6	0.76
	4	68	88.3 ± 32.2	60	51.4 ± 15.7	<0.0001 *
	7	56	98.2 ± 36.5	48	51.7 ± 19.8	<0.0001 *
Infant Serum 25(OH)D nmol/L	1	93	31.9 ± 21.7	94	29.6 ± 16.1	0.41
	4	67	81.4 ± 26.5	60	105.5 ± 50.4	0.001 *
	7	55	92.2 ± 35.5	47	109.1 ± 43.3	0.03 *

++ N = number of observations. * Maternal serum 25(OH)D (nmol/l) and infant serum 25(OH)D (nmol/L) were significantly different between the two groups at visit 4 and visit 7 (Two-sided T-tests).

3.1.2. Secondary Outcome

The percentage of mothers and infants that achieved serum 25(OH)D ≥ 50 nmol/L, considered adequate by the Institute of Medicine based on the needs of 97.5% of the healthy population for bone health [9], were similar in the two groups at baseline; 18% in the 6000 IU group vs. 16% in the 600 IU group (p = 0.70). However, by visit 7, there was a significantly higher percentage of mothers in 6000 IU group with adequate vitamin D status than mothers in 600 IU group (96% vs. 52%, $p < 0.0001$) (Table 4).

Table 4. Categories of maternal and infant serum 25(OH)D status by visit and group.

Variables	Visit	6000 IU Group [n/N (%)]	600 IU Group [n/N (%)]	p-value
Maternal Serum 25(OH)D ≥ 50 nmol/L	1	17/94 (18%)	15/94 (16%)	0.70
	4	64/68 (94%)	30/60 (50%)	<0.0001 *
	7	54/56 (96%)	25/48 (52%)	<0.0001 *
Infant Serum 25(OH)D ≥ 50 nmol/L	1	18/93 (19%)	15/94 (16%)	0.54
	4	59/67 (88%)	53/60 (88%)	0.96
	7	49/55 (89%)	43/47 (91%)	0.75

n = number of observations with serum 25(OH)D value ≥ 50 nmol/L within the group and N is number of observations in each group. (%) is the percentage of serum 25(OH)D ≥ 50 nmol/L within each group. * Significant difference between the two groups of mothers at visits 4 and 7 (Chi-squared test).

For the infants, the percentage of infants with adequate vitamin D status (serum 25(OH)D ≥ 50 nmol/L) in the two groups were similar at all the visits and at visit 7, the end of study, (91% in infants on direct plus maternal supplementation vs. 89% in infants whose mothers alone were supplemented, p = 0.75) (Table 4).

3.1.3. Serum PTH Findings

Serum PTH were evaluated to assess the PTH and vitamin D response to vitamin D supplementation during the intervention. At visit 7, the higher PTH in mothers in 600 IU group was associated with significantly lower serum 25(OH)D than those of mothers in 6000 IU group (51.3 vs. 39.7 pg/mL) ($p < 0.003$) (Table 5). There were no differences in the serum PTH levels of infants in the two groups at any of the visit times (Table 5).

Table 5. Comparison of maternal and infant serum calcium, PTH and maternal urine Ca/Cr ratio and infant serum calcium and PTH by group and visit.

Variables	Visit	N++	6000 IU Group (n = 95) Mean ± SD	N++	600 IU Group (n = 95) Mean ± SD	p-value
Maternal						
Serum Ca (mmol/L)	1	95	3.36 ± 0.08	94	2.33 ± 0.07	0.11
	4	68	2.35 ± 0.08	60	2.33 ± 0.08	0.26
	7	58	2.34 ± 0.08	47	2.34 ± 0.09	0.86
Serum PTH (pg/ml)	1	94	46.4 ± 25.7	93	50.4 ± 25.1	0.29
	4	68	40.1 ± 22.3	61	47.0 ± 20.1	0.06
	7	58	39.7 ± 18.1	48	51.3 ± 25.6	0.003 *
Urine Ca/Cr ratio (mmol/mmol)	1	90	0.16 ± 0.15	90	0.14 ± 12.0	0.24
	4	66	0.24 ± 0.27	60	0.20 ± 0.15	0.24
	7	56	0.24 ± 0.20	49	0.19 ± 0.13	0.13
Infant						
Serum Ca (mmol/L)	1	95	2.69 ± 0.08	94	2.69 ± 0.09	0.31
	4	67	2.62 ± 0.09	60	2.64 ± 0.09	0.31
	7	57	2.57 ± 0.09	48	2.54 ± 0.09	0.15
Serum PTH (pg/ml)	1	91	30.4 ± 21.4	91	31.1 ± 21.8	0.84
	4	64	20.7 ± 12.0	59	21.3 ± 13.0	0.78
	7	57	26.7 ± 28.0	47	26.7 ± 13.2	0.98

++ N = number of observations. * The maternal serum PTH significantly different between the two groups (Two-sided T-tests).

3.1.4. Breast Milk Vitamin D Content

The breast milk vitamin D content in mothers in the two groups was evaluated to compare the effect of maternal vitamin D_3 supplementation of 6000 IU/day and 600 IU/day on milk vitamin D supply to their nursing infants. There was a very significant interaction between the milk vitamin D during the intervention (Figure 2). The mean vitamin D content at baseline were low in both groups of mothers (25 IU/L in 6000 IU group vs. 17.4 IU/L in 600 IU group, $p = 0.36$) (Table 1) and 57% of 182 lactating mothers had values below detection of the assay. After six months of vitamin D supplementation (visit 7), the mothers in 6000 IU group achieved higher mean vitamin D milk content of 202 ± 190 compared with 26.2 ± 38 in mothers in 600 IU group ($p < 0.0001$). The median values of milk vitamin D are compared in Table 6 using nonparametric tests since the data was not normally distributed.

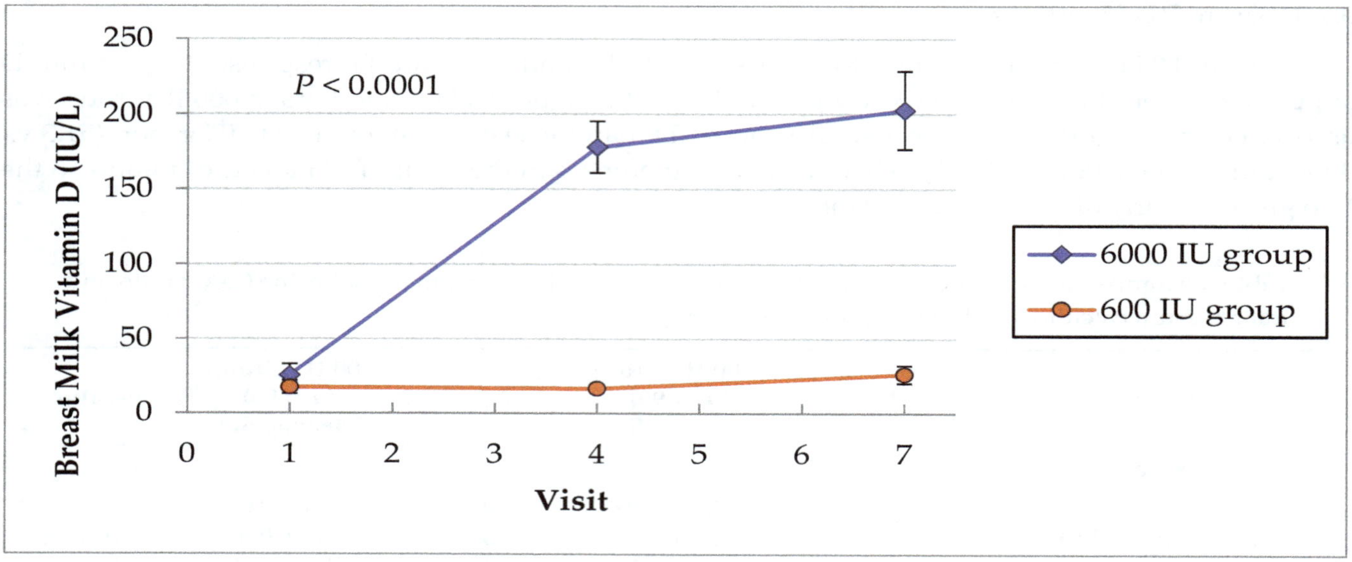

Figure 2. Breast milk vitamin D showed significant interactions between the groups. Mothers in 6000 IU group had substantial higher mean vD milk content of 202 IU/L compared with 26 IU/L in mothers in the 600 IU group at visit 7 ($p < 0.0001$).

Table 6. Comparison of breast milk vitamin D between groups at Visit 1, Visit 4, Visit 7.

Variables	Visit	N++	6000 IU Group ($n = 95$) Median (Range)	N++	600 IU Group ($n = 95$) Median (Range)	p-value
Breast Milk Vitamin D (IU/L)	1	92	8.1 (8.1, 532.0)	90	8.1 (8.1, 379.9)	0.7657
	4	68	185.9 (8.1, 644.0)	60	12.1 (8.1, 70.8)	<0.0001 *
	7	54	143.7 (8.1, 852.5)	41	14.3 (8.1, 203.1)	<0.0001 *

++ N = number of observations. * The median milk vitamin D content were significantly different between the two groups at visits 4 and 7 (Wilcoxon Mann-Whitney Test).

3.1.5. Safety Assessment

Total serum calcium levels were similar at baseline and at visits 4 and 7 in both groups of mothers. Similarly, the mean urine maternal calcium/creatinine ratios were similar at visits 1, 4 and 7 (Table 5) and there were no safety concerns. Serum calcium levels in the two groups of infants were also similar at visits 1, 4 and 7 (Table 5). The Data Safety Monitoring Board (DSMB) monitored the progress of the study and did not identify serious adverse events that warranted stopping the study.

3.1.6. Health Outcomes

A. The mothers on 6000 IU (group 1) had a self-reported health status that was not significantly different than those on 600 IU (group 2) at visit 4 ($p = 0.95$) and at visit 7 ($p = 0.83$).

B. The health status reported for infants of mother in group 1 was not significantly different than those of mothers in group 2 at visit 4 (Fisher's Exact test $p = 0.83$) and at visit 7 ($p = 1.0$).

C. Infant growth parameters, weight, length and head circumference, were also similar at baseline and on follow up between the two groups at visits 4 and 7 (Table 7).

Table 7. Comparison of Infant Birth Weight (g), Length (cm), and Head Circumference (cm) by Visit and Group.

Variables	Visit	N++	6000 IU Group (n = 95) Mean ± SD	N++	600 IU Group (n = 95) Mean ± SD	p-value
Weight (g)		95	3404.7 ± 509.3	95	3338.6 ± 448.4	0.34
Length (cm)	1	95	50.8 ± 2.9	95	50.9 ± 2.1	0.86
Head circumference (cm)		95	34.8 ± 2.2	95	34.7 ± 1.4	0.58
Weight (g)		68	7250.9 ± 849.3	62	7021.2 ± 783	0.11
Length (cm)	4	68	64.3 ± 2.5	62	64.1 ± 2.4	0.72
Head circumference (cm)		68	41.9 ± 1.5	62	41.6 ± 1.1	0.20
Weight (g)		58	8917.0 ± 1085.7	49	8789.0 ± 915.3	0.50
Length (cm)	7	58	70.7 ± 2.8	49	70.8 ± 3.1	0.84
Head circumference (cm)		58	44.8 ± 1.5	49	44.6 ± 1.0	0.32

++ N = number of observations. There were no significant differences between the two groups.

4. Discussion

The high prevalence of vitamin D deficiency in the present study as early as one month postpartum justifies the need for a modified strategy for prevention of vitamin D deficiency in mother–infant dyads in Arab breastfeeding population possibly starting from pregnancy. The severity of vitamin D deficiency suggests that vitamin D deficiency in mothers and infants is an unrecognized public health problem [12] which is detrimental to mothers and their infants.

Based on the definition of vitamin D deficiency, four out of five breastfed infants in this study had vitamin D deficiency at the first month of life, 47% had very low serum 25(OH)D level of <25 nmol/L, and over half (57%) had serum 25(OH)D lower than 30 nmol/L which is consistent with increased risk of rickets and lower respiratory infection without vitamin D supplementation or sunlight exposure [9,15,16]. The findings support the current reports that vitamin D deficiency in infants continues to be a significant global public health problem in low and middle resource countries worldwide [2,7] and warrants heightened attention. The explanations for the high prevalence of vitamin D deficiency in the exclusively breastfeeding infants in this study include lack of sunlight exposure shown by low mean sun index score of 4.52 compared with a mean sun index score of 68 in a cohort of breastfeeding infants in Cincinnati in summer [18], lack of vitamin D supplementation soon after birth due to "delay policy" of the Health Ministry of the country to supplement breastfeeding infants with vitamin D from age 2–12 months, and maternal vitamin D deficiency. Sunshine deprivation is common among mothers and infants in many Middle Eastern countries for cultural reasons and vitamin D supplementation rate of infants is low as in high income countries [18,19]. Since changes in sunlight exposure behavior may be difficult culturally, an alternative approach with high-dose maternal vitamin D supplementation alone was evaluated to optimize maternal vitamin D and milk vitamin D status to improve vitamin D nutrition of the nursing infant. Under research condition, the currently recommended direct supplementation of infants with 400 IU/day plus maternal supplementation of 600 IU achieved a slightly higher mean serum 25(OH)D of 109 nmol/L after 6 months of supplementation (visit 7) than 92 nmol/L in infants whose mothers alone were supplemented with 6000 IU/day and the infant received no supplementation ($p < 0.03$). Nonetheless, the percentage of infants in the two groups that achieved adequate serum 25(OH)D level of ≥50 nmol/L were similar (91% in infants on direct 400 IU/day plus maternal supplementation of 600 IU/day vs. 89% in infants of mothers in 6000 IU group and the infant received no supplementation ($p = 0.75$)) (Table 4). Furthermore, there were no differences in serum PTH response to vitamin D supplementation in the two groups at any of the visit times providing additional evidence of similarity in vitamin D status in response to vitamin D supplementation in both groups of infants (Table 5). Therefore, in the present study, maternal supplementation alone with 6000 IU/day vitamin D_3 achieved adequate infant vitamin D status, similar to direct infant supplementation of 400 IU/day plus maternal supplementation of 600 IU/day vitamin D_3.

A recent large randomized controlled trial indicated that serum 25(OH)D of infants who had direct vitamin D supplementation with 400 IU/day plus maternal supplementation of 400 IU/day and infants of mothers on 6400 IU/day supplementation alone and the infant received no supplementation were similar (108 vs. 98 nmol/L) [24] and our findings in infants are similar to theirs. It is also of interest that mean serum 25(OH)D of 90 nmol/L had been reported among unsupplemented infants of indigenous populations in East Africa who do not lack sunlight exposure [32], supporting a concept that "normal infant vitamin D concentration" could be naturally higher than is currently understood. The finding also suggests that vitamin D status could be "naturally higher" depending on sunshine and limited sun exposure in unsupplemented infants and be a significant contributor to infant vitamin D status.

Addressing maternal findings, the magnitude of vitamin D deficiency in the mothers was similar to those reported from India [11] but higher than 62% in breastfeeding mothers in Mexico City and 52% in mothers from Shanghai or 11% in a cohort of breastfeeding mothers in Cincinnati, USA [13,18]. In addition, the serum 25(OH)D levels of 35 nmol/L in the mothers were low compared with the baseline values of 82–90 nmol/L reported in breastfeeding mothers in a recent study from South Carolina, US [24]. Over one third of the mothers (36%) at baseline had serum 25(OH)D < 30 nmol/L which is consistent with increased risk of osteomalacia and non-skeletal disorders in adults [9,10] and is detrimental to the mothers, and vitamin D nutrition of their infants as referred to in earlier reports [23,24]. After 6 months of vitamin D supplementation, 6000 IU/day vitamin D_3 supplementation was significantly more effective in optimizing maternal vitamin D status than 600 IU/day. Serum 25(OH)D increased by 62 nmol/L between visit 1 and visit 7 in mothers in 6000 IU group compared with only 17.5 nmol/L in mothers in 600 IU group ($p < 0.0001$). In addition, a higher proportion of mothers (96%) in 6000 IU group compared with 52% of mothers in 600 IU group achieved adequate vitamin D status at visit 7 defined a priori as serum 25(OH)D ≥ 50 nmol/L ($p < 0.0001$). PTH levels in mothers in 600 IU group was higher than in mothers in 6000 IU group probably due to significantly lower vitamin D status in 600 IU group following vitamin D supplementation (Table 3). In the randomized controlled trial from the U.S. [24], maternal supplementation alone with 6400 IU/day vitamin D_3 also was more effective in elevating maternal serum 25(OH)D after 6 months of vitamin D supplementation than maternal supplementation with 400 IU/day. In that study there was a decline of 10.5 nmol/L in the 400 IU group but a 52 nmol/L increase after 6 months supplementation in the 6400 IU group ($p < 0.0001$). The increment in the serum 25(OH)D after six months of 6400 IU vitamin D supplementation is similar to the findings in this study. Therefore, the high-dose supplementation is more effective in optimizing maternal vitamin D status and the low dose is inadequate supplementation for high-risk, sunshine deprived population. It is of interest that at the end of the intervention 2% of mothers in the 6400 group and 13% in the 400 group would be considered vitamin D deficient (<50 nmol/L) in the US study [24]. In contrast, 4% of mothers in the 6000 group in the present study and almost half (48%) of those in the 600 group were considered vitamin D deficient. Part of the explanation for the difference in response to supplementation could be related to differences in baseline vitamin D status between mothers in this and the other study which has been shown to affect response to supplementation [25,26]. The mean 25(OH)D level of 98 nmol/L at the end of the study in 6000 IU group is still lower than mean 25(OH)D of 135 nmol/L reported at delivery among unsupplemented traditional female Tanzanian population in East Africa where mothers had no significant sunlight restriction as in breastfeeding mothers in Qatar [32]. Maintaining serum 25(OH)D ≥ 75 nmol/L has been associated with reduced risk of non-skeletal health disorders [10] and may be of theoretical benefit to a higher number of mothers in the 6000 IU group. If the objective of supplementation during lactation is to optimize vitamin D status in mother–infant pairs, then effective high-dose maternal supplementation still needs to be identified especially in high-risk population.

Monitoring of serum calcium, Ca/Cr ratio and serum 25(OH)D in our study did not show any significant difference between the two groups nor any serious adverse events that warrants stopping the study. Two infants had serum 25(OH)D of 94 ng/ml, below the predetermined upper limit of 25(OH)D without any other biochemical or clinical evidence of vitamin D toxicity. Safety parameters in two recent studies from South Carolina, US [23,24], which included serum calcium, and urine Ca/Cr ratios were similar in the two groups of mothers and infants, and revealed no evidence of vitamin D toxicity.

Although it is known that low human milk vitamin D content (range 5–80 IU/L) [24,33] contributes to the low vitamin D nutrition in unsupplemented breastfeeding infants who lack sun exposure, recent studies indicate that maternal vitamin D supplementation of 1000 IU/day would be expected to increase milk vitamin D content by 80 IU/L to improve vitamin D intake of nursing infants [23,28]. In the present study, baseline milk vitamin D levels were within the lower range of previously reported levels but 57% of the mothers in the two groups had undetectable vitamin D content and the milk provided no vitamin D for the nursing infant. After six months of vitamin D supplementation, the mean milk vitamin D level at visit 7 rose to a higher mean value of 202 IU/L in the 6000 IU group (Figure 2) or a median value of 143.7 IU/L (Table 6) than in the 600 group ($p < 0.0001$). The efficacy of the high-dose supplementation of 6000 IU to meet the current recommended infant vitamin D intake was lower than predicted. The lower efficacy may also be related to the effect of limited maternal sun exposure on breast milk vitamin D content as shown in another previous study [23]. It, however, supports our hypothesis that mothers in 6000 IU group would improve milk vitamin D, which would benefit her infant while mothers on 600 IU/day would only have marginal or lack milk vitamin D for their nursing infants. The mean vitamin D content of 202 IU/L in mothers in 6000 IU group was within the lower range of recommended vitamin D intake of 200–400 IU/day for nursing infants [24], while the milk vitamin D content of mothers in 600 IU group was very insufficient without direct vitamin D supplementation to meet the recommended daily intake of nursing infants, as shown in another study [23] in which milk vitamin D was measured. A recent large RCT which compared vitamin D status in infants of the mother who received 6400 IU/day alone with direct infant supplementation of 400 IU plus maternal supplementation of 400 IU/day also found similar vitamin D levels in the two groups of infants but the contribution of milk vitamin D was not compared because vitamin D content in the milk was not measured [24]. To the best of our knowledge, this would be the first study of the effect of high-dose maternal vitamin D supplementation on serum and milk vitamin D status as part of an alternative strategy to prevent vitamin D deficiency in infants in an Arab population with severe magnitude of vitamin D deficiency, and which provided comparison with results of previous landmark US studies [23,24]. Putting all the results together, 6000 IU/day maternal vitamin D supplementation alone appeared safe, optimizes maternal vitamin D status, increased milk vitamin D intake for nursing infants, and achieved similar adequate vitamin D status as in infants on direct 400 IU/day plus maternal 600 IU/day vitamin D supplementation.

There were no differences in the reported health status of the mothers and infants, and in the growth parameters of the infants between the two groups on follow up.

The limitations of our study include moderately adequate sample size, but a high dropout rate among the mothers mostly due to lack of compliance with exclusive breastfeeding and withdrawal from follow up with no specific reasons. Because the study is conducted in Arab breastfeeding mother and infant dyads, we only enrolled Arab mothers for this specific study. The results may be modified in other high-risk populations because of differences in sunlight exposure behavior and dose of vitamin D supplementation.

The present study provided additional valuable data to inform future research in other high-risk populations with similar population characteristics on the effective dose of daily high-dose maternal supplementation alone as an alternative option to reduce global burden of vitamin D deficiency in breastfeeding infants [24]. If successful, the strategy could provide data for health care providers to show that breast milk alone could be a source of vitamin D for breastfeeding infant with appropriate effective maternal high-dose vitamin D supplementation alone (6000–6400 IU or more). This option to prevent vitamin D deficiency in the breastfeeding mother–infant dyads would warrant public health education of health care professionals and providers. It is of interest that a recent study [34] found maternal preference for taking medication themselves as opposed to giving the vitamin D supplement to their infants. The authors suggested that maternal supplementation alone may improve vitamin D intake of the nursing infant in an environment where infant supplementation rate is low.

5. Conclusions

Maternal vitamin D_3 supplementation alone with 6000 IU/day achieved similar adequate vitamin D status as in infants on direct vitamin D_3 supplementation of 400 IU/day plus maternal 600 IU/day supplementation, and safely optimizes maternal vitamin D status with increase in milk vitamin D content. It supports high-dose maternal vitamin D supplementation alone as a possible alternative strategy to reduce the burden of global vitamin D deficiency in breastfeeding infants and their mothers and warrants more studies on appropriate effective dose especially in high-risk populations.

Author Contributions: Conceptualization, A.D., K.M.S., N.S.A.-J. and A.B.; formal analysis, N.E.; funding acquisition, A.D. and A.B.; investigation, A.D. and K.M.S.; methodology, A.D., K.M.S. and A.B.; project administration, A.D. and K.M.S.; software, N.E.; supervision, A.D. and K.M.S.; validation, N.E.; writing—original draft, A.D.; writing—review and editing, A.D., K.M.S., N.S.A.-J., A.B. and N.E.

Acknowledgments: Adriana Reedy and Bin Zhang provided data editing and statistical support; Ghadeer Mustafa provided supervision of data entry; Maram Fakhory and Heba Ibrahim for data collection; Zenica Ramos for project administrative matters; and Donna Bridges for administrative support. Bruce Hollis and Carol Wagner gave expert advice during the implementation of the project.

References

1. Munns, C.F.; Shaw, N.; Kiely, M.; Specker, B.L.; Thacher, T.D.; Ozono, K.; Michigami, T.; Tiosano, D.; Mughal, M.Z.; Makitie, O.; et al. Global consensus recommendations on prevention and management of nutritional rickets. *J. Clin. Endocrinol. Metab.* **2016**, *101*, 394–415. [CrossRef] [PubMed]
2. Creo, A.L.; Thacher, T.D.; Pettifor, J.M.; Strand, M.A.; Fischer, P.R. Nutritional rickets around the world: An update. *Paediatr. Int. Child Health* **2017**, *37*, 84–98. [CrossRef] [PubMed]
3. Bener, A.; Hoffmann, G.F. Nutritional rickets among children in a sun rich country. *Int. J. Pediatr. Endocrinol.* **2010**, *2010*, 410502. [CrossRef] [PubMed]
4. Uush, T. Prevalence of classic signs and symptoms of rickets and vitamin D deficiency in Mongolian children and women. *J. Steroid Biochem. Mol. Biol.* **2013**, *136*, 207–210. [CrossRef] [PubMed]
5. Wheeler, B.J.; Dickson, N.P.; Houghton, L.A.; Ward, L.M.; Taylor, B.J. Incidence and characteristics of vitamin D deficiency rickets in New Zealand children: A New Zealand Paediatric Surveillance Unit study. *Aust. N. Z. J. Public Health* **2015**, *39*, 380–383. [CrossRef]
6. Wagner, C.L.; Greer, F.R. Prevention of rickets and vitamin D deficiency in infants, children, and adolescents. *Pediatrics* **2008**, *122*, 1142–1152. [CrossRef]
7. Roth, D.E.; Abrams, S.A.; Aloia, J.; Bergeron, G.; Bourassa, M.W.; Brown, K.H.; Calvo, M.S.; Cashman, K.D.; Combs, G.; De-Regil, L.M.; et al. Global prevalence and disease burden of vitamin D deficiency: A roadmap for action in low- and middle-income countries. *Ann. N. Y. Acad. Sci.* **2018**, *1430*, 44–79. [CrossRef]
8. Dawodu, A.; Wagner, C.L. Prevention of vitamin D deficiency in mothers and infants worldwide—A paradigm shift. *Paediatr. Int. Child Health* **2012**, *32*, 3–13. [CrossRef]
9. Institute of Medicine. *Dietary Reference Intakes for Calcium and Vitamin D*; The National Academies Press: Washington, DC, USA, 2011.
10. Holick, M.F.; Binkley, N.C.; Bischoff-Ferrari, H.A.; Gordon, C.M.; Hanley, D.A.; Heaney, R.P.; Murad, M.H.; Weaver, C.M. Evaluation, treatment, and prevention of vitamin D deficiency: An Endocrine Society clinical practice guideline. *J. Clin. Endocrinol. Metab.* **2011**, *96*, 1911–1930. [CrossRef]

11. Seth, A.; Marwaha, R.K.; Singla, B.; Aneja, S.; Mehrotra, P.; Sastry, A.; Khurana, M.L.; Mani, K.; Sharma, B.; Tandon, N. Vitamin D nutritional status of exclusively breast fed infants and their mothers. *J. Pediatr. Endocrinol. Metab.* **2009**, *22*, 241–246. [CrossRef]
12. Salameh, K.; Al-Janahi, N.S.; Reedy, A.M.; Dawodu, A. Prevalence and risk factors for low vitamin D status among breastfeeding mother-infant dyads in an environment with abundant sunshine. *Int. J. Womens Health* **2016**, *8*, 529–535. [CrossRef] [PubMed]
13. Dawodu, A.; Davidson, B.; Woo, J.G.; Peng, Y.M.; Ruiz-Palacios, G.M.; de Lourdes Guerrero, M.; Morrow, A.L. Sun exposure and vitamin D supplementation in relation to vitamin D status of breastfeeding mothers and infants in the global exploration of human milk study. *Nutrients* **2015**, *7*, 1081–1093. [CrossRef] [PubMed]
14. Palacios, C.; Gonzalez, L. Is vitamin D deficiency a major global public health problem? *J. Steroid Biochem. Mol. Biol.* **2014**, *144PA*, 138–145. [CrossRef] [PubMed]
15. Wayse, V.; Yousafzai, A.; Mogale, K.; Filteau, S. Association of subclinical vitamin D deficiency with severe acute lower respiratory infection in Indian children under 5 y. *Eur. J. Clin. Nutr.* **2004**, *58*, 563–567. [CrossRef] [PubMed]
16. Roth, D.E.; Shah, R.; Black, R.E.; Baqui, A.H. Vitamin D status and acute lower respiratory infection in early childhood in Sylhet, Bangladesh. *Acta Paediatr.* **2010**, *99*, 389–393. [CrossRef]
17. Hollis, B.W.; Wagner, C.L. Assessment of dietary vitamin D requirements during pregnancy and lactation. *Am. J. Clin. Nutr.* **2004**, *79*, 717–726.
18. Dawodu, A.; Zalla, L.; Woo, J.G.; Herbers, P.M.; Davidson, B.S.; Heubi, J.E.; Morrow, A.L. Heightened attention to supplementation is needed to improve the vitamin D status of breastfeeding mothers and infants when sunshine exposure is restricted. *Matern. Child Nutr.* **2012**. [CrossRef]
19. Perrine, C.G.; Sharma, A.J.; Jefferds, M.E.; Serdula, M.K.; Scanlon, K.S. Adherence to vitamin D recommendations among US infants. *Pediatrics* **2010**, *125*, 627–632. [CrossRef]
20. Hollis, B.W.; Wagner, C.L. Vitamin D requirements during lactation: High-dose maternal supplementation as therapy to prevent hypovitaminosis D for both the mother and the nursing infant. *Am. J. Clin. Nutr.* **2004**, *80*, 1752S–1758S. [CrossRef]
21. Thacher, T.D.; Fischer, P.R.; Strand, M.A.; Pettifor, J.M. Nutritional rickets around the world: Causes and future directions. *Ann. Trop. Paediatr.* **2006**, *26*, 1–16. [CrossRef]
22. Heaney, R.P.; Davies, K.M.; Chen, T.C.; Holick, M.F.; Barger-Lux, M.J. Human serum 25-hydroxycholecalciferol response to extended oral dosing with cholecalciferol. *Am. J. Clin. Nutr.* **2003**, *77*, 204–210. [CrossRef] [PubMed]
23. Wagner, C.L.; Hulsey, T.C.; Fanning, D.; Ebeling, M.; Hollis, B.W. High-dose vitamin D3 supplementation in a cohort of breastfeeding mothers and their infants: A 6-month follow-up pilot study. *Breastfeed Med* **2006**, *1*, 59–70. [CrossRef] [PubMed]
24. Hollis, B.W.; Wagner, C.L.; Howard, C.R.; Ebeling, M.; Shary, J.R.; Smith, P.G.; Taylor, S.N.; Morella, K.; Lawrence, R.A.; Hulsey, T.C. Maternal Versus infant vitamin D supplementation during lactation: A randomized controlled trial. *Pediatrics* **2015**, *136*, 625–634. [CrossRef] [PubMed]
25. Dawodu, A.; Saadi, H.F.; Bekdache, G.; Javed, Y.; Altaye, M.; Hollis, B.W. Randomized controlled trial (RCT) of vitamin D supplementation in pregnancy in a population with endemic vitamin D deficiency. *J. Clin. Endocrinol. Metab.* **2013**, *98*, 2337–2346. [CrossRef] [PubMed]
26. Heaney, R.P. Vitamin D–baseline status and effective dose. *N. Engl. J. Med.* **2012**, *367*, 77–78. [CrossRef] [PubMed]
27. Barger-Lux, M.J.; Heaney, R.P. Effects of above average summer sun exposure on serum 25-hydroxyvitamin D and calcium absorption. *J. Clin. Endocrinol. Metab.* **2002**, *87*, 4952–4956. [CrossRef] [PubMed]
28. Greer, F.R.; Hollis, B.W.; Napoli, J.L. High concentrations of vitamin D2 in human milk associated with pharmacologic doses of vitamin D2. *J. Pediatrics* **1984**, *105*, 61–64. [CrossRef]
29. Wall, C.R.; Stewart, A.W.; Camargo, C.A., Jr.; Scragg, R.; Mitchell, E.A.; Ekeroma, A.; Crane, J.; Milne, T.; Rowden, J.; Horst, R.; et al. Vitamin D activity of breast milk in women randomly assigned to vitamin D3 supplementation during pregnancy. *Am. J. Clin. Nutr.* **2016**, *103*, 382–388. [CrossRef]
30. Hollis, B.W.; Pittard, W.B., 3rd; Reinhardt, T.A. Relationships among vitamin D, 25-hydroxyvitamin D, and vitamin D-binding protein concentrations in the plasma and milk of human subjects. *J. Clin. Endocrinol. Metab.* **1986**, *62*, 41–44. [CrossRef]

31. Vieth, R.; Chan, P.C.; MacFarlane, G.D. Efficacy and safety of vitamin D3 intake exceeding the lowest observed adverse effect level. *Am. J. Clin. Nutr.* **2001**, *73*, 288–294. [CrossRef]
32. Luxwolda, M.F.; Kuipers, R.S.; Kema, I.P.; Van der Veer, E.; Dijck-Brouwer, D.A.; Muskiet, F.A. Vitamin D status indicators in indigenous populations in East Africa. *Eur. J. Nutr* **2013**, *52*, 1115–1125. [CrossRef] [PubMed]
33. Dawodu, A.; Tsang, R.C. Maternal vitamin D status: Effect on milk vitamin D content and vitamin D status of breastfeeding infants. *Adv. Nutr.* **2012**, *3*, 353–361. [CrossRef] [PubMed]
34. Umaretiya, P.J.; Oberhelman, S.S.; Cozine, E.W.; Maxson, J.A.; Quigg, S.M.; Thacher, T.D. Maternal preferences for vitamin D supplementation in breastfed infants. *Ann. Fam. Med.* **2017**, *15*, 68–70. [CrossRef] [PubMed]

16

The Antisecretory Factor in Plasma and Breast Milk in Breastfeeding Mothers

Anna Gustafsson [1,2,*], Elisabeth Granström [3], Christina Stecksén-Blicks [3], Christina E. West [4] and Sven-Arne Silfverdal [4]

1 Department of Clinical Science, Intervention and Technology, Karolinska Institutet, SE 141 86 Stockholm, Sweden
2 Department of Neonatology, Karolinska University Hospital, SE 171 76 Stockholm, Sweden
3 Department of Odontology, Pediatric dentistry, Umeå university, SE 901 87 Umeå, Sweden; elisabeth.granstrom@umu.se (E.G.); christina.stecksen-blicks@umu.se (C.S.-B.)
4 Department of Clinical Sciences, Pediatrics, Umeå University, SE 901 87 Umeå, Sweden; christina.west@umu.se (C.E.W.); sven.arne.silfverdal@umu.se (S.-A.S.)
* Correspondence: anna.gustafsson.1@ki.se

Abstract: Inflammation and infection postpartum threaten the mother and her infant. Human milk provides a defense for the infant, but inflammatory complications like mastitis may lead to the cessation of breastfeeding. Antisecretory factor (AF) has a role in the regulation of secretory processes and inflammation. The objective of the study was to describe AF-levels in plasma and breast milk, and in relation to breast complications. Breastfeeding mothers ($n = 95$) were consecutively recruited at a Well Baby Clinic in Umeå, Sweden. At inclusion four weeks postpartum, samples of venous blood (10 mL) and breast milk (10 mL) were collected. Active AF was analyzed with ELISA using a monoclonal antibody mAb43, and was detected in all samples of plasma and breast milk with a positive correlation (Spearman coefficient = 0.40, $p < 0.001$; Pearson correlation = 0.34, $p < 0.01$). High AF-levels in plasma correlated with high AF-levels in breast milk. The results suggest a co-regulation between active AF in plasma and breastmilk, and/or a local regulation of AF in the breast. Further studies are needed to determine the pathways for the activation of AF-levels in breast milk and plasma.

Keywords: antisecretory factor; human milk; breast milk; breastfeeding; inflammation; lactoferrin; candida

---

1. Introduction

Infection and inflammation constitute a threat to the newborn infant and its mother. The gut of the human newborn infant is susceptible to inflammation and inflammatory conditions that may affect the growth of the infant and cause complications, especially in infants born preterm [1,2]. Human milk provides a broad anti-inflammatory defense [3], but sometimes lactation is threatened by inflammatory complications like mastitis that can lead to the cessation of breastfeeding [4]. Mastitis in lactating women is defined by the World Health Organization (WHO) as an inflammatory condition of the breast, which may or may not be accompanied by infection [5]. It varies in severity, ranging from mild symptoms with local inflammation in the affected breast to more serious symptoms including fever, abscess, and septicemia, requiring interventions [6] that may lead to the cessation of breastfeeding [4]. Recent studies have suggested that inflammation in subclinical mastitis may cause a low milk supply and hence increase the risk of impaired growth of the infant, as well as the cessation of breastfeeding [7].

Human milk contains a variety of biologically active components and is involved in the development of the infant immune system and intestinal microbiota [8,9]. The bioactivity of breast milk has been shown to influence gene expression in the neonatal gastrointestinal tract, with a different expression in formula-fed infants when compared with breast-fed infants [10]. Secretory IgA antibodies bind the microbes on the infant's mucosal membranes, preventing activation of the pro-inflammatory defense. Lactoferrin, a major milk protein, is an important protein for protection against inflammation and disease and reduces inflammatory responses. Additionally, the non-absorbed human milk oligosaccharides block the attachment of microbes to the infant's mucosa, preventing infectious diseases [11]. Transfer of numerous cytokines and growth factors via milk may also activate the infant's immune system. Recent studies have detected a human milk microbiome [12], which is suggested to be influenced by factors like mode of delivery, duration of breastfeeding, and place of habitation.

Antisecretory factor (AF) is a protein which regulates secretory processes and inflammation and that might be of importance not only in animals, but also in infants in the postnatal period [13]. AF is present in most human tissues and body fluids, as well as in the placenta and in breast milk [14,15], with a suggested role in the immune system due to expression on macrophages, B-cells, and dendritic cells, and in all secondary lymphoid organs [16]. A high expression of AF is restricted to specific cell populations, such as certain types of epithelia, neuron, endocrine cells, and subgroups of leukocytes [13]. Cells that store AF also have the capacity to synthesize AF. It probably exerts its effects via nerves, but other mechanisms via receptors, binding proteins, and transport channels in the cellular membrane might be involved. AF can be detected in plasma, and is mostly present in an inactive form in healthy persons [13]. Active endogenous AF in plasma increases by exposure to enterotoxins and certain food constituents. An enhanced activation of endogenous AF synthesis improves the clinical outcome in diseases characterized by inflammation and secretory dysfunction in both humans and animals [13,14,17]. In animals, the levels of active AF in breast milk are positively correlated to the levels in plasma, with a higher concentration in milk than in plasma, probably due to the active transport of active AF across the epithelial lining of the mammary gland [13]. Studies of animals have demonstrated that levels of active AF in plasma and milk can be enhanced through an AF inducing diet, with a protective effect in the offspring related to growth and health [18].

In humans, an intervention study in breastfeeding mothers showed that the induction of endogenous AF in breast milk with specially processed cereals (SPC-flakes®) prevented mastitis [15]. An increased AF plasma level has so far not been reported to induce any form of medical side effects [19].

There is, to our knowledge, no previous descriptive study on the basic levels of active AF in plasma and breast milk in breastfeeding women. An increased knowledge of the basic levels of AF in plasma and breastmilk, and their relation, may be a base for intervention studies, aiming to prevent inflammatory complications in both the mother and infant and promote breastfeeding, as well as infant growth and health. The objective of the study was to describe the basic levels of AF in plasma and breast milk in a cohort of breastfeeding mothers in Sweden.

2. Materials and Methods

2.1. Study Population and Ethical Approvals

This study was prospective, explorative, and descriptive, and a sub-study of an investigation of oral candida infection in infants [20] with 100 mother-infant pairs included. The levels of the outcome parameters, candida colonization in newborns, and antisecretory factor in the mothers were not known. We estimated that in this exploratory study, 100 children needed to be included to obtain an acceptable accuracy. A total of 120 mothers and their four-week old infants were invited to participate in a consecutive order at a single Well Baby Clinic in Umeå, Northern Sweden, between April 2011 and September 2012, of whom 20 did not consent to participate. Samples from plasma and breast milk were collected from 95 of the mothers. The study was approved by the Regional Ethical Review Board in Umeå, Sweden (Dnr 2010-218-31M and 2014-341-32M). Before entry, both parents signed written consent.

2.2. Questionnaire

At inclusion, mothers were asked to fill in a questionnaire about dietary habits on the consumption of an AF-inducing diet consisting of SPC-flakes® and other cereals on the market (i.e., breakfast cereals, grain, porridge) that also might induce/activate AF. Questions were also asked about living conditions, delivery mode, infant weight and length at birth, infant feeding, smoking in the family, and use of antibiotics in the mother and infant. Data on the mother's BMI (kg/m^2) were calculated using data on weight and length collected from charts at the last visit during pregnancy at the maternity clinic, and data were available for 86 mothers. At 12 months postpartum, the mother was asked about a history of maternal infections and inflammation, including mastitis and sore nipples.

2.3. Samplings and Analysis of Antisecretory Factor (AF), Lactoferrin and Calcium

From the mothers, samples of venous blood (10 mL) and breast milk (10 mL) were collected at entry (when the infant was four-weeks old). AF appears in both active and inactive forms [21], which was why it was purified by affinity chromatography for optimal binding sensitivity in the subsequent enzyme-linked immunosorbent assay (ELISA) [22]. In brief, 1 mL of breast milk or plasma was purified by running it through a column of Sepharose 6B CL (GE Healthcare BioSciences AB, Uppsala, Sweden), during which AF binds to the matrix by affinity binding. After washing with physiological phosphate buffered saline (PBS), AF was eluted with 1 $mol{\cdot}L^{-1}$ 1 methyl-alfa-D-glucopyronoside in PBS. The eluate was kept at -20 °C until ELISA was performed. Ass. Prof Ewa Johansson and Prof Stefan Lange (Clinical microbiology, Sahlgrenska University Hospital, Gothenburg, Sweden) provided a monoclonal antibody of the IgM isotype (mAb43) to detect the active form of the protein [22]. All samples were run in duplicate and the mean was calculated. The concentrations of AF were expressed as equivalents against the reference peptide AF1–105, a peptide at the N-terminal part of AF including the active part of the full length protein.

Lactoferrin in breastmilk was analyzed using a Human Lactoferrin Elisa kit, HK329 (Hyocult, Biotec Inc., Uden, The Netherlands). The milk samples were diluted to 1.2×10^5, run in duplicate, and the mean of each sample was calculated.

The analyses of AF (purification and ELISA) and lactoferrin were performed by EG, who is an experienced biomedical analyst at the Biochemical laboratory at the Department of Odontology, Faculty of Medicine at Umeå University.

Calcium in plasma was analyzed at the Department of Clinical Chemistry at Umeå University Hospital according to accredited methods.

2.4. Samplings and Analysis of Oral Candida Colonization in Infants

The inside of the cheeks and tongue of the infants were sampled for Candida using a cotton swab. The samples were then cultivated on a selective media Oricult-N semi-quantitative dipslide (Orion Diagnostica, Espoo, Finland) and scored; Score 0 = no growth, Score 1 = 10^3 CFU mL^{-1}, Score 2 = 10^4 $CFU{\cdot}mL^{-1}$, Score 3 = 10^5 $CFU{\cdot}mL^{-1}$.

2.5. Data Analyzes

AF-levels in plasma and breast milk were analyzed descriptively in relation to each other and to the background factors in the mothers (i.e., age, parity BMI, mode of delivery, vaginal candida infection, and tobacco use) and infants (i.e., gestational age, birth weight, and sex). The distribution of levels of active AF in plasma and breast milk cannot be assumed to be normally distributed, since AF is predominantly present in the inactive form in healthy persons in a healthy environment [13] and the study cohort mainly consisted of healthy mothers. Therefore, we used non-parametric tests

(Spearman's correlation, Wilcoxon signed rank test), as well as both non-parametric and parametric tests after log transformation (Pearson's correlation, Independent t-test, paired samples t-test). The log transformed values were used for the analytical analysis. A p-value of <0.05 was regarded as statistically significant. The Kolmogorov–Smirnov test was used to test for the normality distribution. Fisher's exact test was used in the analysis when the numbers of observations were small. The software SPSS (version 24) was used in the analyses.

3. Results

3.1. Descriptive Results

The characteristics of mothers and infants at entry of the study are shown in Table 1. Fifty-four women were multipara, eleven infants were born by caesarean section, and four were born before gestational week 37. None of the women reported the consumption of an AF-inducing diet consisting of SPC-flakes®.

Table 1. Maternal and infant characteristics.

Factor	Total
	$N = 95$
Maternal characteristics	
Age (years) Mean (SD) (range)	32 (4.5) 21–44
Primiparous, n	44
BMI* (kg/m^2) Median (range)	23 (19.6–30.4)
Cesarean Section, n	9
Vaginal Candida Infection, n	16
Treatment for Candida Infection, n	15
Tobacco Use	
Maternal Smoking, n	2
Paternal Smoking, n	1
Maternal Use of Snuff, n	2
Infant characteristics	
Gestational Age < 37 Weeks	3
Birth Weight, Gram Mean (SD)	3552 (481.5)
Female n	50
Oral Candida, n	11
Breast complications	
Pain in the Breast, n	19
Sore Nipples, n	25
Mastitis, n	17
Infection, n	3

* BMI data were collected from 84 of the mothers.

Active AF was present in all samples of plasma and breast milk. The AF-levels were not normally distributed, neither in the plasma (Figure 1a) nor in breast milk (Figure 1b). Furthermore, there was a wider distribution of the level of active AF in the plasma than in the breast milk (Table 2).

Figure 1a,b show the distribution of AF-levels (arbitrary units) in plasma and breastmilk.

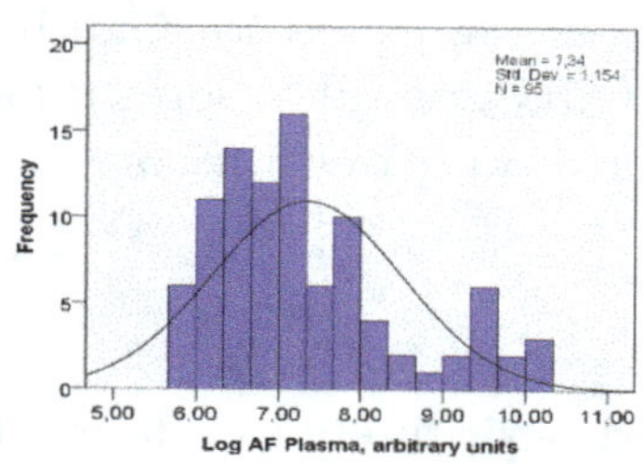

(a)

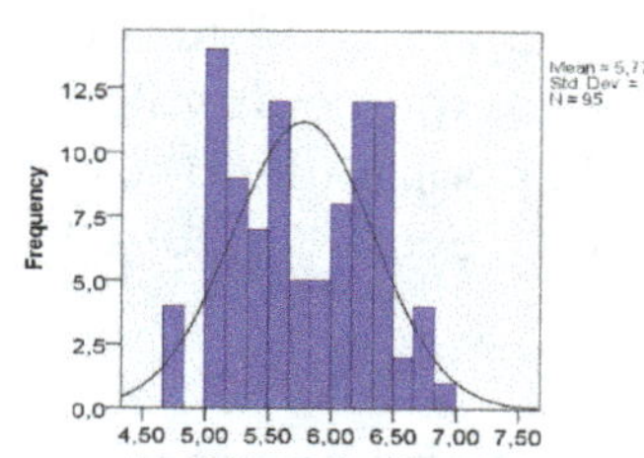

(b)

Figure 1. (**a**) Distribution of log AF-levels (arbitrary units) in the plasma Kolmogorov–Smirnov test of normality, $p < 0.05$. (**b**) Distribution of log AF-levels (arbitrary units) in breastmilk. Kolmogorov–Smirnov test of normality, $p < 0.05$.

Table 2. Distribution of AF (arbitrary units) in plasma and breast milk, before and after log-transformation.

AF Plasma Median (range)	1240 (27,835)
log AF Plasma, Mean (SD)	7.34 (1.15)
AF Breast Milk, Median (range)	293 (904)
log AF Breast Milk, Mean (SD)	5.77 (0.56)

3.2. Analytical Results

There was a positive correlation between the levels of active AF in plasma and breast milk (Spearman's rho = 0.403, $p < 0.001$) (Figure 2).

Figure 2 shows the correlation between AF-levels in the plasma and breast milk.

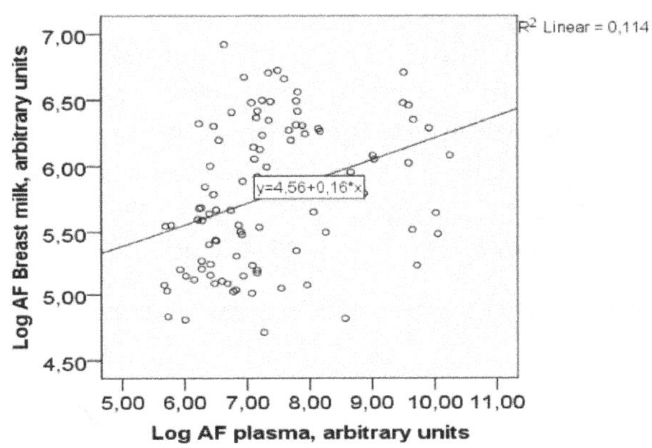

Figure 2. Correlation between the AF-levels (arbitrary units) in plasma and breast milk, Spearman's rho = 0.403, $p < 0.001$.

We found that there was a positive correlation between AF in plasma and the BMI of the mother (Spearman's rho 0.252, $p < 0.05$, Figure 3a), while the correlation to AF in breast milk was not statistically significant (Figure 3b). There were no differences in AF-levels depending on parity, gestational age, or mode of delivery.

None of the mothers reported the intake of specially processed cereals (SPC-Flakes®), and we found no relation between AF and the intake of other cereals on the market (i.e., breakfast cereals, grain, porridge). Seventeen mothers reported a history of vaginal fungal infection during pregnancy and 14 of 17 received anti-fungal treatment. No correlation was found between the level of active AF in plasma or breast milk with neither vaginal fungal infection during pregnancy nor treatment. Furthermore, there was no correlation between infant Candida colonization and AF-levels in plasma or breastmilk ($p > 0.05$).

Twenty-five women reported having had sore nipples. There was a positive correlation between having had sore nipples and pain in the breast (Spearman's rho 0.387, $p < 0.01$), inflammatory mastitis (Spearman's rho 0.443, $p < 0.01$), and breast infection (Spearman's rho 0.302, $p < 0.01$), but no correlation was demonstrated between having had sore nipples or pain in the breast and AF-level in plasma or breast milk.

Figure 3a,b show the AF-levels in plasma and breastmilk in correlation to maternal BMI.

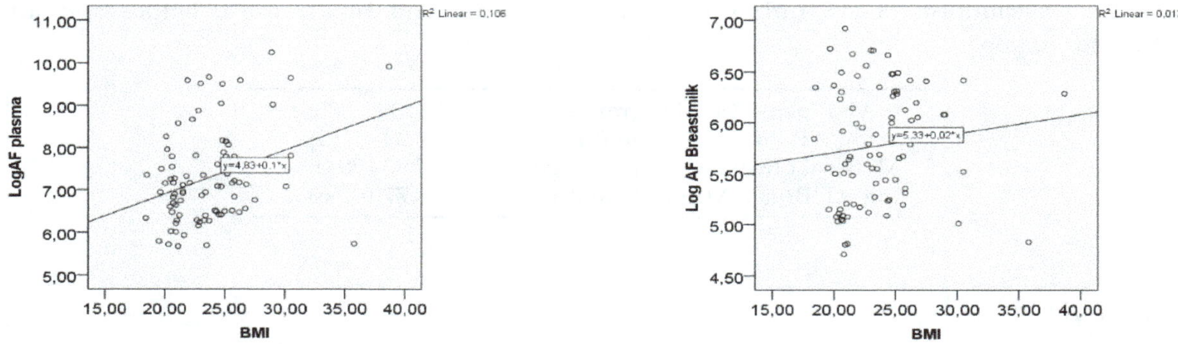

(a) (b)

Figure 3. (**a**) AF-levels in plasma correlating to BMI, Spearman's rho 0.252, $p < 0.05$; (**b**) AF-levels in breast milk in correlation to BMI, Spearman's rho 0.193, $p = 0.08$.

Three women reported having had a history of breast infection, and there was a correlation between breast-infection and low levels of active AF in plasma (Pearson's correlation coefficient 0.220, $p < 0.05$ Pearson correlation), but not in breast milk (Pearson correlation coefficient 0.065, $p > 0.05$). In women who experienced a breast infection, the AF-levels in plasma were lower when compared to those without a history of infection ($p < 0.05$, independent samples t-test) (Figure 4a), while there was no difference in breast milk ($p > 0.05$) (Figure 4b). All three women with breast infections had AF-levels in plasma below the 25th percentile ($p < 0.05$, independent samples t-test).

Figure 4a,b show the AF-levels and reported breast infection.

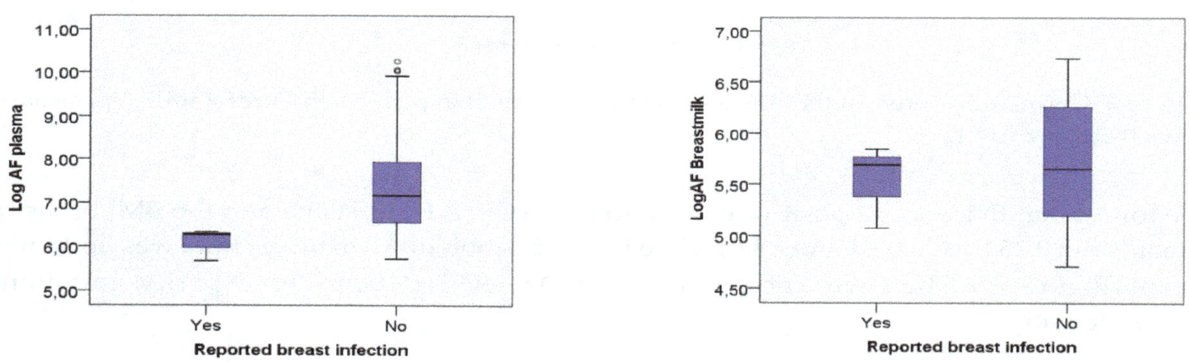

(a) (b)

Figure 4. (**a**) Lower AF-levels in plasma related to having reported a breast infection ($n = 3$) compared with not reporting a breast infection ($p < 0.05$), unfilled circles indicate values 1.5 × IQR or more above the third quartile; (**b**) AF-levels in breast milk related to having reported breast infection ($n = 3$) compared with not reporting a breast infection ($p > 0.05$).

There was a positive correlation between the calcium levels in plasma and having had a breast infection (Spearman's rho—0.255, $p = 0.05$). Figure 5 displays the elevated calcium levels in mothers with a history of breast infection.

Furthermore, we found no association between reported breast complications and oral Candida colonization of the infant (Chi-Square test and Fischer exact test, $p > 0.05$) (Table 3).

Figure 5 shows the reported breast infection and calcium-levels.

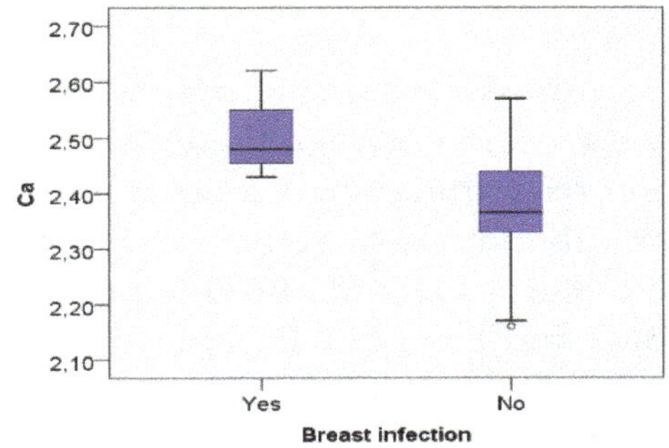

Figure 5. Calcium-levels related to reported breast infection, t-test, independent samples $p < 0.01$, unfilled circle indicates a value 1.5 × *IQR* or more below the third quartile.

Table 3. Maternal breast complication and infant oral Candida colonization.

Maternal Breast Complication		Infant Oral Candida Colonization No Candida	Candida	p-Value
		N	*N*	
Mastitis	yes	17	0	>0.05
	no	56	9	
Breast Infection	yes	3	0	>0.05
	no	69	9	
Sore Nipples	yes	23	2	>0.05
	no	50	6	
Pain in Breast/Nipples	yes	17	2	>0.05
	no	56	7	

The mean lactoferrin level in breastmilk was 2.19 g/L, SD 0.68. A positive correlation was demonstrated between the AF-levels in breast milk and lactoferrin levels (Spearman's rho 0.341, $p < 0.01$, Figure 6a). There was also a positive correlation between the AF-levels in plasma and lactoferrin; however, it did not reach statistical significance (Spearman's rho 0.193, $p = 0.06$, Figure 6b).

Figure 6 shows the correlations between lactoferrin and AF-levels in breast milk and plasma.

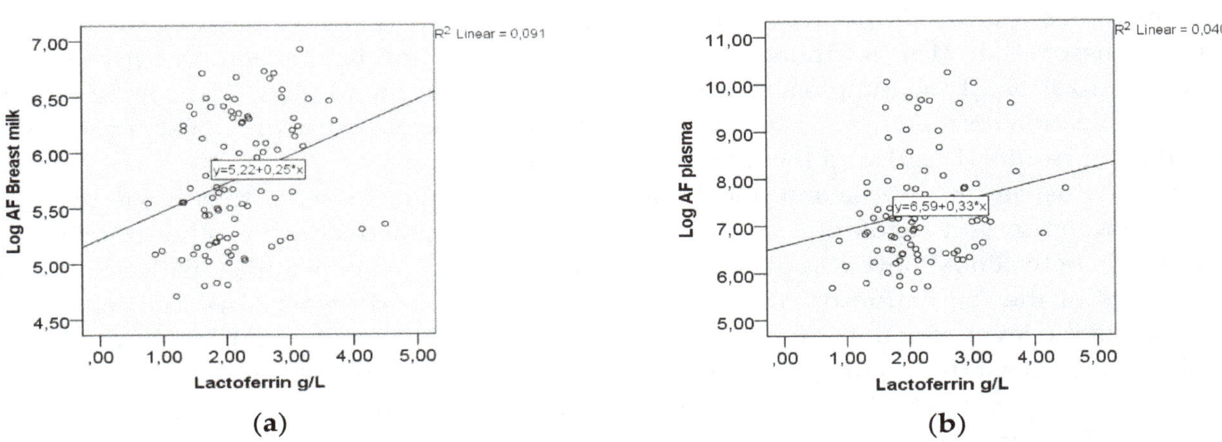

Figure 6. (**a**) Correlation between the AF-levels in breast milk and lactoferrin, Spearman's rho 0.341, $p < 0.01$; (**b**) Correlation between the AF-levels in plasma and lactoferrin, Spearman's rho 0.193, $p = 0.06$.

4. Discussion

Active AF was present in all samples of plasma and breast milk from the mothers at one month post-partum. A positive relation was found between the levels of active AF in plasma and in breast milk, generally with lower levels in breast milk when compared to plasma.

In the majority of the mothers, the levels of active AF in plasma were low, possibly due to a generally healthy population with a high standard of living in an industrialized setting. We found a positive correlation between the BMI and level of AF in plasma. A higher BMI had previously been associated with an increased level of inflammation [23], and a higher AF-level might be a feed-back response to a higher degree of inflammation in general. However, we found no correlation between the AF-levels in breast milk and maternal BMI.

Furthermore, the levels of active AF in breast milk were also low in the majority of mothers. These results were consistent with the results from the intervention study by Svensson et al. [15]. The difference between the factors that correlated with the AF-levels in plasma and breast milk may suggest a local regulation of the AF-levels in the breast due to the health status of the breast and/or the infant. A relationship between the health status of both the mother and the infant and leucocyte count in breast milk has previously been described [24,25], where there were low baseline levels of leukocytes with increasing leukocyte levels, a proxy for the immune response, if the mother or infant had an infection. When the mother and infant are healthy, the origin of maternal cells in human milk is mainly from the mammary epithelium. However, during the first days postpartum and during periods of infection in either the mother or the infant, the human milk cells are dominated by immune cells from the maternal circulation [24,26,27].

The level of active AF was higher in the breast milk from mothers of infants colonized with Candida when compared to mothers of non-colonized infants, but the difference did not reach statistical significance [20]. Active AF in breast milk and lactoferrin were significantly correlated, as demonstrated by a weakly positive correlation between the AF in plasma and lactoferrin, but did not reach statistical significance. Lactoferrin has a role in the innate immunity. A study has shown enhanced levels of lactoferrin, expressed by endothelial cells and activated neutrophils, in breast milk from mothers breastfeeding sick infants [27]. The increased levels of AF in the present study did not protect the infant from Candida colonization [20], but the higher AF-level in breast milk may be due to the colonialization itself and might protect the infant and the mother from active disease.

Three women reported having experienced breast infection, and also had low AF-levels in plasma. The correlation between breast infection and low AF-levels in plasma may indicate an increased risk of breast infection in mothers with low AF-levels. However, there were only three mothers with a breast infection in our material, which is why larger and more detailed studies are needed before firm conclusions can be drawn, although our finding was consistent with the result from the intervention study by Svensson et al. [15]. Furthermore, in this study, we found no correlation between the oral Candida colonization of the infants and breast complications in the mother. The role of infant oral Candida colonization for maternal breast complications during lactation has previously been described with conflicting results [28,29], and there are ongoing studies [30].

Hence, AF is present in plasma and breast milk. Our hypothesis is that AF is involved in the immune defense and regulation of inflammation in the breastfeeding mother and her infant. The correlation between AF-levels in plasma and breast milk was positive and statistically significant. The pathways of the regulation of AF-levels between plasma and breast milk are yet to be fully understood. Is the level of active AF regulated by both the level in maternal plasma and by a local regulation in the breast due to the presence of colonization and/or infection in the breast or infant? Further studies are needed to determine the relation of AF in plasma and AF in breast milk, and the pathways of influence between them.

This study adds to the knowledge about AF in lactating mothers and how it associates with background factors, which has previously been very sparsely studied. The study was performed from 2011 to 2012, and the AF-levels demonstrated in it may be different in a different cohort or time period.

However, in this cohort, the results demonstrated the basic levels of generally healthy woman in an industrialized setting. No consumption of specially processed cereals (SPC-flakes®) was reported and we found no relationship between the AF-levels and intake of other cereals on the market.

The ELISA method we used was a non-commercial, in house version, which has now been further developed as a sandwich ELISA. Basic levels of AF may differ between individuals, and longitudinal studies with repeated measurements may show individual variability. Furthermore, the variability of AF in lactating mothers is unknown. Blood samples were only collected once in the study, at four weeks postpartum. Unfortunately, information on breast complications was not collected at the time of blood sampling, only at 12 months postpartum, and changes in AF-levels may have happened several times during this period of time. However, samples of plasma and samples of breast milk were collected at the same time, and breast complications most commonly appeared in the first weeks to months postpartum. The exact time for reported breast complications and relation in time to the collection of breast milk and plasma samples is unknown, which makes it difficult to establish firm conclusions about the causality between mastitis or sore nipples and AF-levels. Only three mothers in the cohort reported having had a breast infection, which is a low prevalence. However, all three mothers who experienced a breast infection during the first year after pregnancy had low AF-levels in plasma at one month post-partum. Furthermore, we found a positive correlation between calcium in plasma and having experienced a breast infection, which was consistent with the results from the study by Li et al. [31], who showed higher levels of calcium related to subclinical mastitis. They also demonstrated a positive correlation between calcium and the pro-inflammatory cytokine IL-6. Calcium is known to be involved in the recruitment of neutrophils to sites of inflammation. Changes in intracellular calcium levels play an important role in neutrophil activation and function [32].

5. Conclusions

Active AF was present in plasma and breast milk in all mothers and their levels were positively correlated. Active AF was predominantly low in both plasma and breast milk, but there was a broader distribution of AF-levels in plasma when compared with the AF-levels in breast milk. The results suggest a possible local regulation of AF-levels in the breast, as well as a co-regulation with AF-levels in plasma. This study contributes to the knowledge regarding the basic patterns of active AF in plasma and breastmilk. The study was explorative and further longitudinal studies on active AF in breast milk and plasma are needed.

Author Contributions: C.S.-B., CW., and S.-A.S. planned and designed the study and performed the data collection. E.G. performed the laboratory analysis. AG performed the statistical analysis, prepared tables and figures, and wrote the first draft of the manuscript. C.S.-B., C.E.W., A.G., and S.-A.S. reviewed and edited the manuscript. S.-A.S. supervised the process.

Acknowledgments: We express our gratitude to the parents and their children for their participation, and the nurses at Teg Child Health Centre/Well Baby Clinic, Umeå who recruited and sampled the children: Birgitta Isaksson, Ann-Sofie Gustafsson, Britt Stenmark, and Åsa Granberg. We also thank Prof. Lange and Ass. Prof Johansson of Gothenburg University for providing the monoclonal antibody against AF.

References

1. Goldenberg, R.L.; Culhane, J.F.; Iams, J.D.; Romero, R. Epidemiology and causes of preterm birth. *Lancet* **2008**, *371*, 75–84. [CrossRef]
2. Blencowe, H.; Cousens, S.; Chou, D.; Oestergaard, M.; Say, L.; Moller, A.B.; Kinney, M.; Lawn, J.; Born Too Soon Preterm Birth, A. Born too soon: The global epidemiology of 15 million preterm births. *Reprod. Health* **2013**, *10*, S2. [CrossRef] [PubMed]

3. Ballard, O.; Morrow, A.L. Human milk composition: Nutrients and bioactive factors. *Pediatr. Clin. N. Am.* **2013**, *60*, 49–74. [CrossRef] [PubMed]
4. Berens, P.D. Breast pain: Engorgement, nipple pain, and mastitis. *Clin. Obstet. Gynecol.* **2015**, *58*, 902–914. [CrossRef] [PubMed]
5. Inch, S.; Fisher, C. Breastfeeding: Early problems. *Pract. Midwife* **2000**, *3*, 12–15. [PubMed]
6. Jahanfar, S.; Ng, C.J.; Teng, C.L. Antibiotics for mastitis in breastfeeding women. *Cochrane Database Syst. Rev.* **2009**. [CrossRef]
7. Ingman, W.V.; Glynn, D.J.; Hutchinson, M.R. Inflammatory mediators in mastitis and lactation insufficiency. *J. Mammary Gland Biol. Neoplasia* **2014**, *19*, 161–167. [CrossRef] [PubMed]
8. Andreas, N.J.; Kampmann, B.; Mehring Le-Doare, K. Human breast milk: A review on its composition and bioactivity. *Early Hum. Dev.* **2015**, *91*, 629–635. [CrossRef] [PubMed]
9. Lonnerdal, B. Bioactive proteins in breast milk. *J. Paediatr. Child Health* **2013**, *49* (Suppl. 1), 1–7. [CrossRef] [PubMed]
10. Donovan, S.M.; Wang, M.; Li, M.; Friedberg, I.; Schwartz, S.L.; Chapkin, R.S. Host-microbe interactions in the neonatal intestine: Role of human milk oligosaccharides. *Adv. Nutr.* **2012**, *3*, 450s–455s. [CrossRef] [PubMed]
11. Hanson, L.A. Session 1: Feeding and infant development breast-feeding and immune function. *Proc. Nutr. Soc.* **2007**, *66*, 384–396. [CrossRef] [PubMed]
12. Cabrera-Rubio, R.; Collado, M.C.; Laitinen, K.; Salminen, S.; Isolauri, E.; Mira, A. The human milk microbiome changes over lactation and is shaped by maternal weight and mode of delivery. *Am. J. Clin. Nutr.* **2012**, *96*, 544–551. [CrossRef] [PubMed]
13. Lange, S.; Lönnroth, I. The antisecretory factor: Synthesis, anatomical and cellular distribution, and biological action in experimental and clinical studies. *Int. Rev. Cytol.* **2001**, *210*, 39–75. [PubMed]
14. Zaman, S.; Aamir, K.; Lange, S.; Jennische, E.; Silfverdal, S.A.; Hanson, L.A. Antisecretory factor effectively and safely stops childhood diarrhoea: A placebo-controlled, randomised study. *Acta Paediatr.* **2014**, *103*, 659–664. [CrossRef] [PubMed]
15. Svensson, K.; Lange, S.; Lönnroth, I.; Widström, A.M.; Hanson, L. Induction of anti-secretory factor in human milk may prevent mastitis. *Acta Paediatr.* **2004**, *93*, 1228–1231. [CrossRef] [PubMed]
16. Davidson, T.S.; Hickey, W.F. Distribution and immunoregulatory properties of antisecretory factor. *Lab. Investig.* **2004**, *84*, 307–319. [CrossRef] [PubMed]
17. Ulgheri, C.; Paganini, B.; Rossi, F. Antisecretory factor as a potential health-promoting molecule in man and animals. *Nutr. Res. Rev.* **2010**, *23*, 300–313. [CrossRef] [PubMed]
18. Lange, S.; Martinsson, K.; Lonnroth, I.; Goransson, L. Plasma level of antisecretory factor (ASF) and its relation to post-weaning diarrhoea in piglets. *J. Vet. Med. Ser. B* **1993**, *40*, 113–118. [CrossRef]
19. Bjorck, S.; Bosaeus, I.; Ek, E.; Jennische, E.; Lonnroth, I.; Johansson, E.; Lange, S. Food induced stimulation of the antisecretory factor can improve symptoms in human inflammatory bowel disease: A study of a concept. *Gut* **2000**, *46*, 824–829. [CrossRef] [PubMed]
20. Stecksen-Blicks, C.; Granstrom, E.; Silfverdal, S.A.; West, C.E. Prevalence of oral candida in the first year of life. *Mycoses* **2015**, *58*, 550–556. [CrossRef] [PubMed]
21. Johansson, E.; Lange, S.; Lonnroth, I. Identification of an active site in the antisecretory factor protein. *Biochim. Biophys. Acta* **1997**, *1362*, 177–182. [CrossRef]
22. Johansson, E.; Lonnroth, I.; Jonson, I.; Lange, S.; Jennische, E. Development of monoclonal antibodies for detection of antisecretory factor activity in human plasma. *J. Immunol. Methods* **2009**, *342*, 64–70. [CrossRef] [PubMed]
23. Cox, A.J.; West, N.P.; Cripps, A.W. Obesity, inflammation, and the gut microbiota. *Lancet Diabetes Endocrinol.* **2015**, *3*, 207–215. [CrossRef]
24. Hassiotou, F.; Hartmann, P.E. At the dawn of a new discovery: The potential of breast milk stem cells. *Adv. Nutr.* **2014**, *5*, 770–778. [CrossRef] [PubMed]
25. Bode, L.; McGuire, M.; Rodriguez, J.M.; Geddes, D.T.; Hassiotou, F.; Hartmann, P.E.; McGuire, M.K. It's alive: Microbes and cells in human milk and their potential benefits to mother and infant. *Adv. Nutr.* **2014**, *5*, 571–573. [CrossRef] [PubMed]
26. Hassiotou, F.; Hepworth, A.R.; Metzger, P.; Tat Lai, C.; Trengove, N.; Hartmann, P.E.; Filgueira, L. Maternal and infant infections stimulate a rapid leukocyte response in breastmilk. *Clin. Transl. Immunol.* **2013**, *2*, e3. [CrossRef] [PubMed]

27. Riskin, A.; Almog, M.; Peri, R.; Halasz, K.; Srugo, I.; Kessel, A. Changes in immunomodulatory constituents of human milk in response to active infection in the nursing infant. *Pediatr. Res.* **2012**, *71*, 220–225. [CrossRef] [PubMed]
28. Andrews, J.I.; Fleener, D.K.; Messer, S.A.; Hansen, W.F.; Pfaller, M.A.; Diekema, D.J. The yeast connection: Is candida linked to breastfeeding associated pain? *Am. J. Obstet. Gynecol.* **2007**, *197*, 424. [CrossRef] [PubMed]
29. Jimenez, E.; Arroyo, R.; Cardenas, N.; Marin, M.; Serrano, P.; Fernandez, L.; Rodriguez, J.M. Mammary candidiasis: A medical condition without scientific evidence? *PLoS ONE* **2017**, *12*, e0181071. [CrossRef] [PubMed]
30. Amir, L.H.; Cullinane, M.; Garland, S.M.; Tabrizi, S.N.; Donath, S.M.; Bennett, C.M.; Cooklin, A.R.; Fisher, J.R.; Payne, M.S. The role of micro-organisms (staphylococcus aureus and candida albicans) in the pathogenesis of breast pain and infection in lactating women: Study protocol. *BMC Pregnancy Childbirth* **2011**, *11*, 54. [CrossRef] [PubMed]
31. Li, C.; Solomons, N.W.; Scott, M.E.; Koski, K.G. Subclinical mastitis (SCM) and proinflammatory cytokines are associated with mineral and trace element concentrations in human breast milk. *J. Trace Elem. Med. Biol.* **2018**, *46*, 55–61. [CrossRef] [PubMed]
32. Immler, R.; Simon, S.I.; Sperandio, M. Calcium signaling and related ion channels in neutrophil recruitment and function. *Eur. J. Clin. Investig.* **2018**, e12964. [CrossRef] [PubMed]

Permissions

All chapters in this book were first published by MDPI; hereby published with permission under the Creative Commons Attribution License or equivalent. Every chapter published in this book has been scrutinized by our experts. Their significance has been extensively debated. The topics covered herein carry significant findings which will fuel the growth of the discipline. They may even be implemented as practical applications or may be referred to as a beginning point for another development.

The contributors of this book come from diverse backgrounds, making this book a truly international effort. This book will bring forth new frontiers with its revolutionizing research information and detailed analysis of the nascent developments around the world.

We would like to thank all the contributing authors for lending their expertise to make the book truly unique. They have played a crucial role in the development of this book. Without their invaluable contributions this book wouldn't have been possible. They have made vital efforts to compile up to date information on the varied aspects of this subject to make this book a valuable addition to the collection of many professionals and students.

This book was conceptualized with the vision of imparting up-to-date information and advanced data in this field. To ensure the same, a matchless editorial board was set up. Every individual on the board went through rigorous rounds of assessment to prove their worth. After which they invested a large part of their time researching and compiling the most relevant data for our readers.

The editorial board has been involved in producing this book since its inception. They have spent rigorous hours researching and exploring the diverse topics which have resulted in the successful publishing of this book. They have passed on their knowledge of decades through this book. To expedite this challenging task, the publisher supported the team at every step. A small team of assistant editors was also appointed to further simplify the editing procedure and attain best results for the readers.

Apart from the editorial board, the designing team has also invested a significant amount of their time in understanding the subject and creating the most relevant covers. They scrutinized every image to scout for the most suitable representation of the subject and create an appropriate cover for the book.

The publishing team has been an ardent support to the editorial, designing and production team. Their endless efforts to recruit the best for this project, has resulted in the accomplishment of this book. They are a veteran in the field of academics and their pool of knowledge is as vast as their experience in printing. Their expertise and guidance has proved useful at every step. Their uncompromising quality standards have made this book an exceptional effort. Their encouragement from time to time has been an inspiration for everyone.

The publisher and the editorial board hope that this book will prove to be a valuable piece of knowledge for researchers, students, practitioners and scholars across the globe.

List of Contributors

Zainab Taha, Ludmilla Wikkeling-Scott and Dimitrios Papandreou
Department of Health Sciences, College of Natural and Health Sciences, Zayed University, Abu Dhabi, UAE

Ahmed Ali Hassan
Taami for Agricultural and Animal Production, Khartoum, Sudan

Stefanie N. Hinkle, Aiyi Liu and Cuilin Zhang
Epidemiology Branch, Division of Intramural Population Health Research, Eunice Kennedy Shriver National Institute of Child Health and Human Development, National Institutes of Health, Bethesda, MD 20817, USA

Pranati L. Panuganti
Epidemiology Branch, Division of Intramural Population Health Research, Eunice Kennedy Shriver National Institute of Child Health and Human Development, National Institutes of Health, Bethesda, MD 20817, USA
The Warren Alpert Medical School of Brown University, Providence, RI 02903, USA

Shristi Rawal
Epidemiology Branch, Division of Intramural Population Health Research, Eunice Kennedy Shriver National Institute of Child Health and Human Development, National Institutes of Health, Bethesda, MD 20817, USA
Department of Nutritional Sciences, School of Health Professions, Rutgers University, Newark, NJ 07107, USA

Sjurdur F. Olesen
Centre for Fetal Programming, Department of Epidemiology Research, Statens Serum Institut, DK 2300 Copenhagen, Denmark

Anne C. B. Thuesen
Department of Endocrinology, Rigshospitalet University Hospital, DK-2200 Copenhagen, Denmark

Louise G. Grunnet
Centre for Fetal Programming, Department of Epidemiology Research, Statens Serum Institut, DK 2300 Copenhagen, Denmark
Department of Endocrinology, Rigshospitalet University Hospital, DK-2200 Copenhagen, Denmark
The Danish Diabetes Academy, DK-5000 Odense, Denmark

Yuan Lin
Epidemiology Branch, Division of Intramural Population Health Research, Eunice Kennedy Shriver National Institute of Child Health and Human Development, National Institutes of Health, Bethesda, MD 20817, USA
Department of Epidemiology, Richard M. Fairbanks School of Public Health, Indiana University, Indianapolis, IN 46202, USA

Sylvia H. Ley
Harvard T.H. Chan School of Public Health, Harvard University, Boston, MA 02115, USA
Channing Division of Network Medicine, Harvard Medical School and Brigham and Women's Hospital, Boston, MA 02115, USA

Mohèb Elwakiel
Food Quality and Design Group, Wageningen University & Research, Bornse Weilanden 9, 6708 WG Wageningen, The Netherlands
Laboratory of Food Chemistry, Wageningen University & Research, Bornse Weilanden 9, 6708 WG Wageningen, The Netherlands

Kasper A. Hettinga
Food Quality and Design Group, Wageningen University & Research, Bornse Weilanden 9, 6708 WG Wageningen, The Netherlands

Henk A. Schols
Laboratory of Food Chemistry, Wageningen University & Research, Bornse Weilanden 9, 6708 WG Wageningen, The Netherlands

Sjef Boeren
Laboratory of Biochemistry, Wageningen University & Research, Stippeneng 4, 6708 WE Wageningen, The Netherlands

Jos A. Hageman
Biometris-Applied Statistics, Wageningen University & Research, Droevendaalsesteeg 1, 6708 PB Wageningen, The Netherlands

Ignatius M. Szeto
Inner Mongolia Yili Industrial Group Co., Ltd., Jinshan Road 8, Hohhot 010110, China

Roser Porta
Neonatal Unit, Dexeus University Hospital, 5 Sabino Arana st, 08028 Barcelona, Spain

Eva Capdevila
Pediatric Unit, Department of Primary Care, Catalonia Health Authority, Balmes st, 08007 Barcelona, Spain

Gemma Ginovart and Elisenda Moliner
Neonatal Unit, Santa Creu i Sant Pau University Hospital, 87 mSant Quinti st. 08041 Barcelona, Spain

Marta Nicolàs
Neonatal Unit, Germans Trias i Pujol University Hospital, Canyet Road, 08916 Badalona, Spain

Antonio Gutiérrez
Department of Hematology, Son Espases University Hospital. IdISBa Balearic Medical Research Council, Valldemossa Road, 79, 07010 Palma de Mallorca, Spain
COMIB Advisory, Passeig de Mallorca, 42, 07012 Palma de Mallorca, Spain

Jaume Ponce-Taylor
Urgent Care Centre, Department of Primary Care, Balearic Health Authority, 1 Illes Balears st. 07014 Palma de Mallorca, Spain

Sergio Verd
Pediatric Unit, Department of Primary Care, Balearic Health Authority, Matamusinos st. 07013 Palma de Mallorca, Spain

Francesc Botet
Neonatal Unit, University Maternity Hospital, 5 Sabino Arana st. 08028 Barcelona, Spain

Zoya Gridneva, Wan Jun Tie, Ching Tat Lai, Peter E. Hartmann and Donna T. Geddes
School of Molecular Sciences, M310, The University of Western Australia, Crawley, Perth, WA 6009, Australia

Alethea Rea
Centre for Applied Statistics, The University of Western Australia, Crawley, Perth, WA 6009, Australia

Leigh C. Ward
School of Chemistry and Molecular Biosciences, The University of Queensland, St. Lucia, Brisbane, QLD 4072, Australia

Kevin Murray
School of Population and Global Health, The University of Western Australia, Crawley, Perth, WA 6009, Australia

Therese A. O'Sullivan
School of Medical and Health Sciences, Edith Cowan University, 270 Joondalup Drive, Joondalup, WA 6027, Australia

Joy Cooke
Maternity Unit, Glengarry Private Hospital, Duncraig, WA 6023, Australia

Chris McCafferty
School of Nursing and Midwifery, Edith Cowan University, Joondalup,WA 6027, Australia

Roslyn Giglia
Telethon Kids Institute, University of Western Australia, Subiaco,WA 6008, Australia

Matylda Czosnykowska-Łukacka, Barbara Broers and Barbara Królak-Olejnik
Neonatology Department, Wroclaw Medical University, Borowska 213, 50-556 Wroclaw, Poland

Magdalena Orczyk-Pawiłowicz
Department of Chemistry and Immunochemistry, Wroclaw Medical University, M. Skłodowskiej-Curie 48/50, 50-369 Wrocław, Poland

Zhaoming Xu, David D. Kitts and Susan I. Barr
Food, Nutrition, and Health Program, The University of British Columbia, Vancouver, BC V6T 1Z4, Canada

Roger A. Dyer and Sheila M. Innis
BC Children's Hospital Research Institute, Vancouver, BC V5Z 4H4, Canada

Alejandra M. Wiedeman, Kaitlin M. March and Nancy N. Chen
Food, Nutrition, and Health Program, The University of British Columbia, Vancouver, BC V6T 1Z4, Canada
BC Children's Hospital Research Institute, Vancouver, BC V5Z 4H4, Canada

Kyly C. Whitfield
Food, Nutrition, and Health Program, The University of British Columbia, Vancouver, BC V6T 1Z4, Canada
BC Children's Hospital Research Institute, Vancouver, BC V5Z 4H4, Canada
Department of Applied Human Nutrition, Mount Saint Vincent University, Halifax, NS B3M 2J6, Canada

Hou Kroeun and Ly Sokhoing
Helen Keller International—Cambodia Country Office, Phnom Penh 12301, Cambodia

Prak Sophonneary
National Nutrition Programme, Maternal and Child Health Centre, Ministry of Health, Phnom Penh 12202, Cambodia

Timothy J. Green
Food, Nutrition, and Health Program, The University of British Columbia, Vancouver, BC V6T 1Z4, Canada
BC Children's Hospital Research Institute, Vancouver, BC V5Z 4H4, Canada
South Australia Health and Medical Research Institute, Adelaide, SA 5000, Australia

Jiahui Yu, Tinglan Yuan, Xinghe Zhang, Qingzhe Jin, Wei Wei and Xingguo Wang
State Key Lab of Food Science and Technology, Jiangnan University, Wuxi 214122, China
International Joint Research Laboratory for Lipid Nutrition and Safety, Collaborative Innovation Center of Food Safety and Quality Control in Jiangsu Province, School of Food Science and Technology, Jiangnan University, Wuxi 214122, China

Jessica P. Riedstra and Nicki L. Aubuchon-Endsley
Department of Psychology, Idaho State University, Pocatello, ID 83209, USA

Kirsty V. Biggs
Brighton and Sussex Medical School, Brighton BN2 5BE, UK

Katherine Hurrell
Royal United Hospital, Combe Park, Bath BA1 3NG, UK

Robert J. Boyle
Department of Paediatrics, Imperial College Healthcare NHS Trust, London W2 1NY, UK
inVIVO Planetary Health, Group of the Worldwide Universities Network (WUN), 6010 Park Ave, West New York, NJ 07093, USA

Eleanor Matthews
Department of Paediatrics, Imperial College Healthcare NHS Trust, London W2 1NY, UK

Ekaterina Khaleva
Department of Paediatrics, Saint-Petersburg State Paediatric Medical University, 194353 Saint Petersburg, Russia
inVIVO Planetary Health, Group of the Worldwide Universities Network (WUN), 6010 Park Ave, West New York, NJ 07093, USA

Daniel Munblit
Department of Paediatrics, Imperial College Healthcare NHS Trust, London W2 1NY, UK
inVIVO Planetary Health, Group of the Worldwide Universities Network (WUN), 6010 Park Ave, West New York, NJ 07093, USA
Faculty of Pediatrics, I. M. Sechenov First Moscow State Medical University, 119991 Moscow, Russia

Alexandre G. Torres
Laboratory of Food Science and Nutritional Biochemistry, Institute of Chemistry, Federal University of Rio de Janeiro, Rio de Janeiro 21941-909, Brazil

Michele R. Machado
Laboratory of Food Science and Nutritional Biochemistry, Institute of Chemistry, Federal University of Rio de Janeiro, Rio de Janeiro 21941-909, Brazil
School of Nutrition, Faculdade Arthur Sa Earp Neto (FMP/FASE), Petropolis, Rio de Janeiro 25680 120, Brazil

Fernanda Kamp
Laboratory of Food Science and Nutritional Biochemistry, Institute of Chemistry, Federal University of Rio de Janeiro, Rio de Janeiro 21941-909, Brazil
Biochemistry Core, Federal Institute of Education, Science and Technology of Rio de Janeiro, Rio de Janeiro 20270-021, Brazil

Juliana C. Nunes
Laboratory of Food Science and Nutritional Biochemistry, Institute of Chemistry, Federal University of Rio de Janeiro, Rio de Janeiro 21941-909, Brazil
School of Nutrition, Federal University of the State of Rio de Janeiro, Rio de Janeiro 22290-250, Brazil

Tatiana El-Bacha
Laboratory of Food Science and Nutritional Biochemistry, Institute of Chemistry, Federal University of Rio de Janeiro, Rio de Janeiro 21941-909, Brazil
Institute of Nutrition, Federal University of Rio de Janeiro, Rio de Janeiro 21941-902, Brazil
Department of Physiology, Development and Neuroscience, University of Cambridge, Cambridge CB2 3EL, UK

Thomas Sevrin
Laboratoire FRANCE Bébé Nutrition, 53000 Laval, France
Nantes Université, INRA, UMR 1280 PhAN, CRNHOuest, IMAD, F-44000 Nantes, France

Marie-Cécile Alexandre-Gouabau, Blandine Castellano, Audrey Aguesse, Khadija Ouguerram and Clair-Yves Boquien
Nantes Université, INRA, UMR 1280 PhAN, CRNHOuest, IMAD, F-44000 Nantes, France

Patrick Ngyuen
ONIRIS, NP3, CRNH-Ouest, F-44000 Nantes, France

Dominique Darmaun
Nantes Université, INRA, UMR 1280 PhAN, CRNHOuest, IMAD, F-44000 Nantes, France
CHU Nantes, F-44000 Nantes, France

Agnieszka Bzikowska-Jura, Aneta Czerwonogrodzka-Senczyna, Dorota Szostak-Węgierek and Halina Weker
Department of Clinical Dietetics, Faculty of Health Science, Medical University of Warsaw, E Ciolka Str. 27, 01-445 Warsaw, Poland

Gabriela Olędzka
Department of Medical Biology, Faculty of Health Science, Medical University of Warsaw, Nowogrodzka Str. 73, 02-018Warsaw, Poland

Aleksandra Wesołowska
Laboratory of Human Milk and Lactation Research at Regional Human Milk Bank in Holy Family Hospital, Faculty of Health Science, Department of Neonatology, Medical University of Warsaw, Zwirki I Wigury Str. 63A, 02-091Warsaw, Poland

Adekunle Dawodu
Department of Pediatrics, College of Medicine, University of Cincinnati, Cincinnati, OH 45267, USA

Khalil M. Salameh
Division of Pediatrics, Al-Wakra Hospital, Hamad Medical Corporation, Doha, Qatar

Najah S. Al-Janahi
Department of Obstetrics and Gynecology, Women's Hospital, Hamad Medical Corporation, Doha, Qatar

Abdulbari Bener
Department of Biostatistics and Medical Informatics, Cerrahpasa Faculty of Medicine, Istanbul University Cerrahpasa and Istanbul Medipol University, 34098 Cerrahpasa-Istanbul, Turkey

Naser Elkum
Sidra Medicine, Doha, Qatar

Anna Gustafsson
Department of Clinical Science, Intervention and Technology, Karolinska Institutet, SE 141 86 Stockholm, Sweden
Department of Neonatology, Karolinska University Hospital, SE 171 76 Stockholm, Sweden

Elisabeth Granström and Christina Stecksén-Blicks
Department of Odontology, Pediatric dentistry, Umeå university, SE 901 87 Umeå, Sweden

Christina E. West and Sven-Arne Silfverdal
Department of Clinical Sciences, Pediatrics, Umeå University, SE 901 87 Umeå, Sweden

Index

www.ingramcontent.com/pod-product-compliance
Lightning Source LLC
LaVergne TN
LVHW060517210926
848485LV00005B/1096

* 9 7 8 1 6 3 9 2 7 6 0 8 0 *